Pocket Atlas
of Radiographic Anatomy

Pocket Atlas of Radiographic Anatomy

Torsten B. Möller, Emil Reif, and Paul Stark

348 illustrations

1993

Georg Thieme Verlag
Stuttgart · New York

Thieme Medical Publishers, Inc.
New York

Torsten B. Möller, M. D.
Emil Reif, M. D.
Am Caritas-Krankenhaus,
6638 Dillingen/Saar, Germany

Paul Stark, M. D.
Dept. of Radiology,
Brigham and Womens Hospital
Harvard Medical School,
Boston, MA 02115, USA

Translated by

Michael Robertson, D. Phil.
Feuerdornweg 25, 8900 Augsburg 1,
Germany

Thieme Medical Publishers, Inc., 381 Park Avenue South, New York, N.Y. 10016

Typesetting by Setzerei Lihs, Ludwigsburg
(Linotype System 4 – Linotronic 300)
Printed in Germany by
K. Grammlich, D-7401 Pliezhausen

ISBN 3-13-784201-8 (GTV, Stuttgart)
ISBN 0-86577-459-5 (TMP, New York)

Library of Congress Cataloging-in-Publication Data

Möller, Torsten B.
[Taschenatlas der Röntgenanatomie. English]
Pocket Atlas of Radiographic Anatomy / Torsten B. Möller, Emil Reif, and Paul Stark : [Translated by Michael Robertson].
p. cm.
Includes bibliographical references and index.
1. Human anatomy-Atlases. 2. Radiography, Medical-Atlases.
I. Reif, Emil. II. Stark, Paul, 1944 –. III. Title. [DNLM: 1. Anatomy-atlases. 2. Radiography-atlases. QS 17 M726t]
QM25·M55413 1993
611'.0022'2--dc20
DNLM/DLC
for Library of Congress 92-49310

Für
Barbara und Doris

This book deals with the normal radiographic anatomy and its details needed to interpret radiographs.
The book concentrates strictly on "normal" radiographic findings. Each radiograph is supplemented on the opposite page by a drawing with detailed markings. These are numbered from top to bottom, to facilitate finding the captions. Where necessary, several diagrams were added. In addition to anatomical terminology, specialized radiological terms (radiology "slang") are used.
The majority of the radiographs illustrated in this book were provided by the Department of Clinical Radiology, Aachen (Chairman: Prof. R. W. Günter, M. D.). Our thanks go to the radiologic technologists, and to our friends and colleagues. Thanks are also due to Dr. C. Weller-Schweitzer of the Radiology Department of the Caritas Hospital, Dillingen (Chairman: Dr. D. Gerstner) for allowing us to use a few of their excellent images. We would like to express our deepest thanks to Christoph Buntru, M. D., for his outstanding support and assistance.

Dillingen and Boston,
November 1992

Torsten B. Möller,
Emil Reif, Paul Stark

Skeletal Imaging

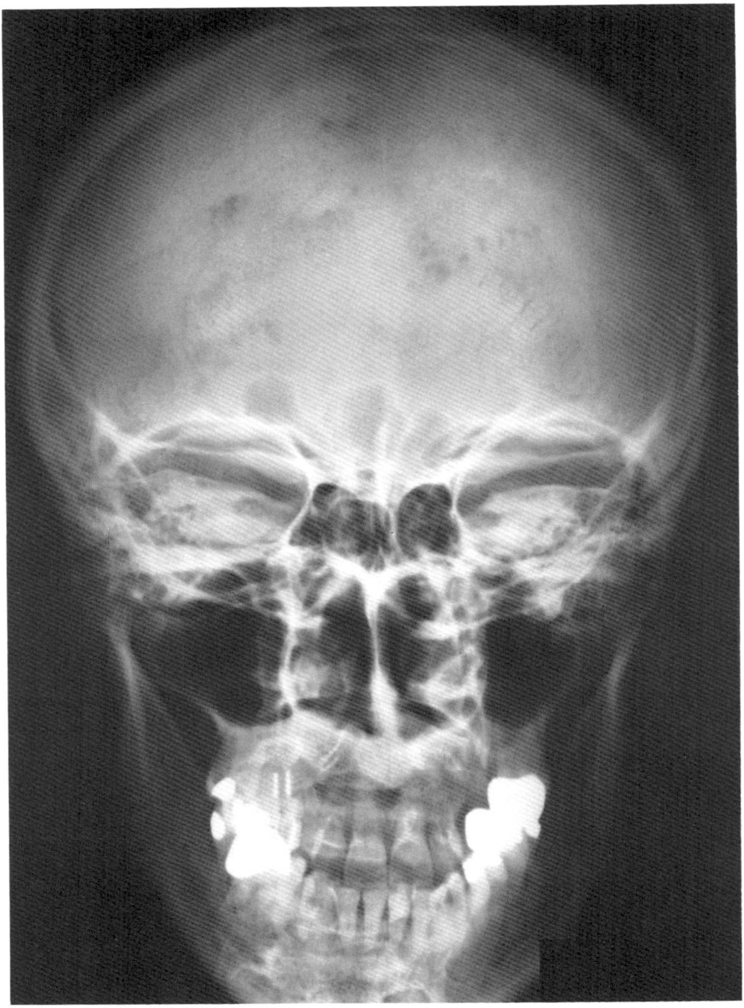

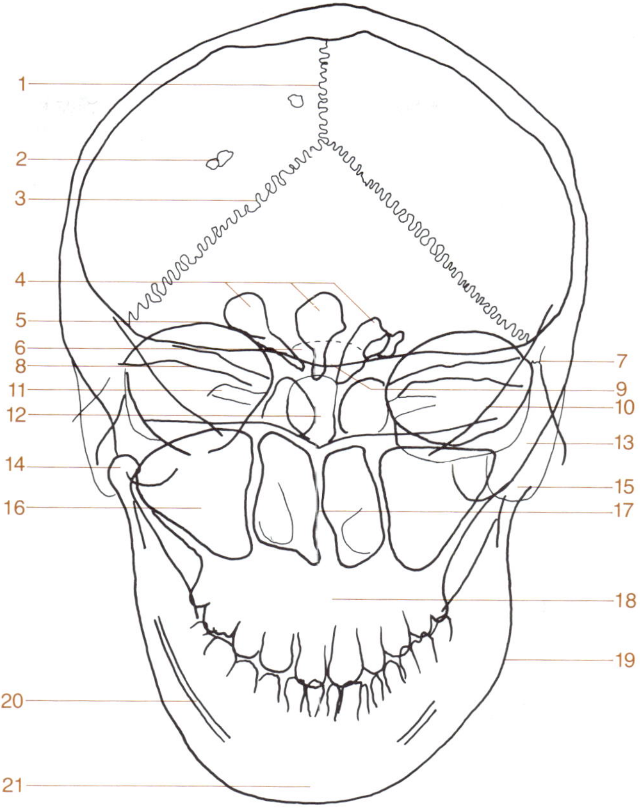

1 Sagittal suture
2 Pacchioni's granulations
3 Lambdoid suture
4 Frontal sinus
5 Roof of the orbit
6 Dorsum sellae
7 Frontozygomatic suture
8 Superior margin of the petrous pyramid
9 Planum sphenoidale
10 Innominate line
11 Internal auditory canal
12 Sphenoid sinus
13 Zygomatic arch
14 Condylar process of the mandible
15 Mastoid process
16 Maxillary sinus
17 Nasal septum
18 Maxilla
19 Angle of the mandible
20 Mandibular canal
21 Mental protuberance

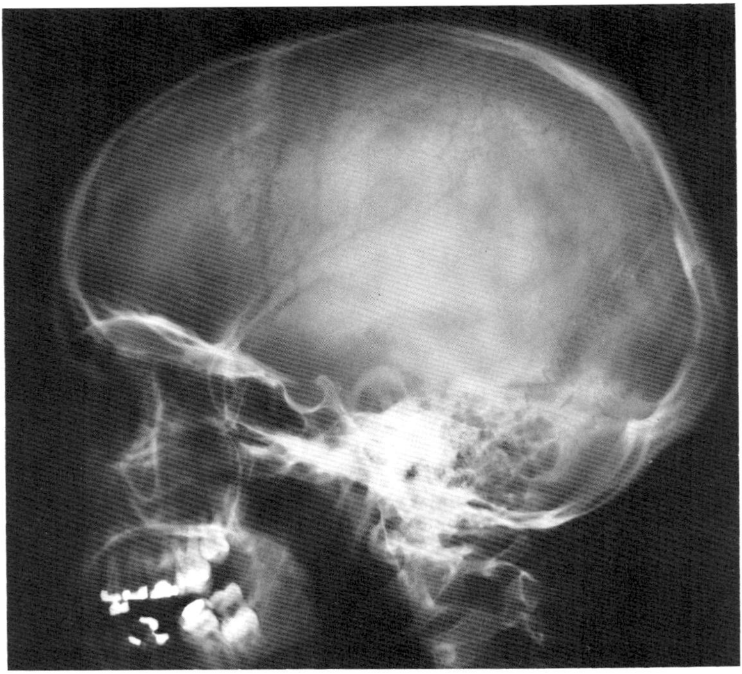

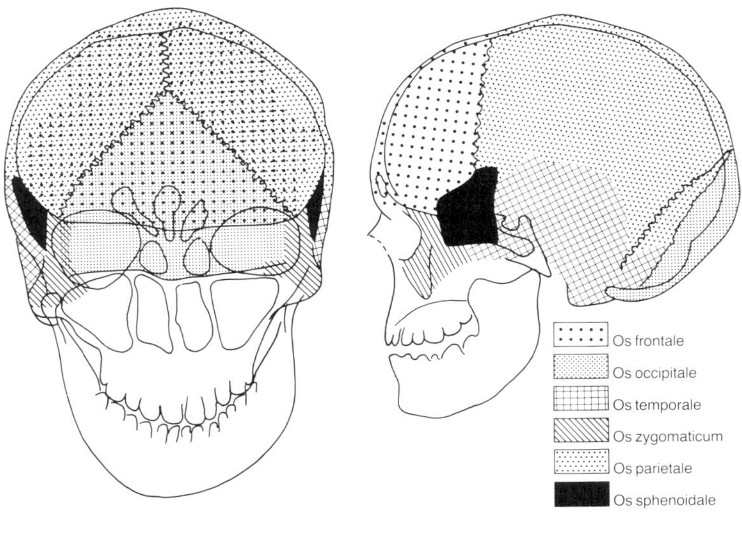
Os frontale
Os occipitale
Os temporale
Os zygomaticum
Os parietale
Os sphenoidale

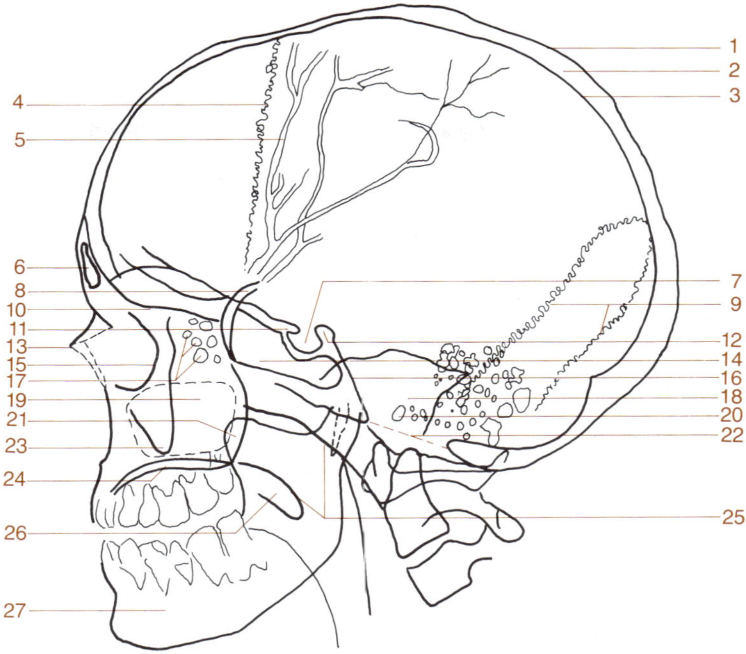

1 Outer table of the skull
2 Diploic space
3 Inner table of the skull
4 Coronal suture
5 Middle meningeal artery groove
6 Frontal sinus
7 Pituitary fossa
8 Greater wing of the sphenoid bone
9 Lambdoid suture
10 Cribriform plate
11 Anterior clinoid process
12 Posterior clinoid process
13 Nasal bone
14 Sphenoid sinus
15 Zygomatic bone (lateral wall of the orbit)
16 Clivus
17 Ethmoidal cells
18 Petrous portion of the temporal bone
19 Maxillary sinus
20 Porus acusticus externus (outer end of the external auditory canal)
21 Coronoid process of the mandible
22 Foramen magnum
23 Zygomatic process
24 Hard palate
25 Nasopharynx
26 Soft palate
27 Mandible

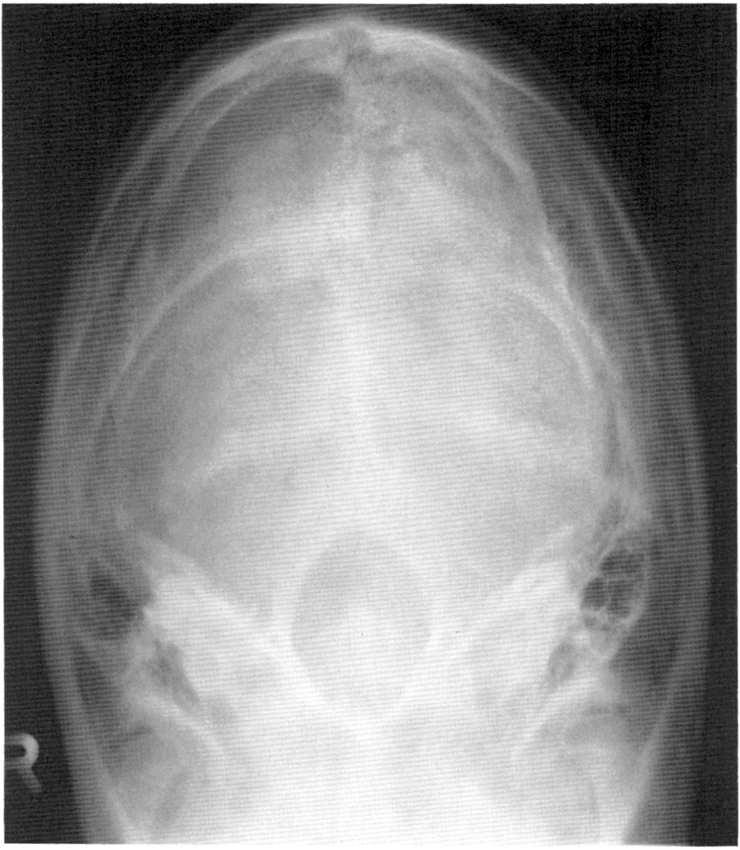
R

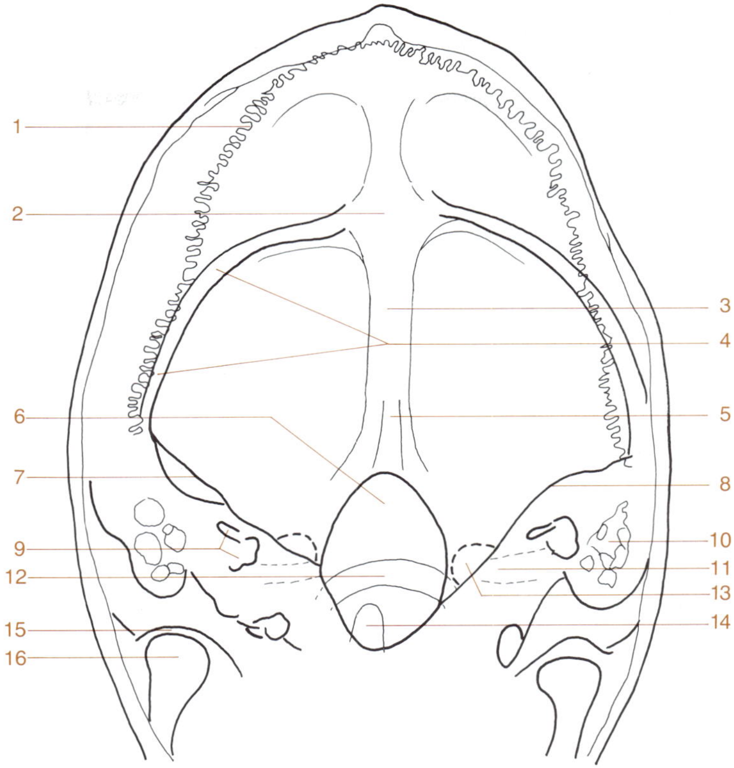

1 Lambdoid suture
2 Occipital protuberances (external and internal)
3 Occipital bone
4 Sulcus of transverse sinus
5 Occipital crest
6 Foramen magnum
7 Petrous bone
8 Arcuate eminence
9 Semicircular canals
10 Mastoid air cells
11 Internal auditory canal
12 Posterior arch of the atlas
13 Jugular foramen
14 Tooth
15 Temporomandibular joint
16 Head of the mandible

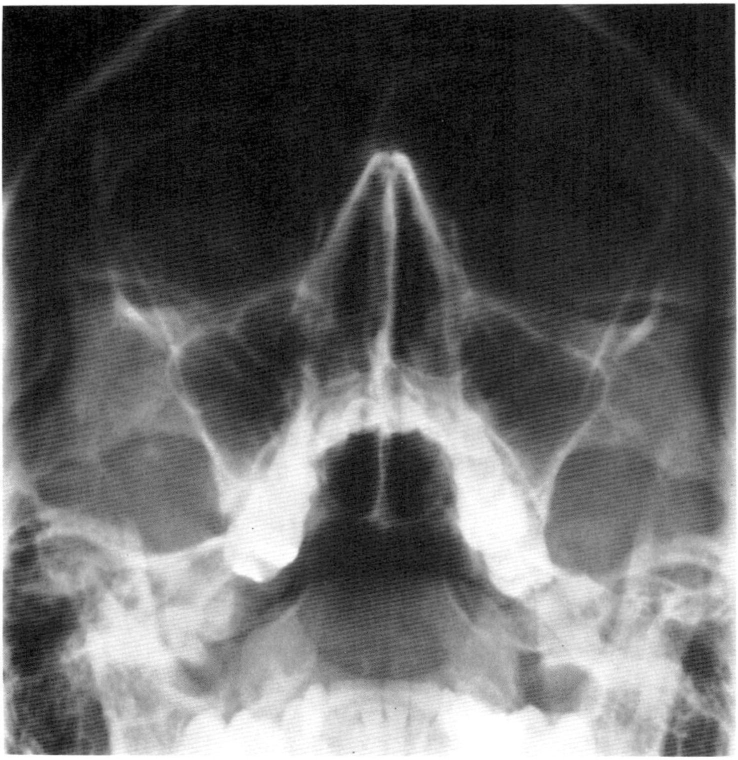

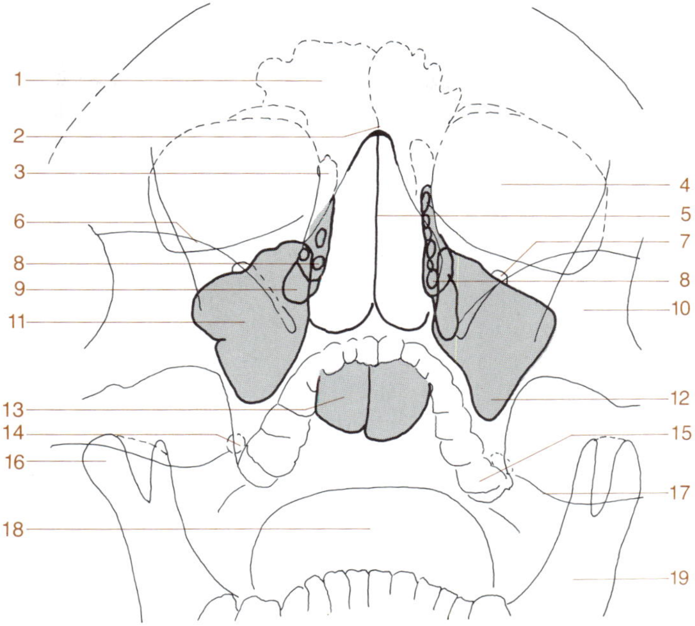

1 Frontal sinus
2 Nasal bone
3 Anterior ethmoidal cells
4 Orbit
5 Nasal septum
6 Greater wing of the sphenoid bone
7 Infraorbital foramen
8 Foramen rotundum
9 Posterior ethmoidal cells
10 Zygomatic bone
11 Maxillary sinus
12 Recessus alveolaris maxillae
13 Sphenoid sinus
14 Foramen ovale
15 Alveolar process of the maxilla
16 Head of the mandible
17 Superior margin of the petrous pyramid
18 Tongue
19 Mandible

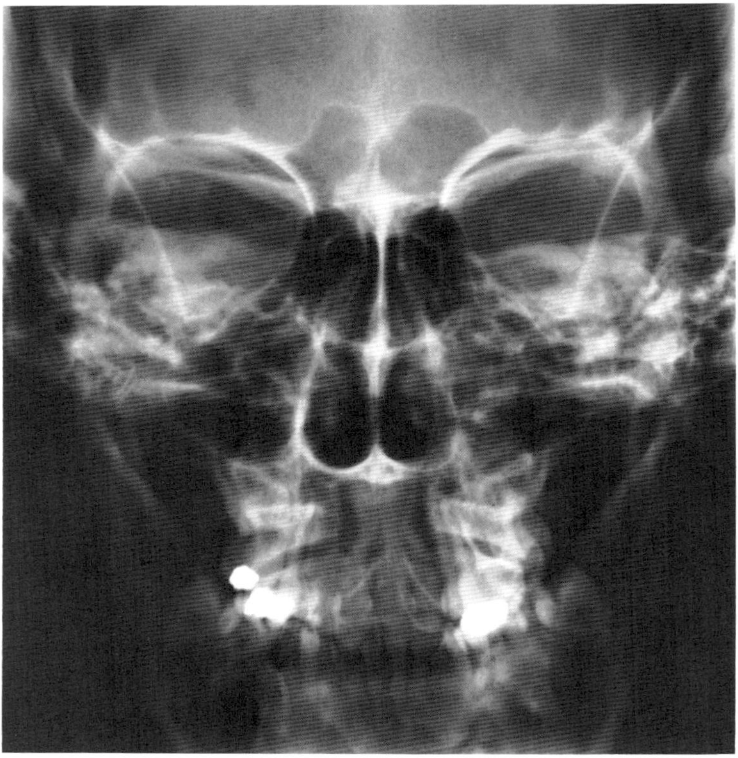

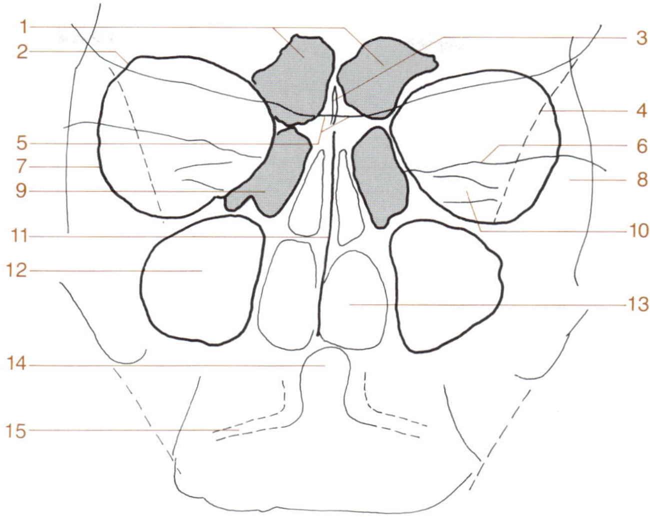

1 Frontal sinus
2 Roof of the orbit
3 Crista galli
4 Innominate line
5 Planum sphenoidale
6 Superior margin of the petrous pyramid
7 Lateral wall of the orbit
8 Zygomatic bone
9 Anterior ethmoidal cells
10 Internal auditory canal
11 Nasal septum
12 Maxillary sinus
13 Nasal cavity
14 Tooth
15 Atlantoaxial joint

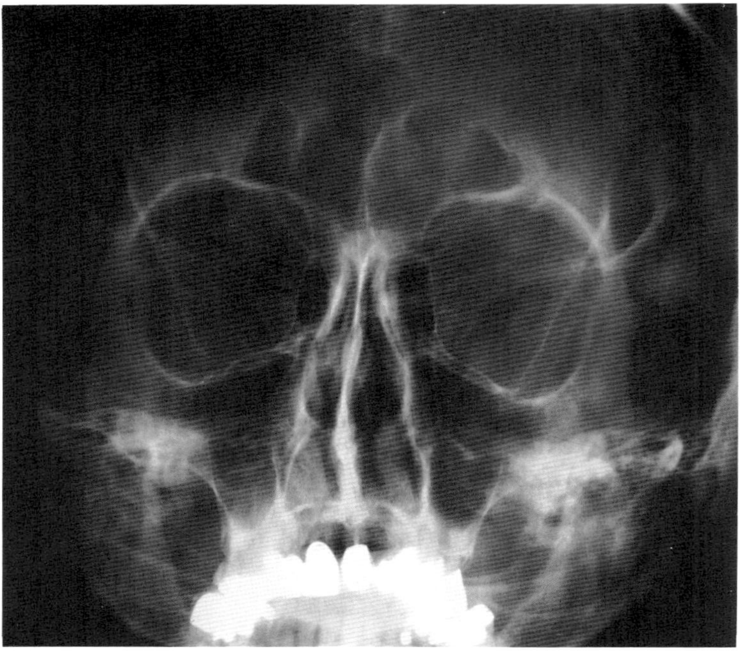

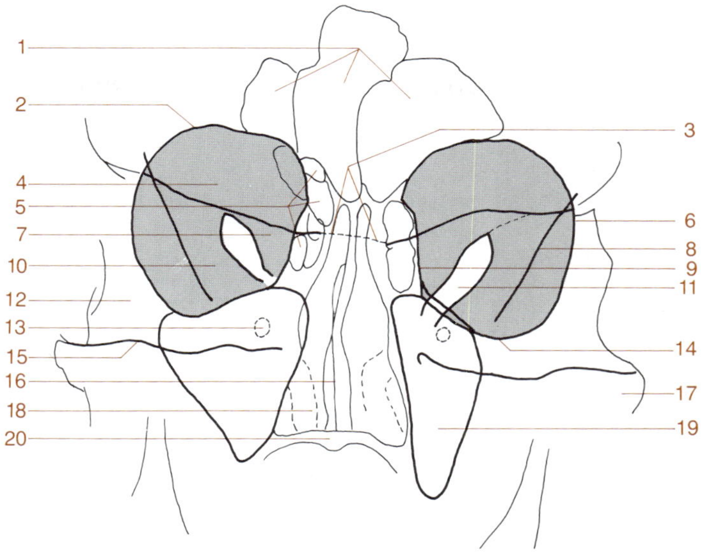

1 Frontal sinus
2 Roof of the orbit
3 Planum sphenoidale
4 Orbit (gray background)
5 Ethmoidal cells
6 Lateral wall of the orbit
7 Lesser wing of the sphenoid bone
8 Innominate line
9 Lamina papyracea
10 Greater wing of the sphenoid bone
11 Superior orbital fissure
12 Frontal process of zygomatic bone
13 Foramen rotundum
14 Floor of the orbit
15 Superior margin of the petrous pyramid
16 Nasal septum
17 Zygomatic arch
18 Inferior turbinate
19 Maxillary sinus
20 Hard palate

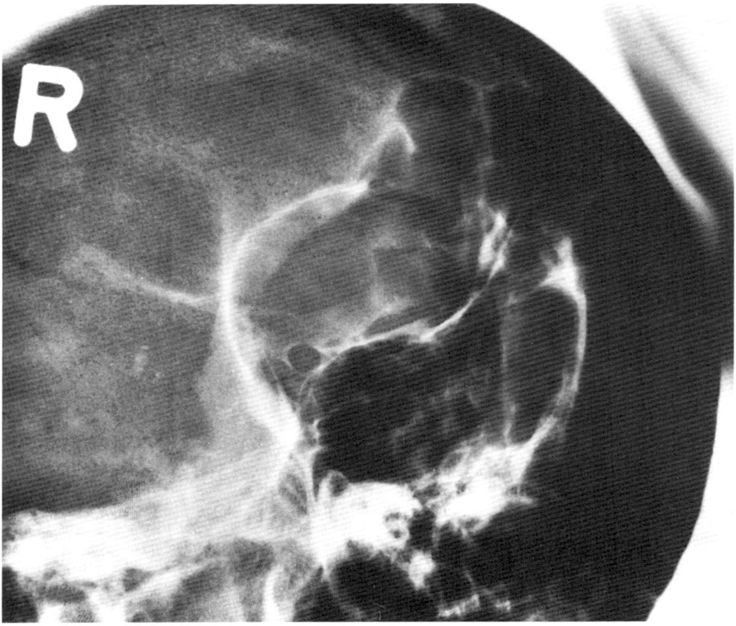
R

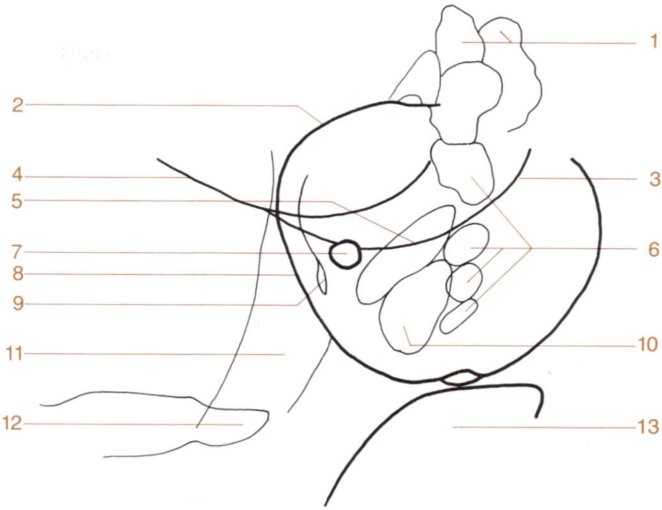

1 Frontal sinus
2 Roof of the orbit
3 Lesser wing of the sphenoid bone, left
4 Lesser wing of the sphenoid bone, right
5 Planum sphenoidale
6 Ethmoidal air cells
7 Optic canal
8 Lateral wall of the orbit
9 Superior orbital fissure
10 Sphenoid sinus
11 Zygomatic arch
12 Petrous portion of the temporal bone
13 Maxillary sinus

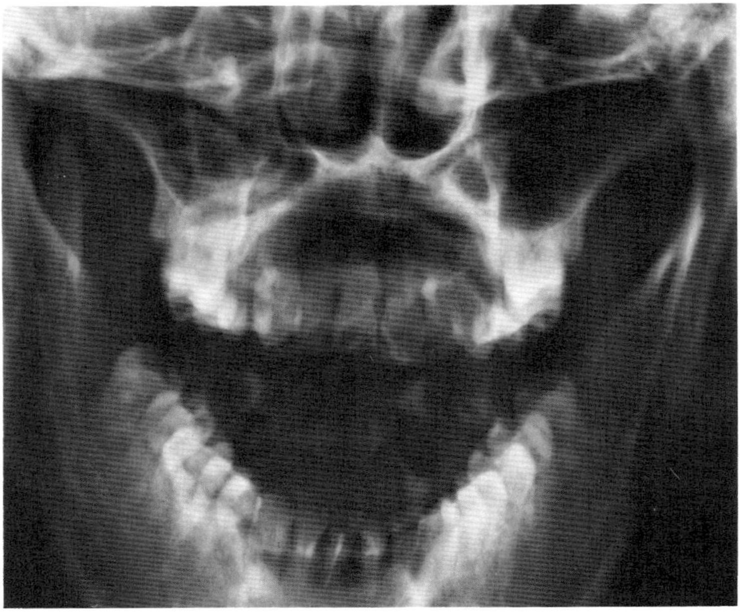

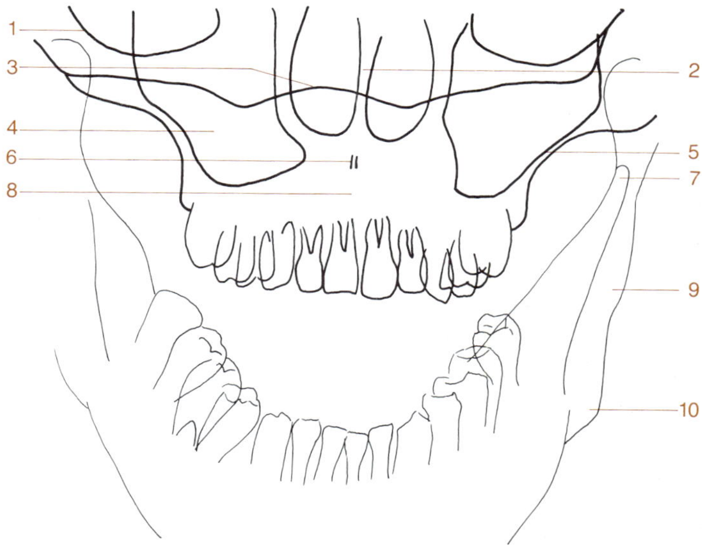

1 Floor of the orbit
2 Nasal septum
3 Base of the skull
4 Maxillary sinus
5 Lateral wall of the maxilla
6 Anterior nasal spine
7 Coronoid process
8 Maxilla
9 Ramus of the mandible
10 Angle of the mandible

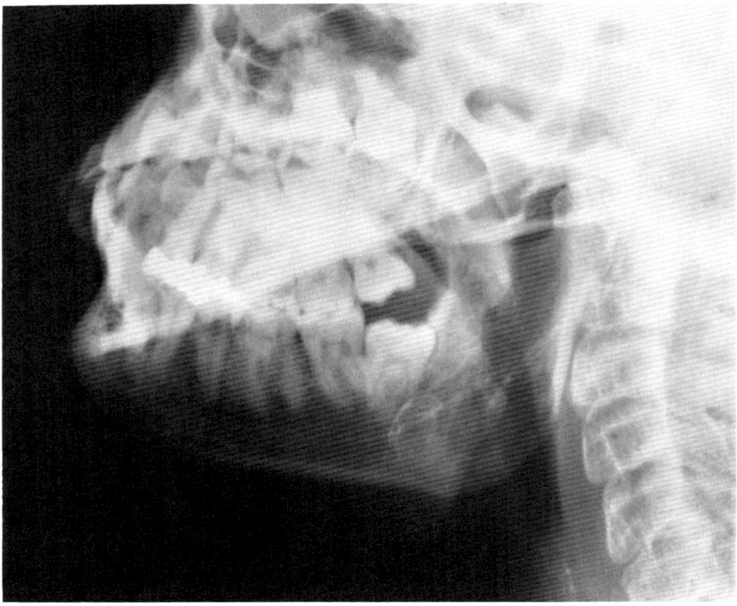

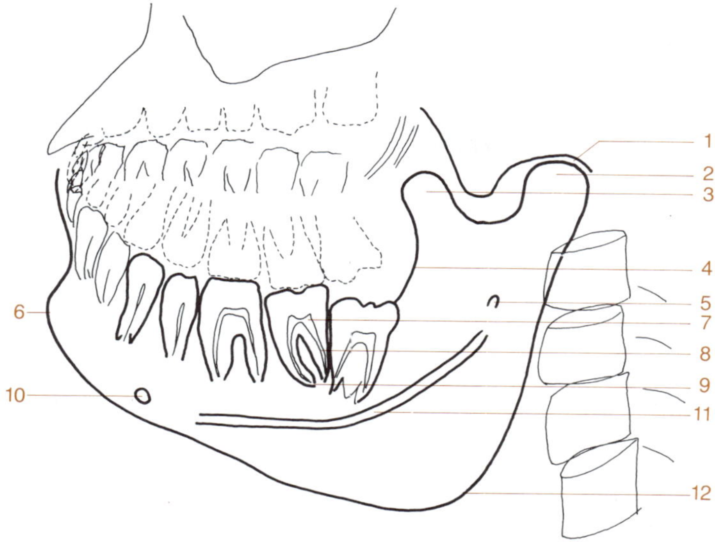

1 Temporomandibular joint
2 Head of the mandible
3 Coronoid process
4 Cortex of mandibular ramus
5 Mandibular foramen
6 Mental protuberance
7 Pulp cavity
8 Dental root canal
9 Apical foramen of the tooth
10 Mental foramen
11 Mandibular canal
12 Angle of the mandible

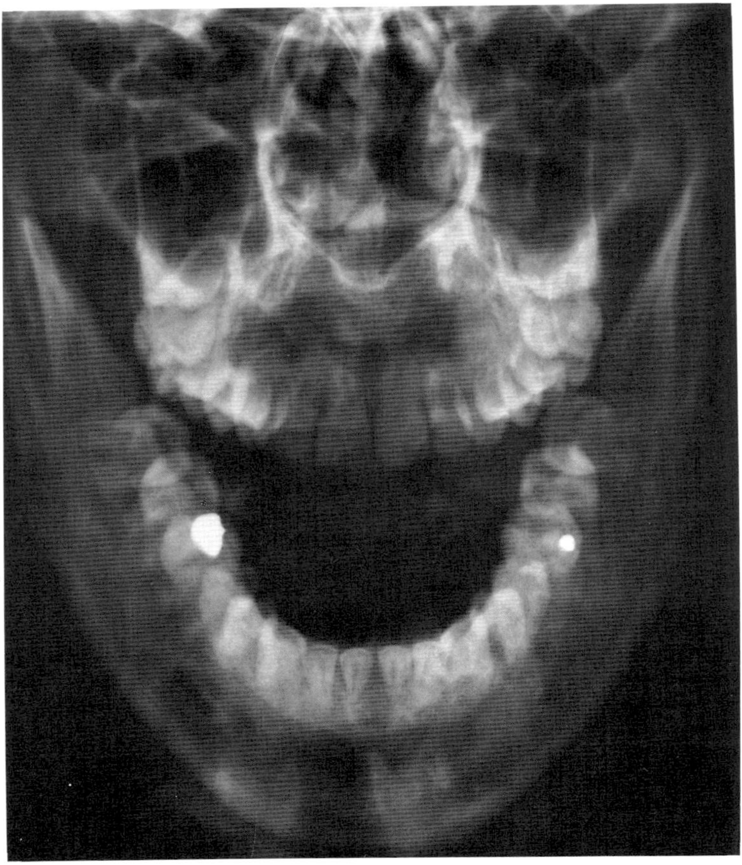

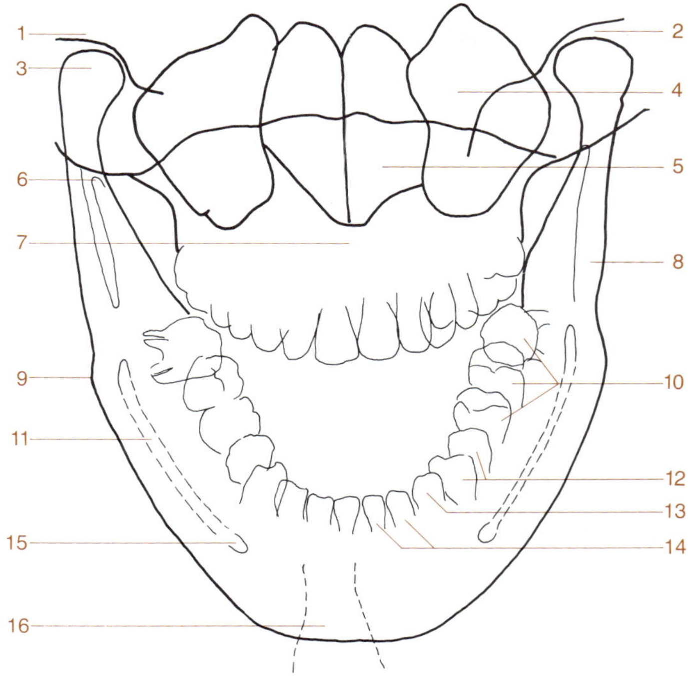

1 Temporal bone
2 Temporomandibular joint
3 Condyle
4 Maxillary sinus
5 Nasal cavity
6 Coronoid process
7 Maxilla
8 Mandibular ramus
9 Angle of the mandible
10 Molar teeth
11 Mandibular canal
12 Premolar teeth
13 Canine teeth
14 Incisor teeth
15 Mental foramen
16 Mental tubercle (tracheal air column superimposed on bone)

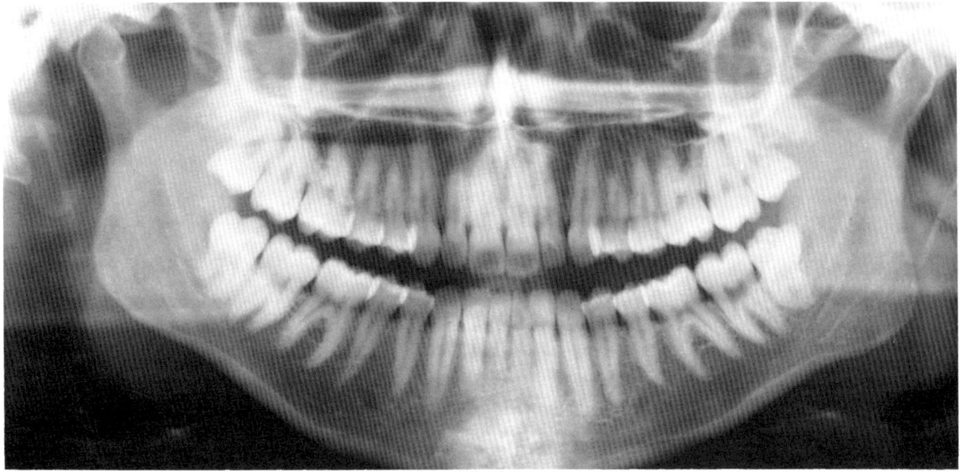

1 Styloid process
2 Soft palate
3 Head of the mandible
4 Condylar process
5 Zygomatic arch
6 Coronoid process
7 Floor of the orbit
8 Nasal cavity

11 Maxillary sinus
12 Pterygopalatine fossa
13 Pterygoid process
14 Angle of the mandible
15 Shadow of the tongue
16 Mandibular canal
17 Hyoid bone
18 Apical foramen of the tooth

21 Dentin
22 Enamel
23 Mental foramen
24 Root of the tooth
25 Incisor teeth
26 Canine tooth
27 Premolar teeth
28 Molar teeth

9 Hard palate
10 Recessus alveolaris (floor of the maxillary sinus)

19 Root canal
20 Pulp cavity

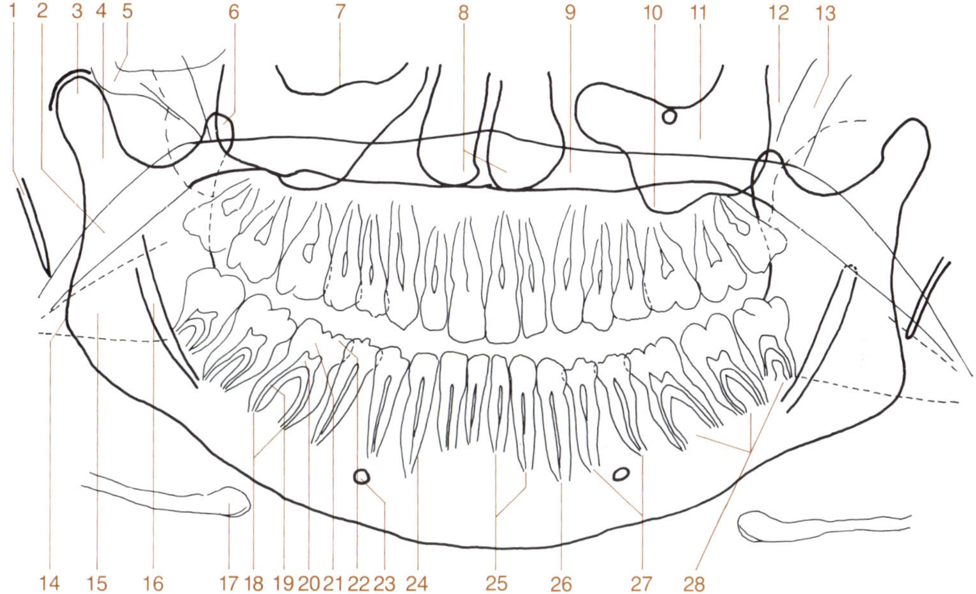

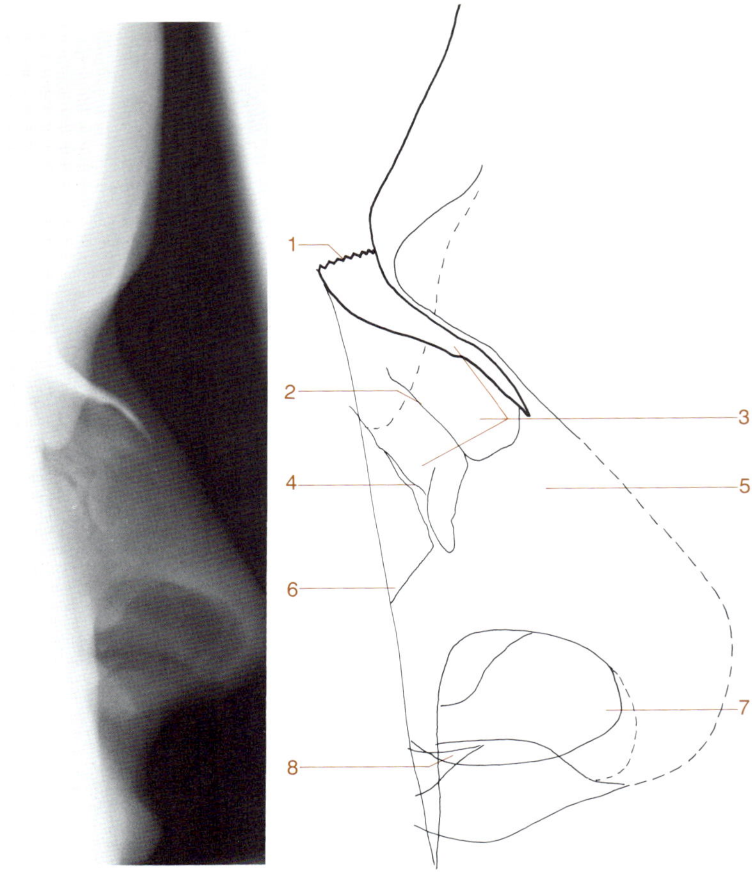

1 Nasofrontal suture
2 Groove for ciliary vessels
3 Nasal bone
4 Nasomaxillary suture
5 Nasal cartilage
6 Maxilla
7 Vestibule of the nose
8 Anterior nasal spine

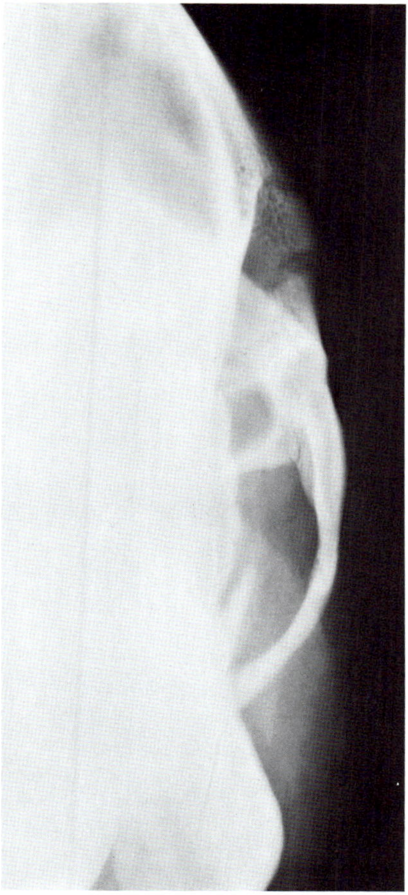

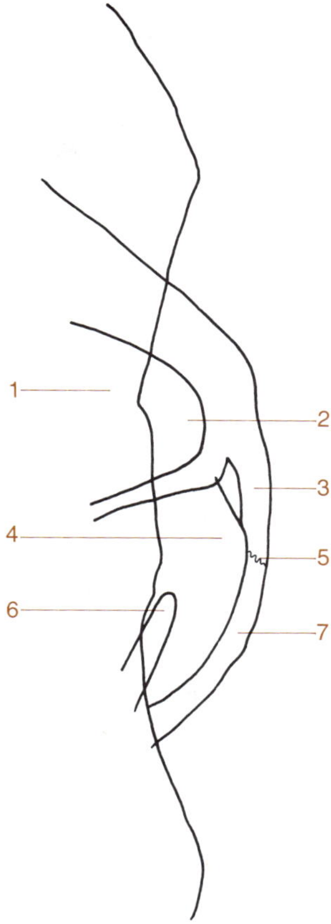

1 Maxillary sinus
2 Zygomatic recess (of the maxillary sinus)
3 Zygomatic arch
4 Temporal fossa
5 Temporozygomatic suture
6 Coronoid process (end on)
7 Zygomatic process of the temporal bone

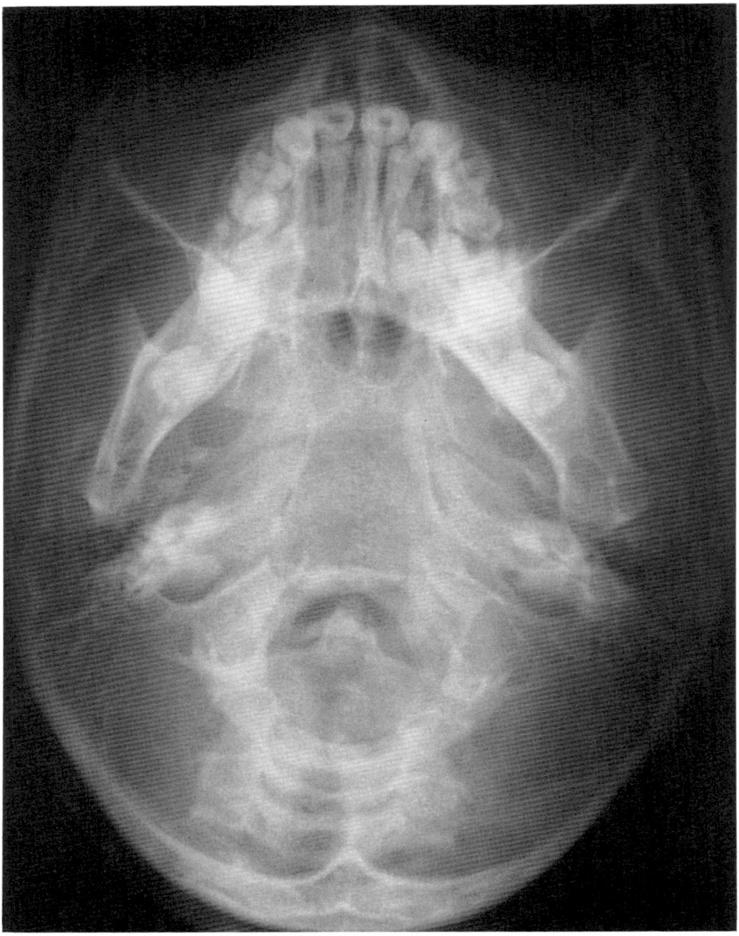

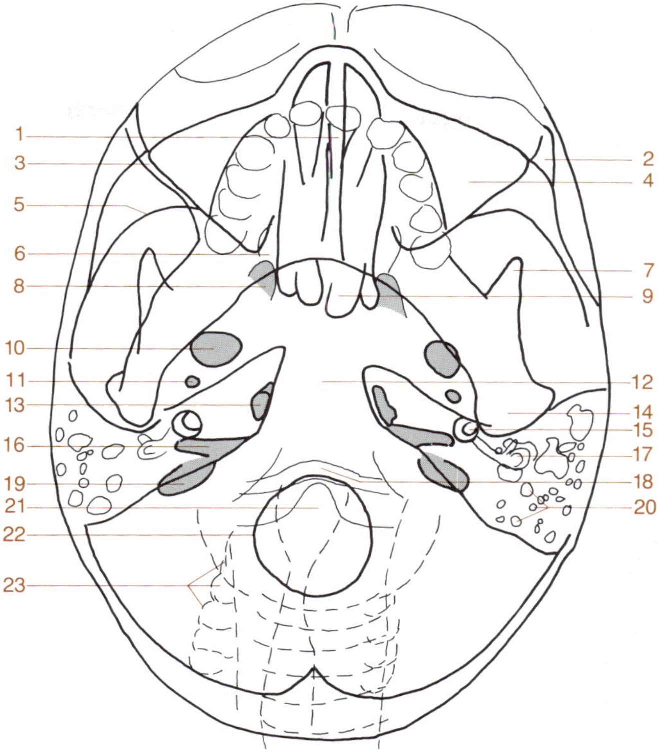

1 Nasal septum
2 Zygomatic bone
3 Posterior wall of maxillary sinus
4 Maxillary sinus (with orbit, partially superimposed)
5 Middle cranial fossa, greater wing (anterior wall of middle cranial fossa)
6 Pterygopalatine fossa
7 Coronoid process
8 Pterygoid fossa
9 Sphenoid sinus
10 Foramen ovale
11 Foramen spinosum
12 Clivus
13 Foramen lacerum
14 Head of the mandible
15 Cochlea
16 Internal auditory canal
17 Semicircular canals
18 Anterior arch of the atlas
19 Jugular foramen
20 Mastoid air cells
21 Odontoid
22 Foramen magnum
23 Cervical spine

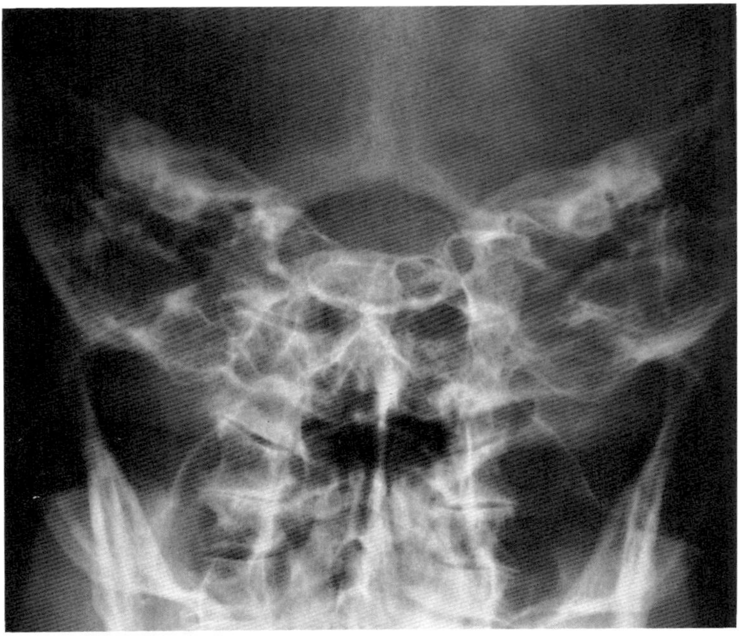

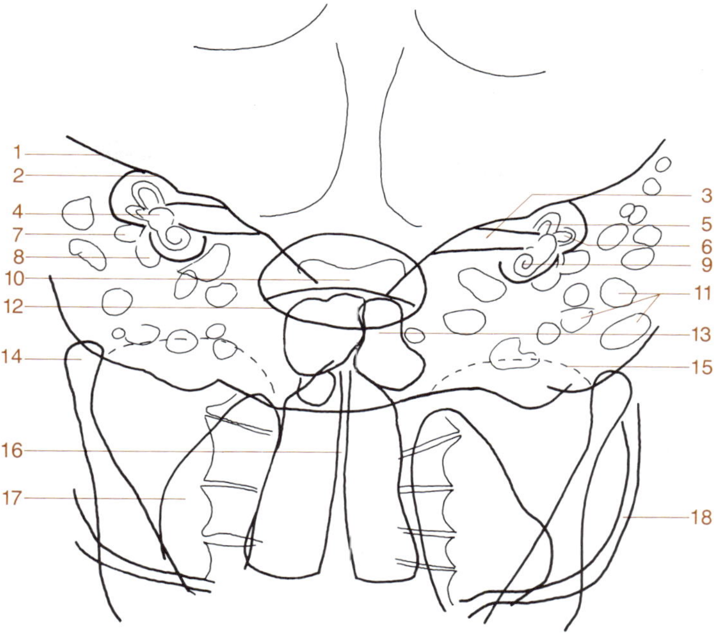

1 Superior margin of the petrous pyramid
2 Arcuate eminence
3 Internal auditory canal
4 Vestibule
5 Anterior semicircular canal
6 Lateral semicircular canal
7 Mastoid antrum
8 Tympanic cavity
9 Cochlea
10 Dorsum sellae
11 Mastoid air cells
12 Foramen magnum
13 Frontal sinus
14 Head of the mandible
15 Roof of the orbit
16 Nasal septum and nasal cavities
17 Maxillary sinus
18 Zygomatic arch

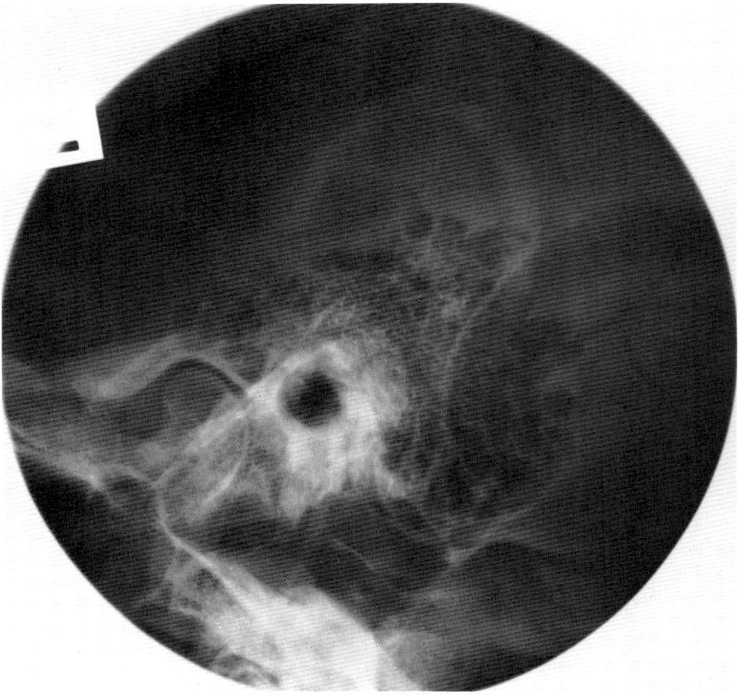

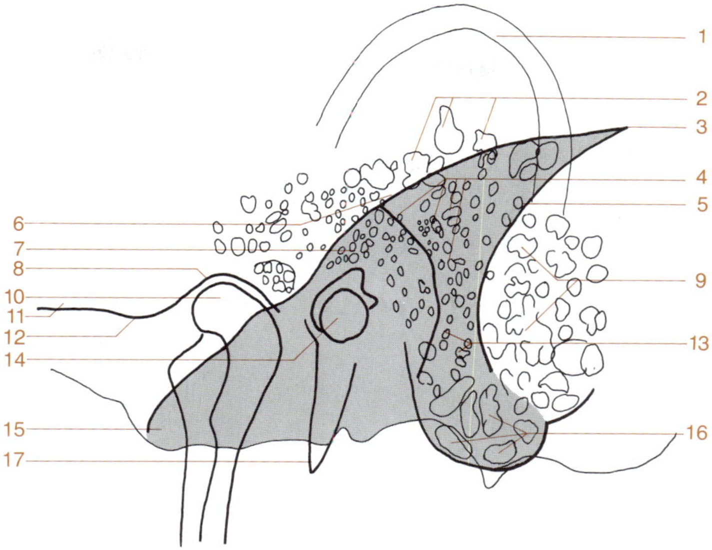

1 External ear
2 Squamal air cells
3 Citelli's angle
4 Periantral air cells
5 Sulcus of the sigmoid sinus
6 Anterior margin of the petrous pyramid
7 Mastoid antrum
8 Temporomandibular joint, articular fossa
9 Marginal air cells
10 Head of the mandible
11 Zygomatic process of the temporal bone
12 Articular eminence
13 Retrofacial air cells
14 Internal and external auditory canal
15 Apex of the petrous pyramid
16 Air cells in the tip of the mastoid process
17 Styloid process

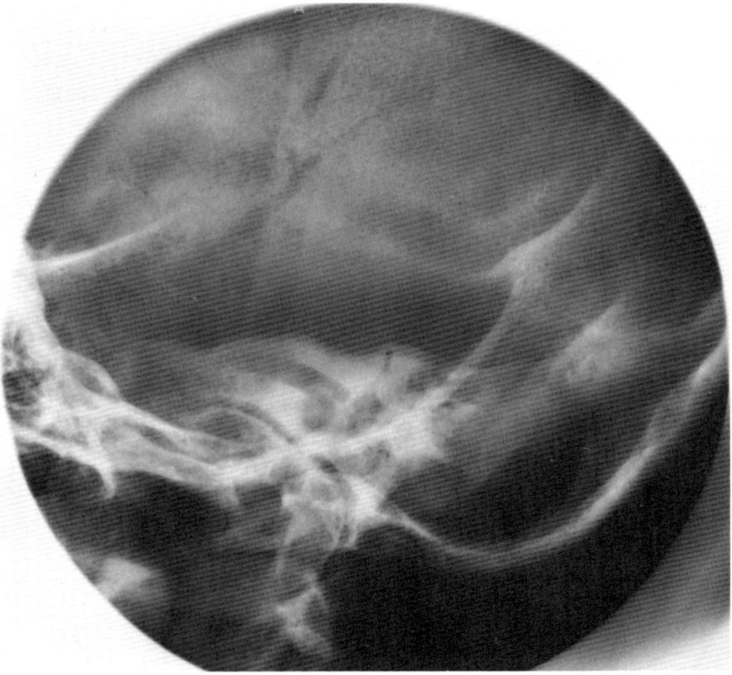

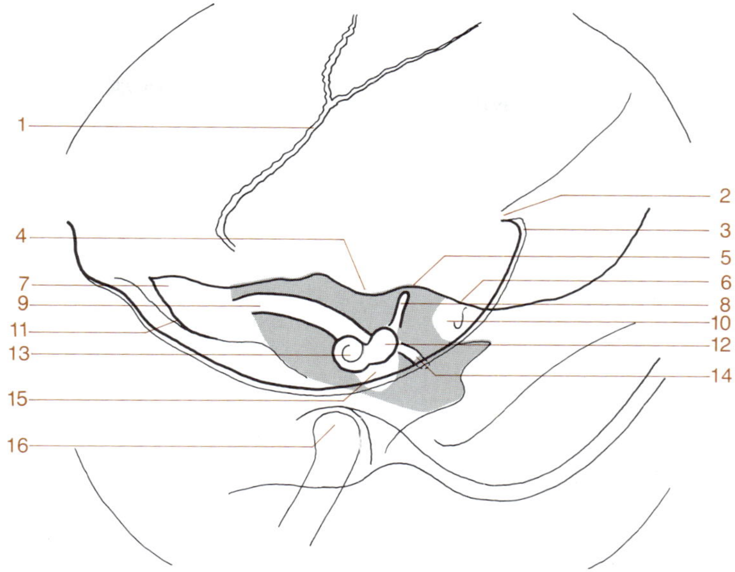

1 Sphenosquamous suture
2 Internal occipital protuberance
3 Internal occipital crest
4 Subarcuate fossa
5 Arcuate eminence
6 Tegmen tympani
7 Apex of the petrous pyramid
8 Anterior semicircular canal
9 Internal auditory canal
10 Antrum
11 Sphenopetrosal fissure
12 Vestibule
13 Cochlea
14 Lateral semicircular canal
15 Tympanic cavity
16 Condyle of the mandible

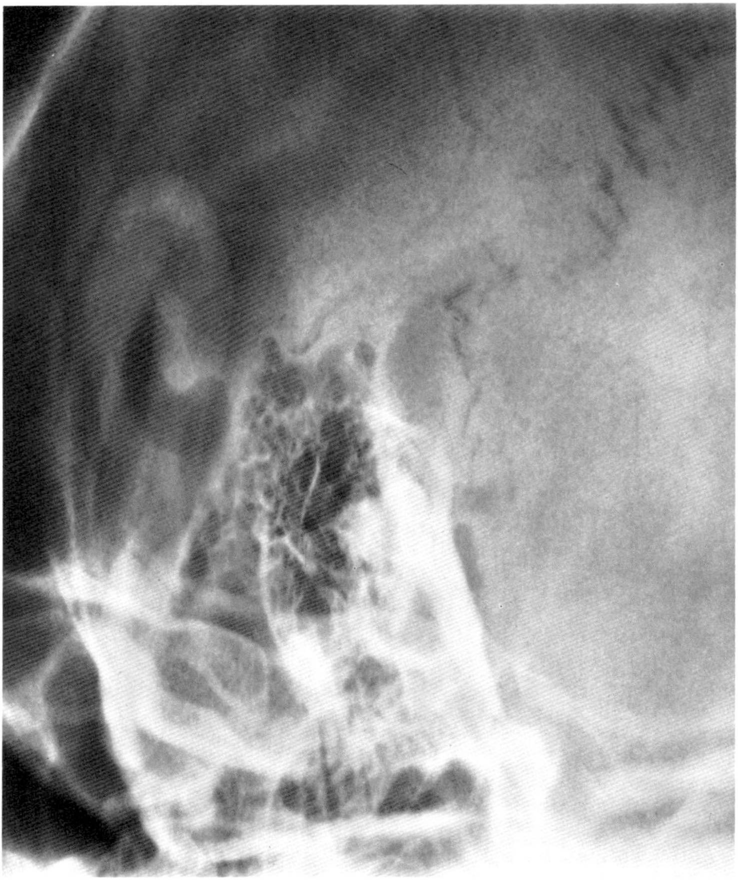

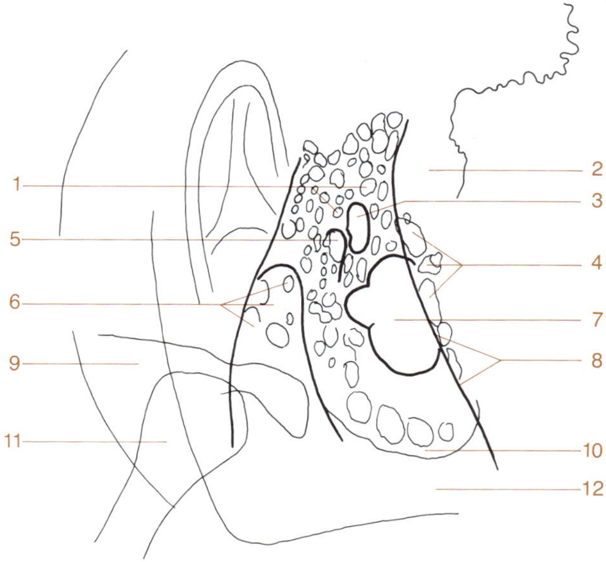

1 Periantral air cells
2 Sigmoid sinus
3 Antrum
4 Retrosinous air cells
5 Aditus ad antrum
6 External auditory canal and tympanic cavity
7 Osseous labyrinth
8 Osseous sinus wall (posterior margin of the petrous pyramid)
9 Zygomatic bone
10 Apex of the mastoid
11 Condyle of the mandible
12 Apex of the petrous pyramid

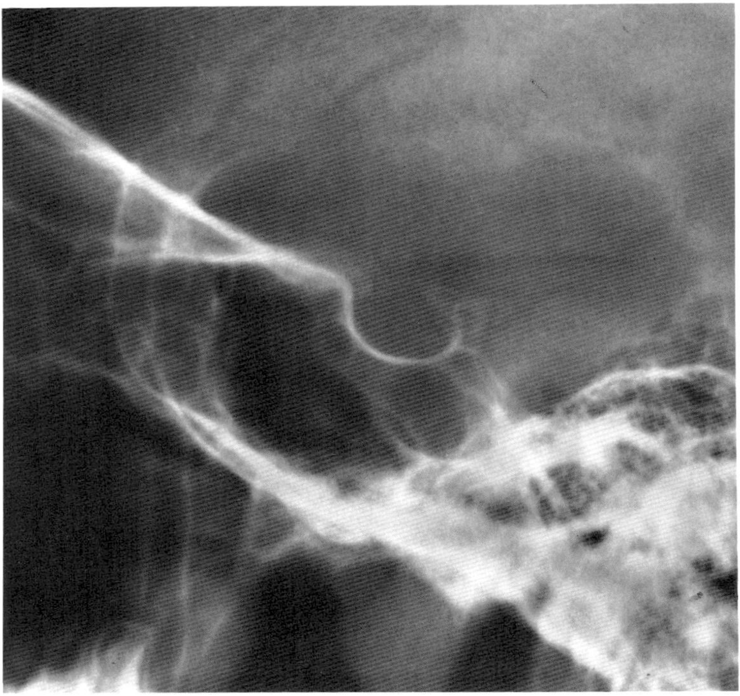

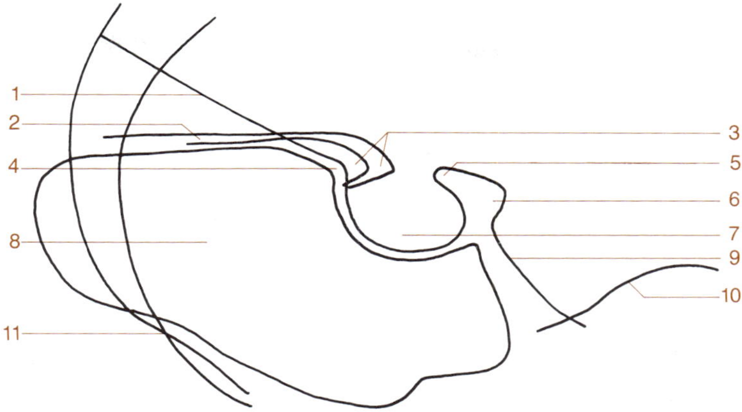

1 Floor of anterior cranial fossa and roof of orbits
2 Planum sphenoidale
3 Anterior clinoid process
4 Tuberculum sellae
5 Posterior clinoid process
6 Dorsum sellae
7 Pituitary fossa
8 Sphenoid sinus
9 Clivus
10 Crista pyramidalis
11 Greater wing of the sphenoid bone (anterior wall of middle cranial fossa)

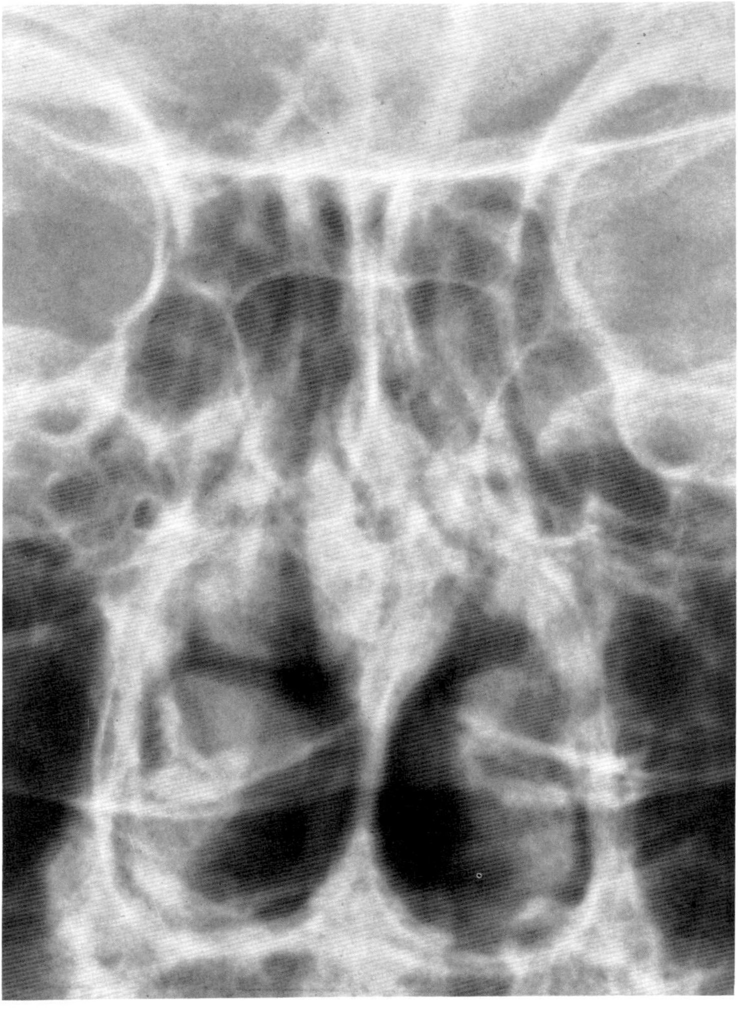

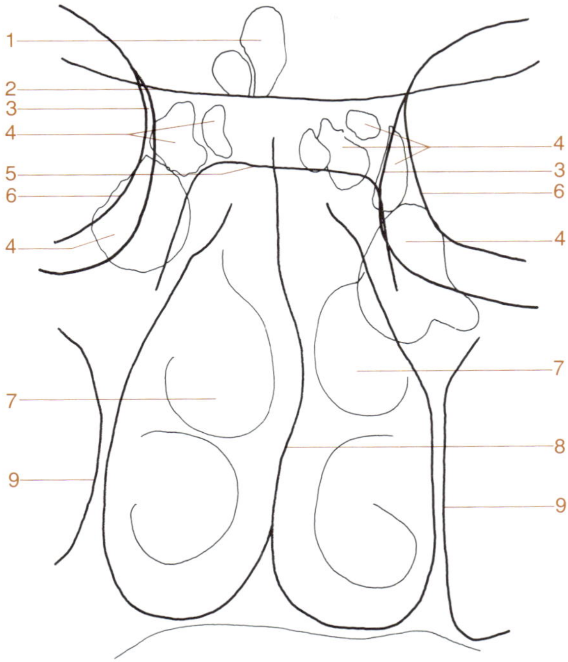

1 Frontal sinuses
2 Planum sphenoidale
3 Medial wall of orbit
4 Ethmoidal cells
5 Pituitary fossa (floor of the sella turcica)
6 Lamina papyracea
7 Nasal turbinates
8 Nasal septum
9 Medial wall of the maxillary sinus

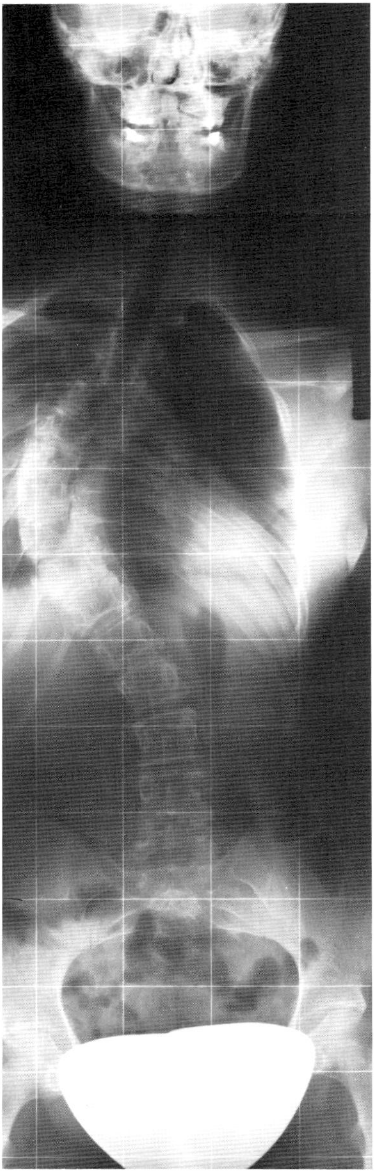

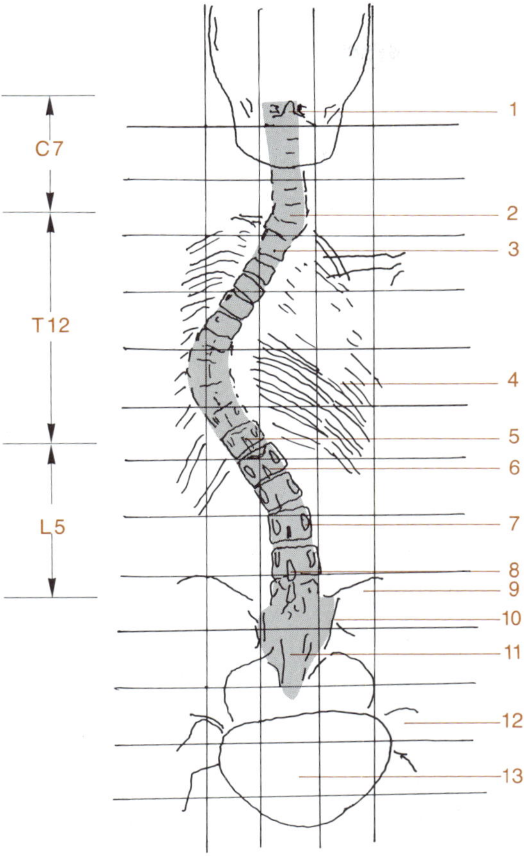

1 Odontoid
2 C7
3 T2
4 Ribcage
5 T12
6 L1
7 Pedicle, L3
8 Spinous process, L6
9 Iliac bone
10 Sacroiliac joint
11 Sacrum
12 Hip joint
13 Gonadal shield

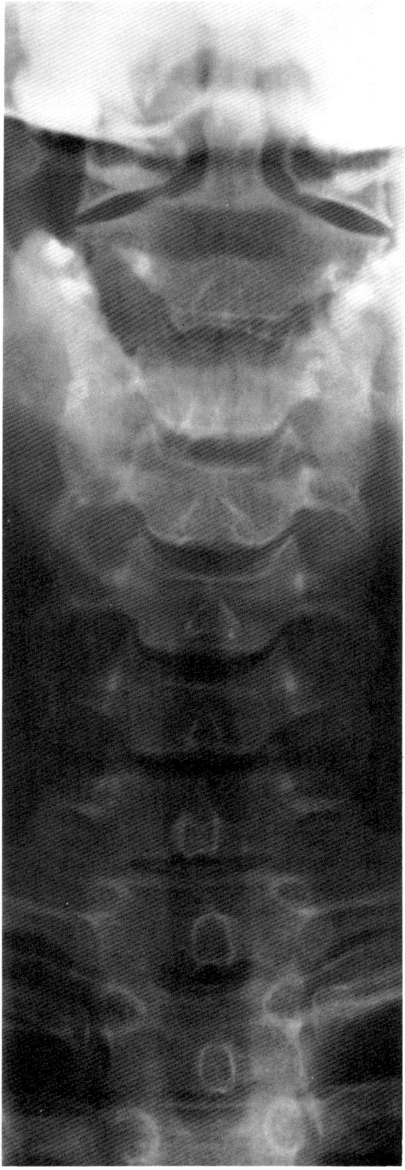

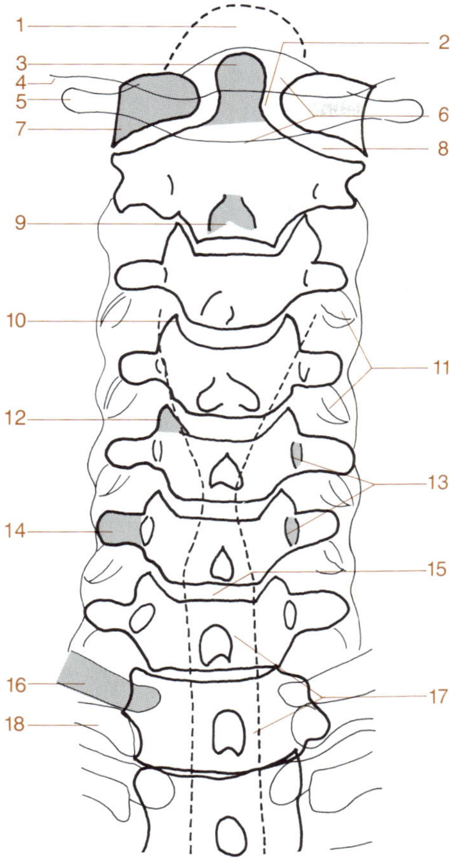

1 Foramen magnum
2 Atlantoaxial joint
3 Odontoid
4 Occipital bone
5 Transverse process
6 Vertebral arch
7 Lateral mass (C1)
8 Atlantoaxial joint
9 Spinous process (bifid)
10 Uncovertebral joint
11 Overlapping articular processes (of the facet joints)
12 Uncinate process
13 Pedicle of the vertebral arch
14 Transverse process
15 Intervertebral disk space
16 Transverse process (T1)
17 Tracheal air column
18 First rib

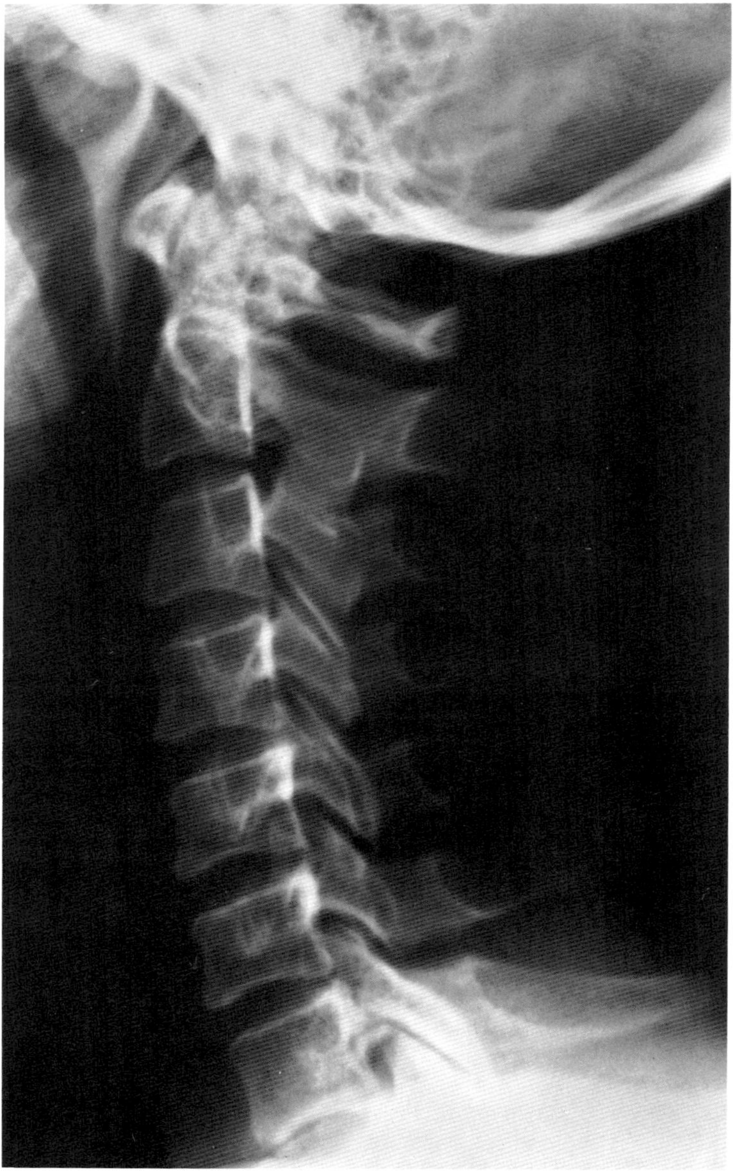

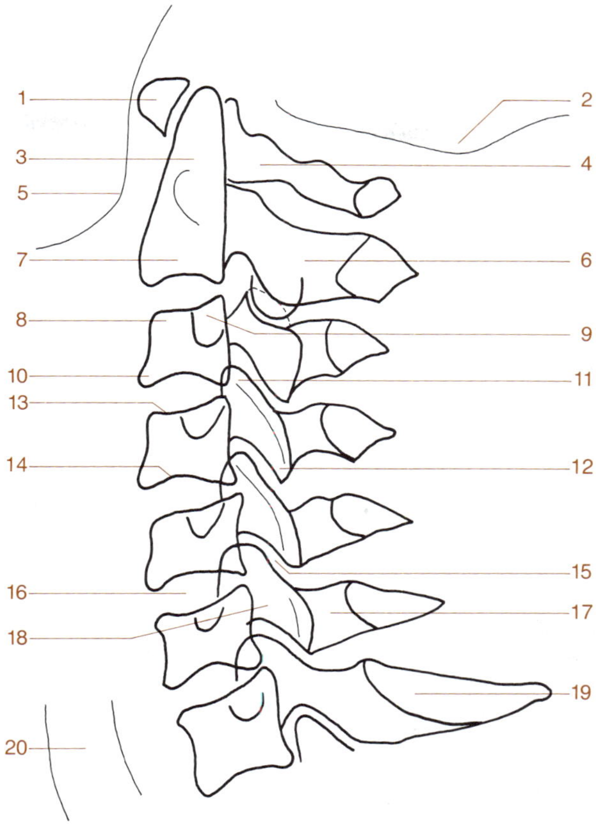

1 Anterior arch of the atlas
2 Base of the skull
3 Odontoid process
4 Posterior arch of the atlas
5 Mandible
6 Spinous process
7 Body of C2
8 Anterior superior vertebral margin
9 Transverse process
10 Anterior inferior vertebral margin
11 Superior articular facet
12 Inferior articular facet
13 Superior vertebral endplate
14 Inferior vertebral endplate
15 Intervertebral facet joint
16 Intervertebral disk space
17 Lamina
18 Articular pillar
19 Spinous process
20 Trachea

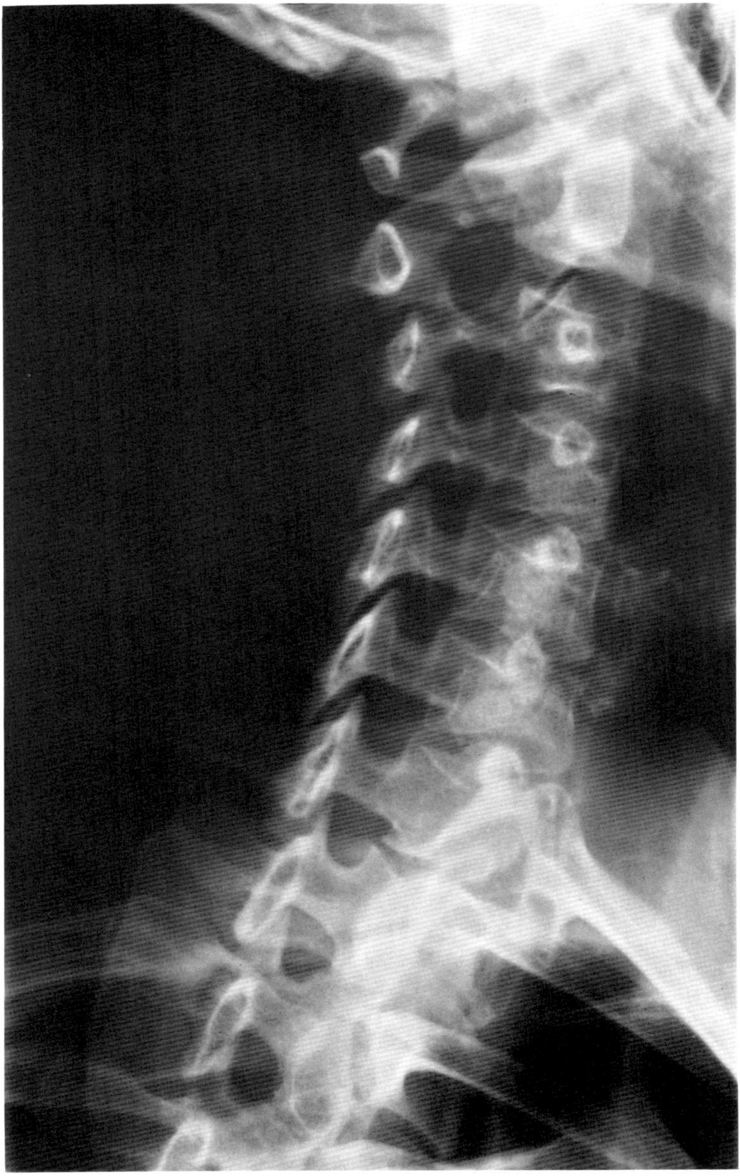

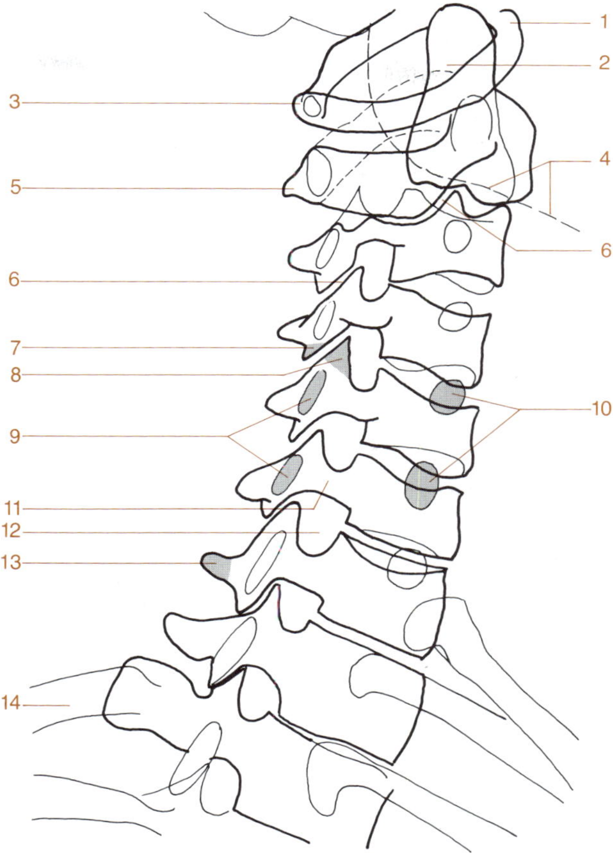

1 Anterior arch
2 Odontoid process
3 Atlas
4 Mandible
5 Body of C2
6 Facet joint
7 Inferior articular facet
8 Superior articular facet
9 Transverse process
10 Contralateral pedicle
11 Pedicle of the vertebral arch
12 Intervertebral foramen
13 Spinous process
14 Ribs

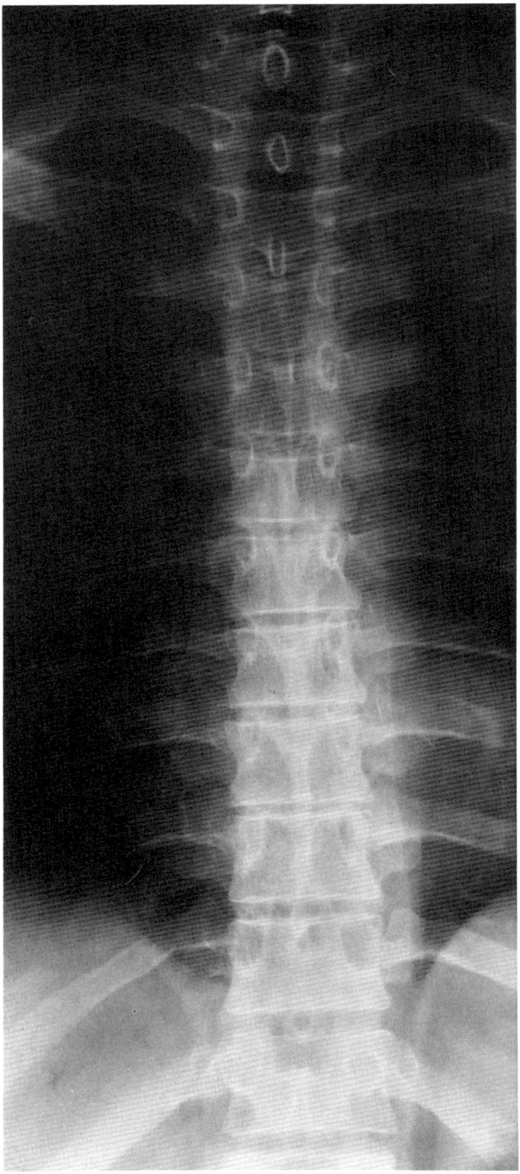

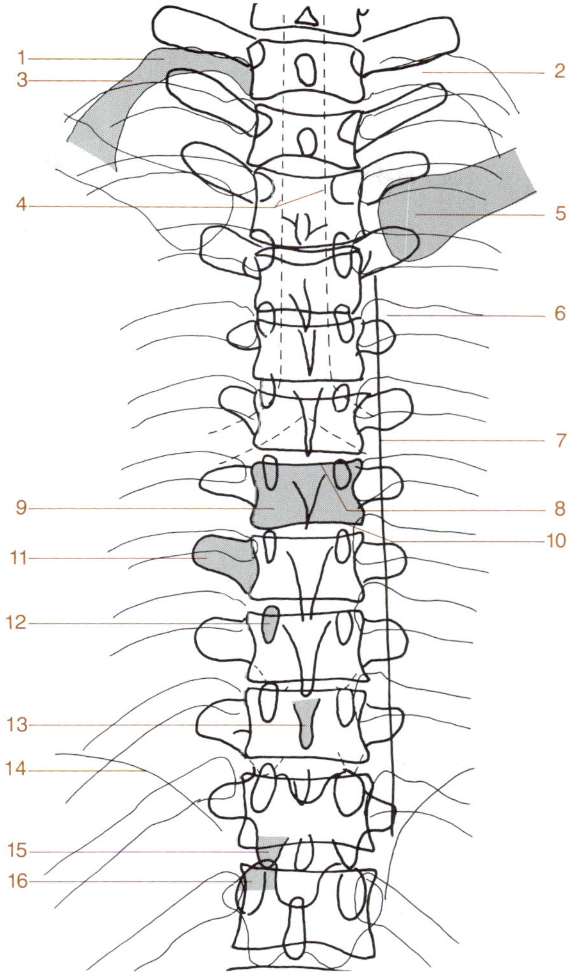

1 Tubercle of rib I
2 Neck of the rib
3 Rib I
4 Trachea
5 Clavicle
6 Head of the rib
7 Paraspinal line
8 Superior vertebral endplate
9 Vertebral body
10 Inferior vertebral endplate
11 Transverse process
12 Pedicle of the vertebral arch
13 Spinous process
14 Diaphragm
15 Inferior articular process
16 Superior articular process

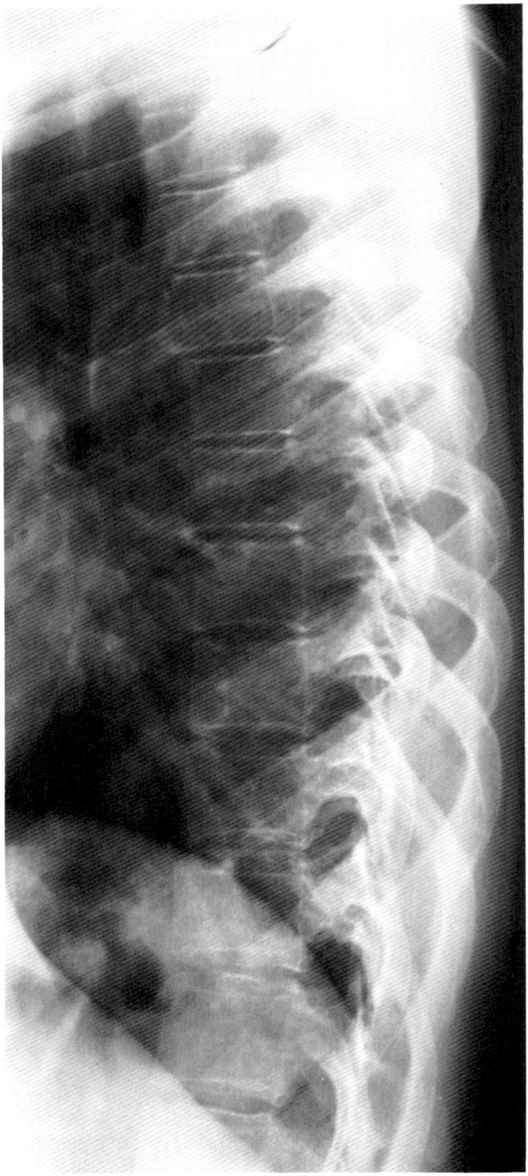

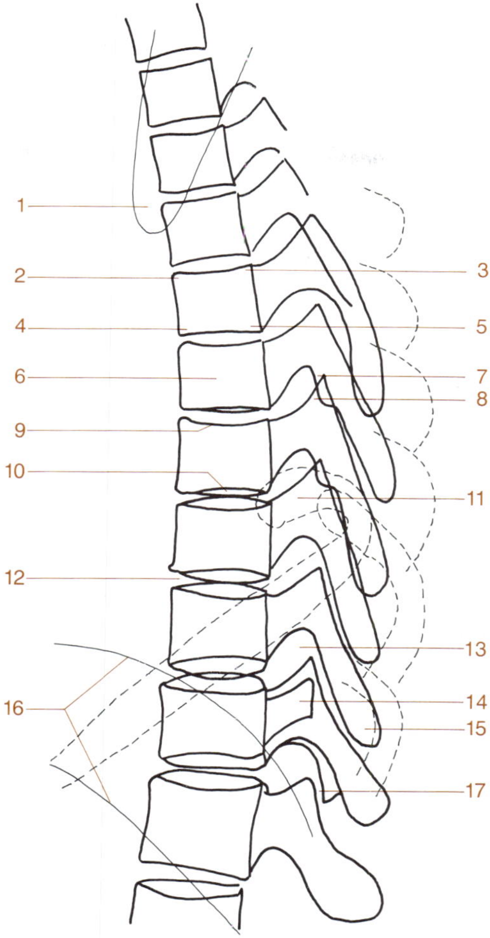

1 Scapula
2 Anterior superior margin
3 Posterior superior margin
4 Anterior inferior margin
5 Posterior inferior margin
6 Vertebral body
7 Superior articular process
8 Inferior articular process
9 Superior vertebral endplate
10 Inferior vertebral endplate
11 Head of the rib
12 Intervertebral disk space
13 Intervertebral foramen
14 Transverse process
15 Spinous process
16 Dome of the diaphragm
17 Intervertebral facet joint

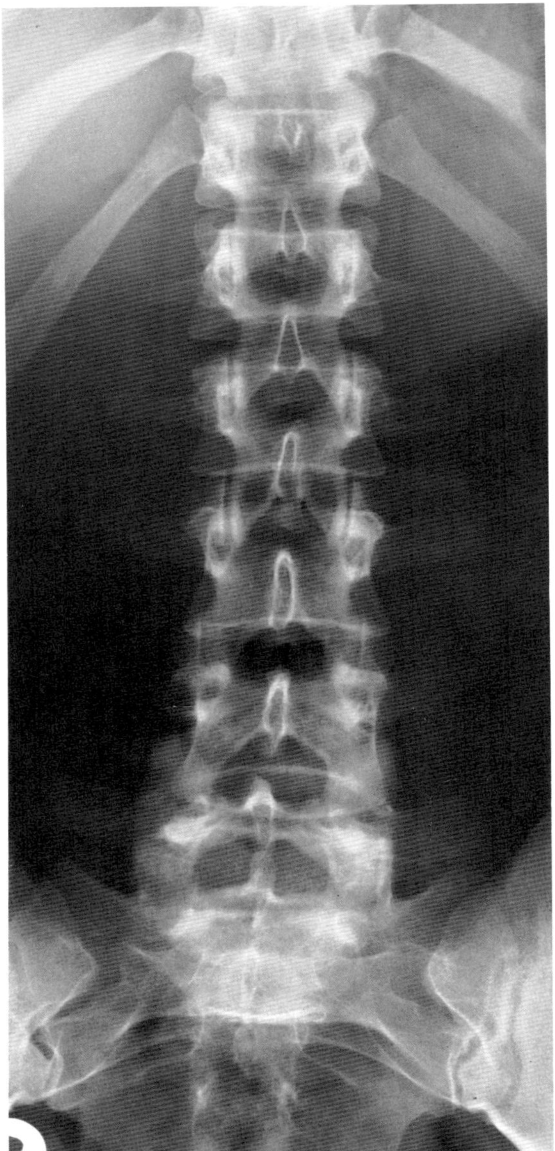

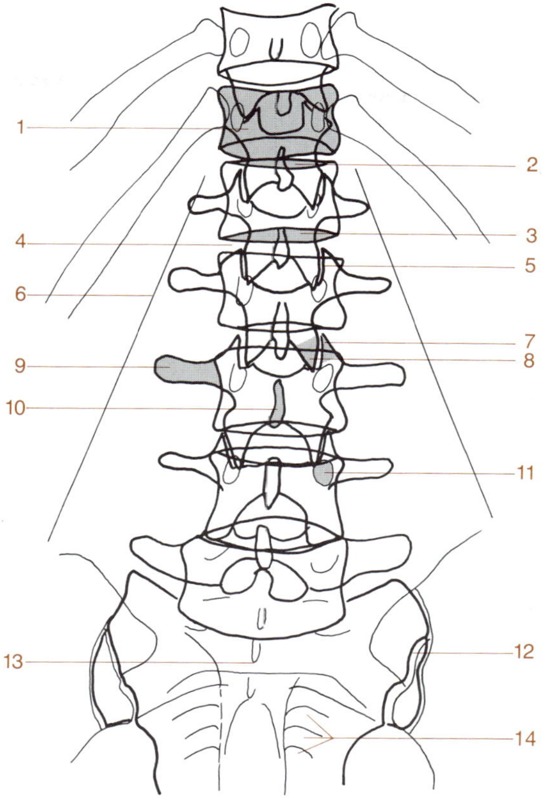

1 Vertebral body
2 Superior vertebral endplate
3 Inferior vertebral endplate
4 Intervertebral disk space
5 Intervertebral facet joint
6 Psoas muscle
7 Superior articular process
8 Inferior articular process
9 Transverse process
10 Spinous process
11 Pedicle of the vertebral arch
12 Sacroiliac joint
13 Sacrum
14 Sacral foramina

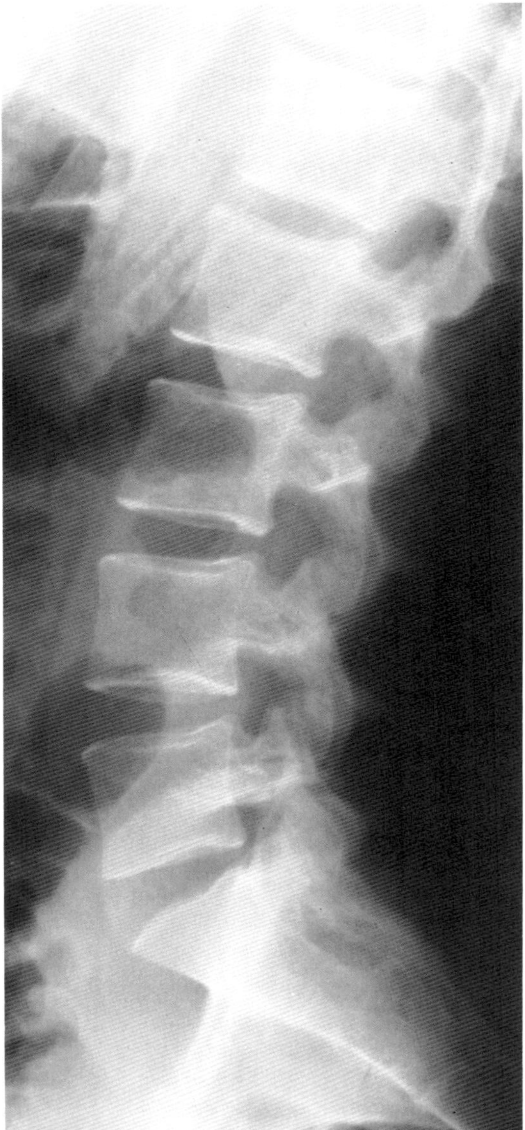

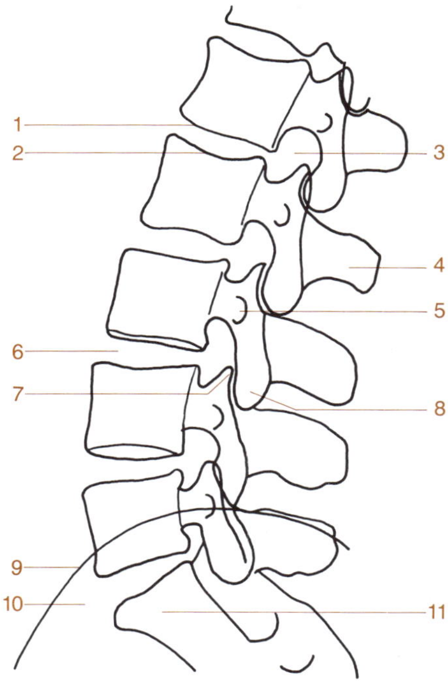

1 Superior vertebral endplate
2 Inferior vertebral endplate
3 Intervertebral foramen
4 Spinous process
5 Transverse process
6 Intervertebral disk space
7 Superior articular process
8 Inferior articular process
9 Iliac crest
10 Promontory
11 Sacrum

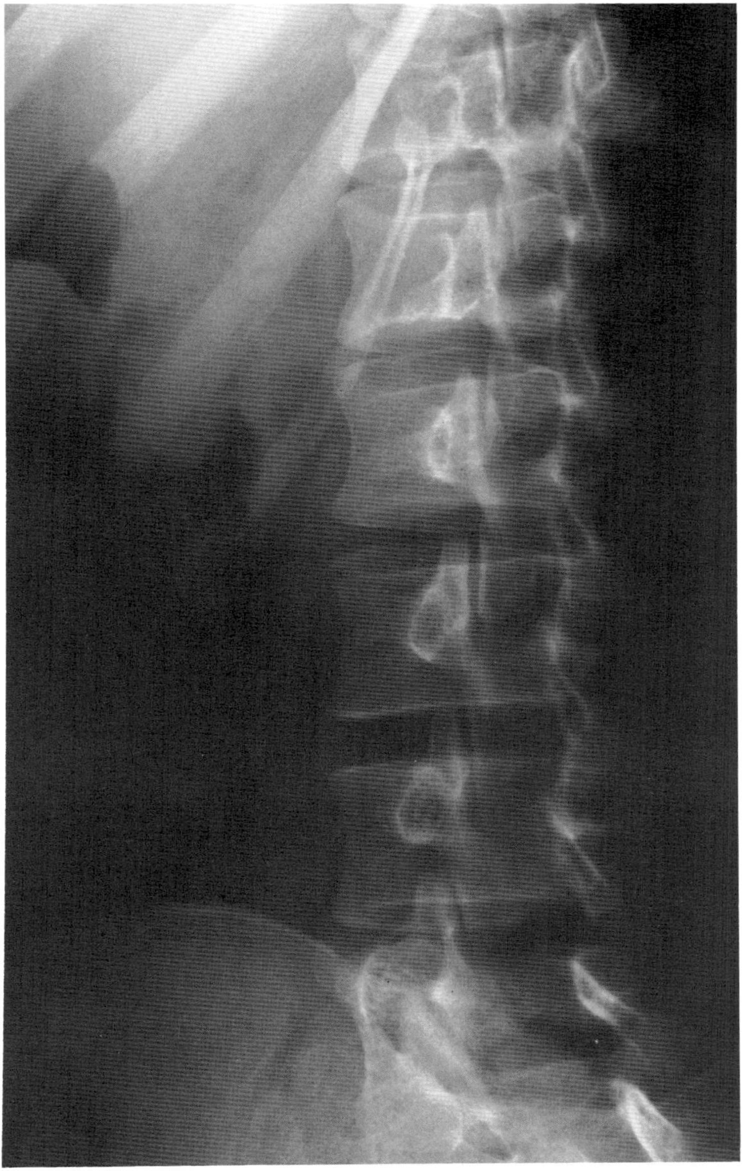

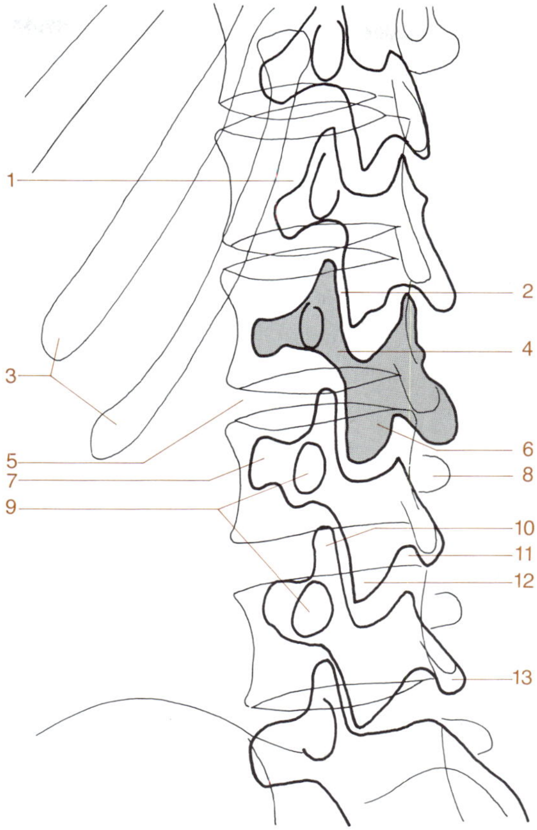

1 Vertebral body
2 Intervertebral disk space
3 Ribs
4 Pars interarticularis
5 Intervertebral disk space
6 Lamina of the vertebral arch
7 Transverse process (ipsilateral)
8 Transverse process (contralateral)
9 Pedicle of the vertebral arch
10 Superior articular process
11 Intervertebral foramen
12 Inferior articular process
13 Spinous process

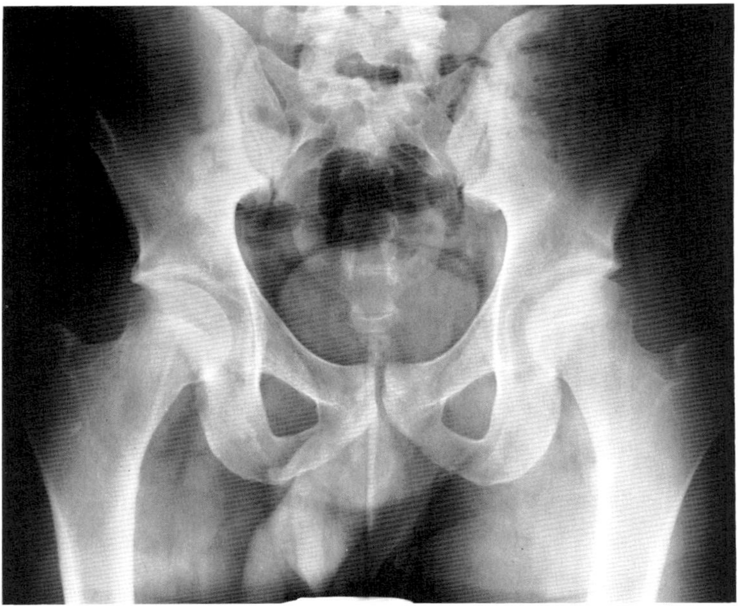

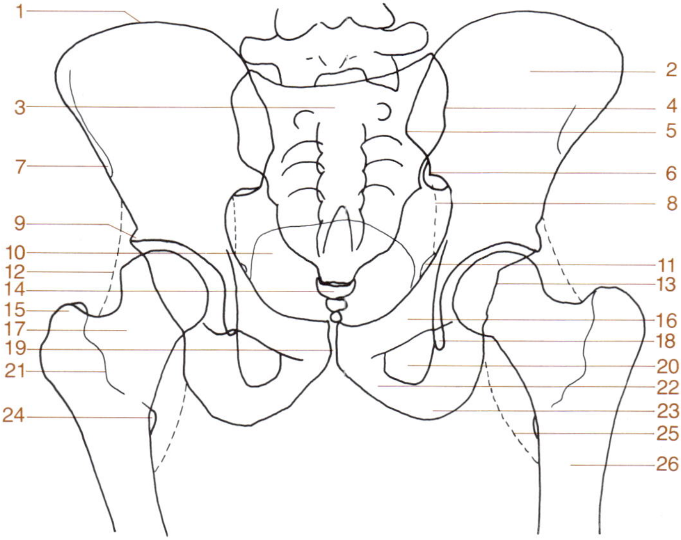

1 Iliac crest
2 Iliac wing
3 Sacrum
4 Sacroiliac joint
5 Posterior superior iliac spine
6 Posterior inferior iliac spine
7 Superior anterior iliac spine
8 Internal obturator muscle
9 Acetabular roof
10 Urinary bladder
11 Ischial spine
12 Fat plane medial to the gluteus minimus muscle
13 Posterior acetabular rim
14 Coccygeal bone
15 Greater trochanter
16 Superior pubic ramus
17 Femoral neck
18 Köhler's teardrop
19 Symphysis pubis
20 Obturator foramen
21 Intertrochanteric line
22 Inferior pubic ramus
23 Ischial tuberosity
24 Lesser trochanter
25 Fat plane medial to the ilio-psoas muscle
26 Femur

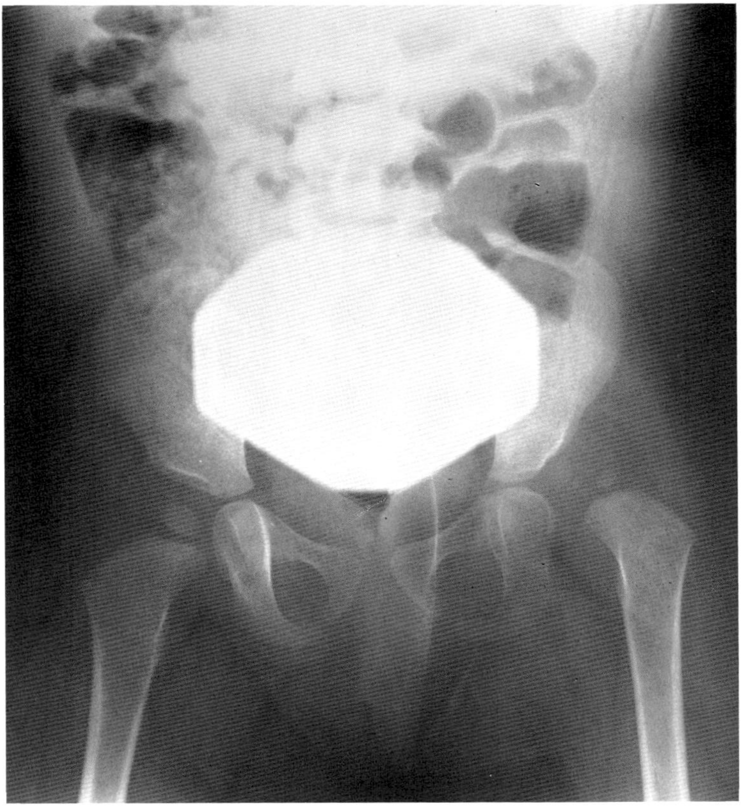

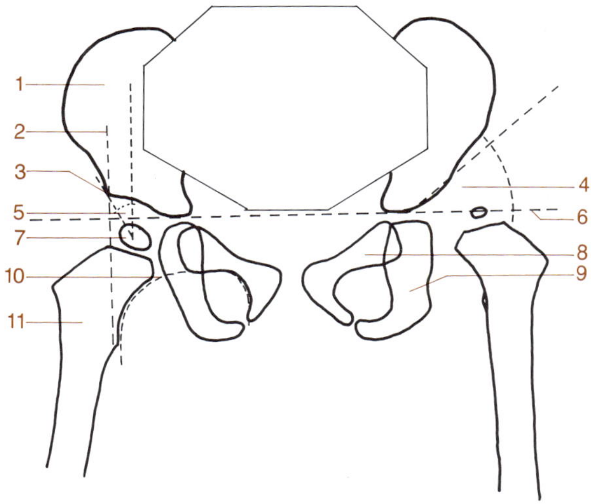

1 Iliac bone
2 Perkin's line (vertical from the roof of the acetabulum to Hilgenreiner's Y–Y line)
3 Roof of the acetabulum
4 Acetabular angle
5 Wiberg's center-to-corner angle (the angle between a vertical rising from the center of the epiphysis and a line running from the roof of the acetabulum to the center of the epiphysis)
6 Hilgenreiner's line (Y–Y line)
7 Femoral head epiphysis
8 Pubic bone
9 Ischial bone
10 Shenton's line (curvilinear connection between the upper margin of the obturator foramen and the neck of the femur)
11 Femur

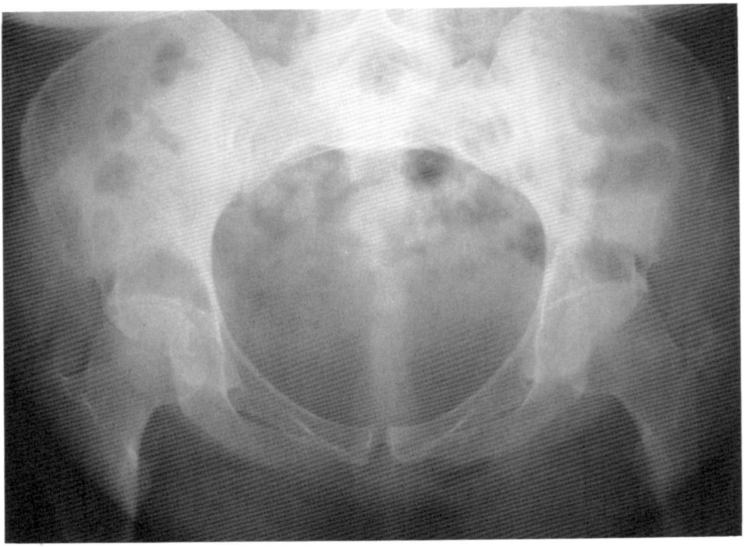

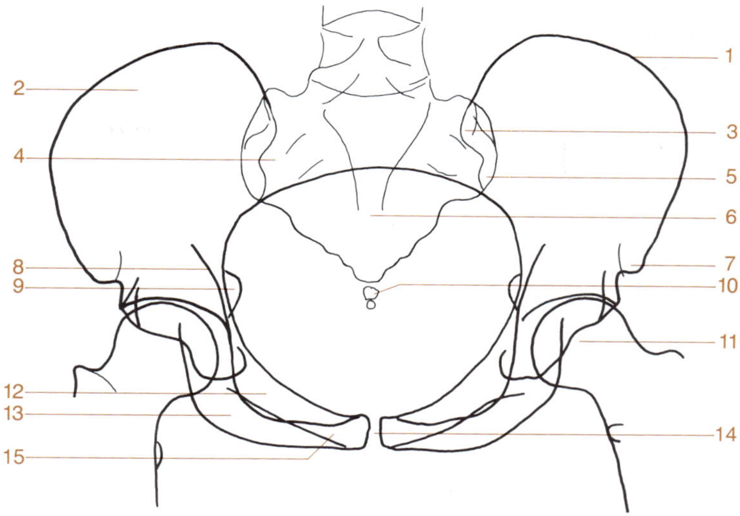

1 Iliac crest
2 Iliac wing
3 Posterior superior iliac spine
4 Sacral wing
5 Posterior inferior iliac spine
6 Sacrum
7 Anterior superior iliac spine
8 Iliopubic line or column
9 Ischial spine
10 Coccygeal bone
11 Femoral head
12 Superior pubic ramus
13 Ischial tuberosity
14 Symphysis pubis
15 Inferior pubic ramus

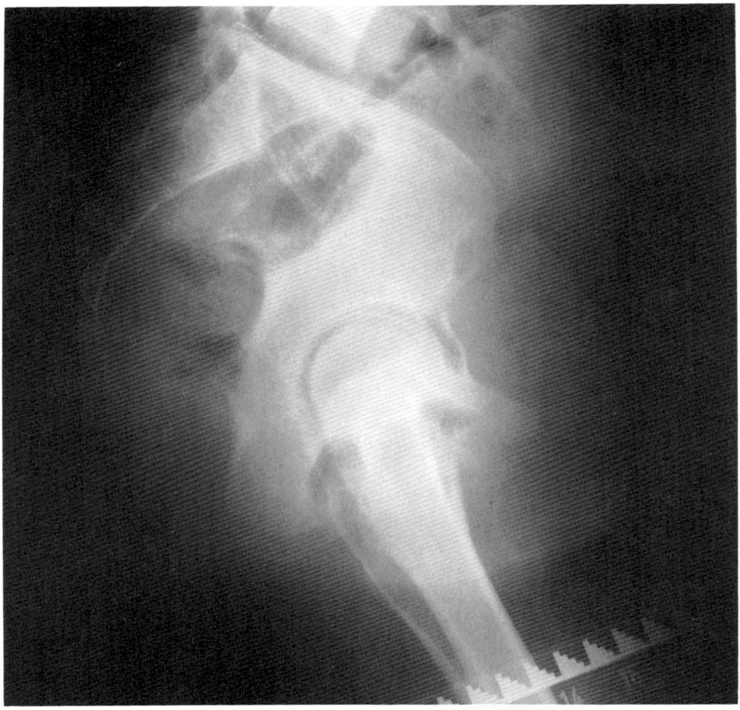

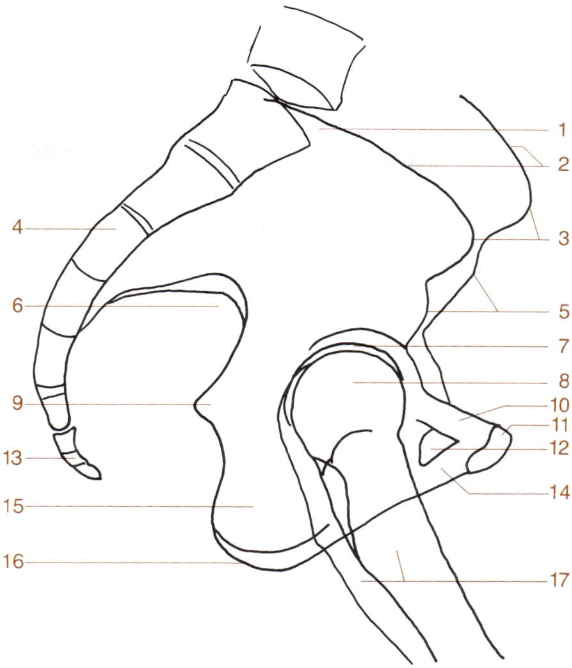

1 Promontory
2 Iliac crest
3 Anterior superior iliac spine
4 Sacrum
5 Anterior inferior iliac spine
6 Greater sciatic notch
7 Hip-joint space
8 Femoral head
9 Ischial spine
10 Superior pubic ramus
11 Symphysis pubis
12 Obturator foramen
13 Coccygeal bone
14 Inferior pubic ramus
15 Ischial body
16 Ischial tuberosity
17 Femur

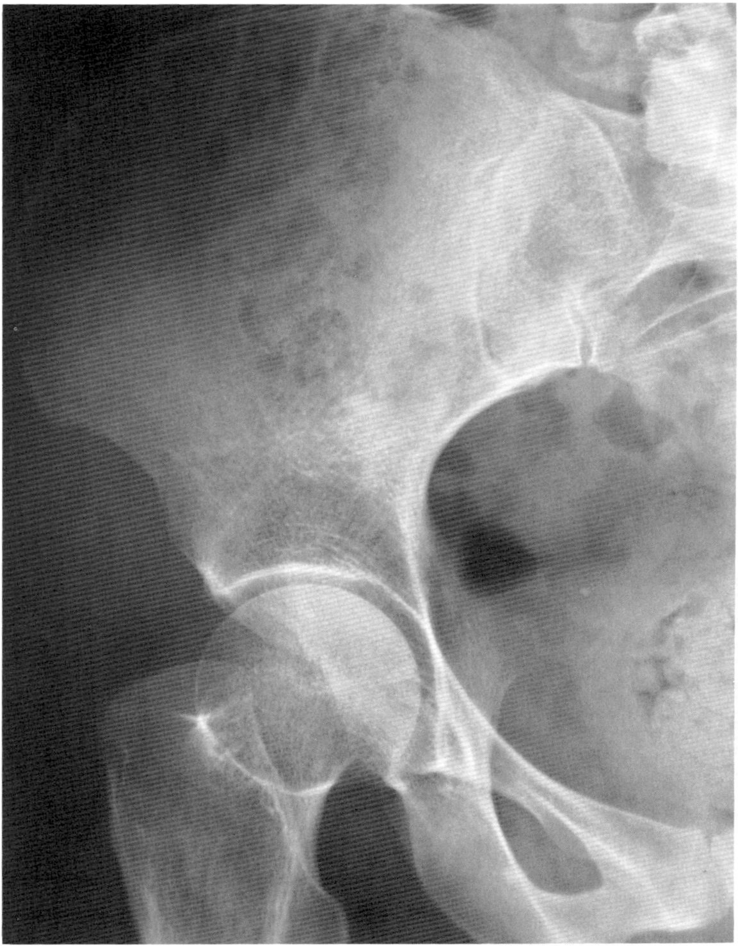

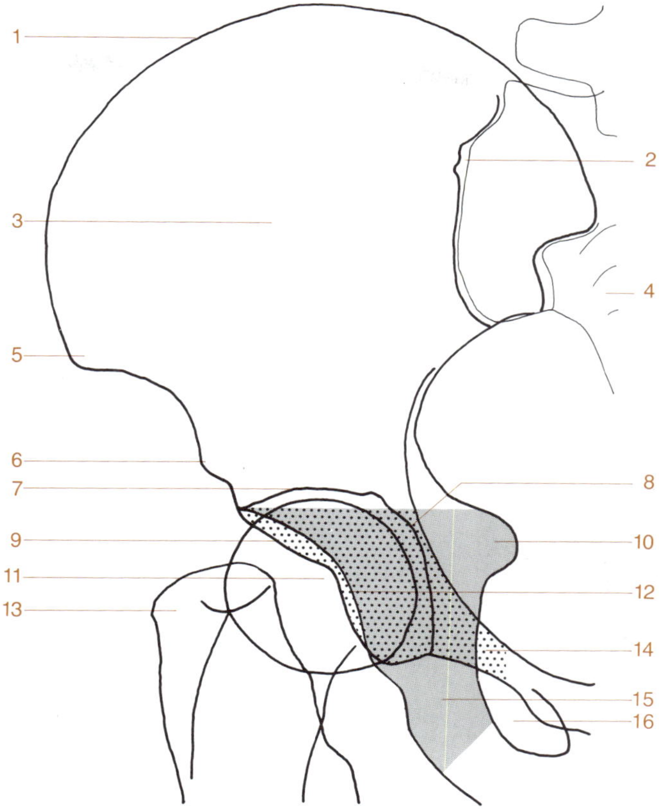

1 Iliac crest
2 Sacroiliac joint
3 Iliac wing
4 Sacrum
5 Anterior superior iliac spine
6 Anterior inferior iliac spine
7 Acetabular roof
8 Floor of the acetabulum
9 Anterior acetabular rim
10 Ischial spine
11 Femoral head
12 Posterior acetabular rim
13 Greater trochanter
14 Pubic bone, anterior column (iliopubic column)
15 Ischial bone, posterior column (ilioischial column)
16 Obturator foramen

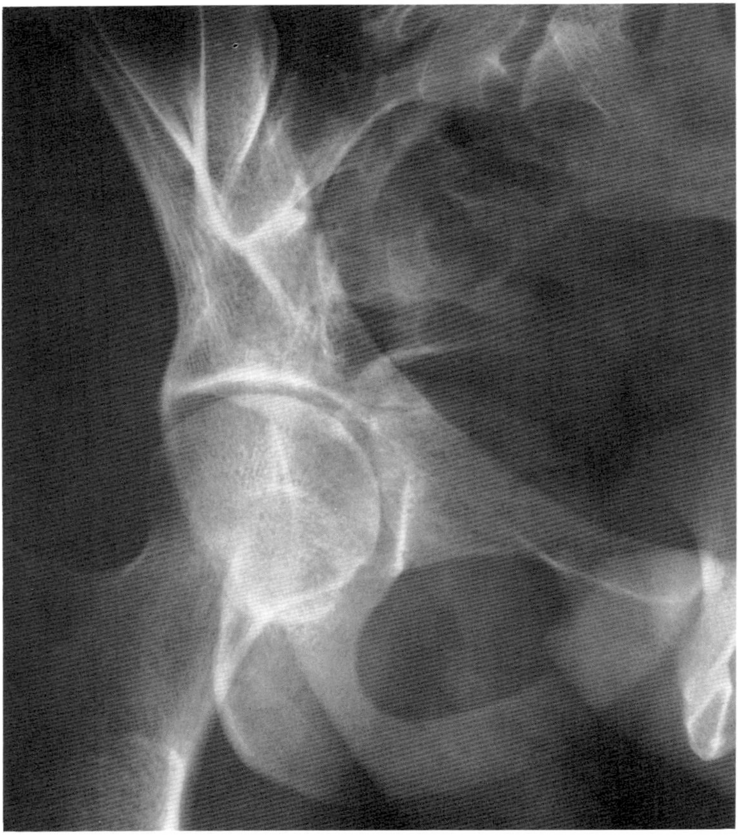

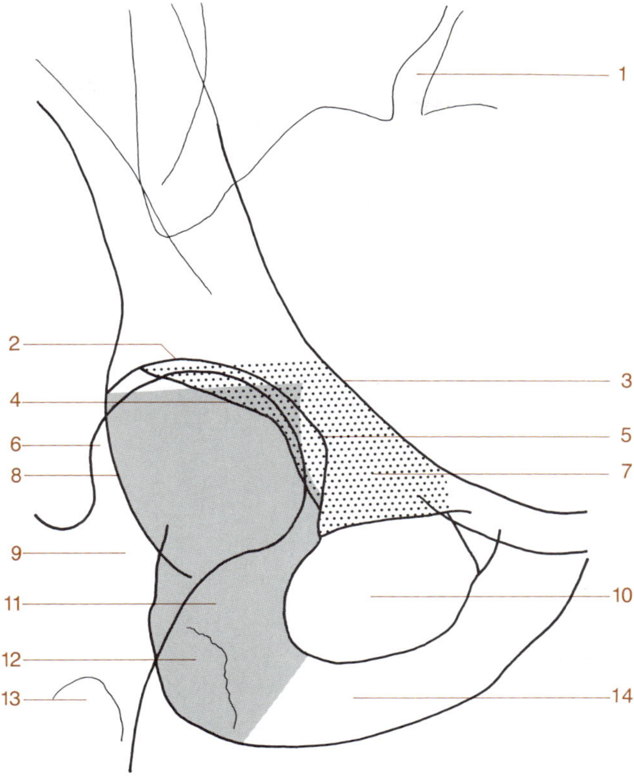

1 Sacroiliac joint
2 Roof of the acetabulum
3 Iliopubic line
4 Anterior acetabular rim
5 Anterior acetabular floor
6 Femoral head
7 Pubic bone, anterior column
8 Posterior acetabular rim
9 Femoral neck
10 Obturator foramen
11 Ischial bone, posterior column
12 Ischial tuberosity
13 Lesser trochanter
14 Inferior pubic ramus

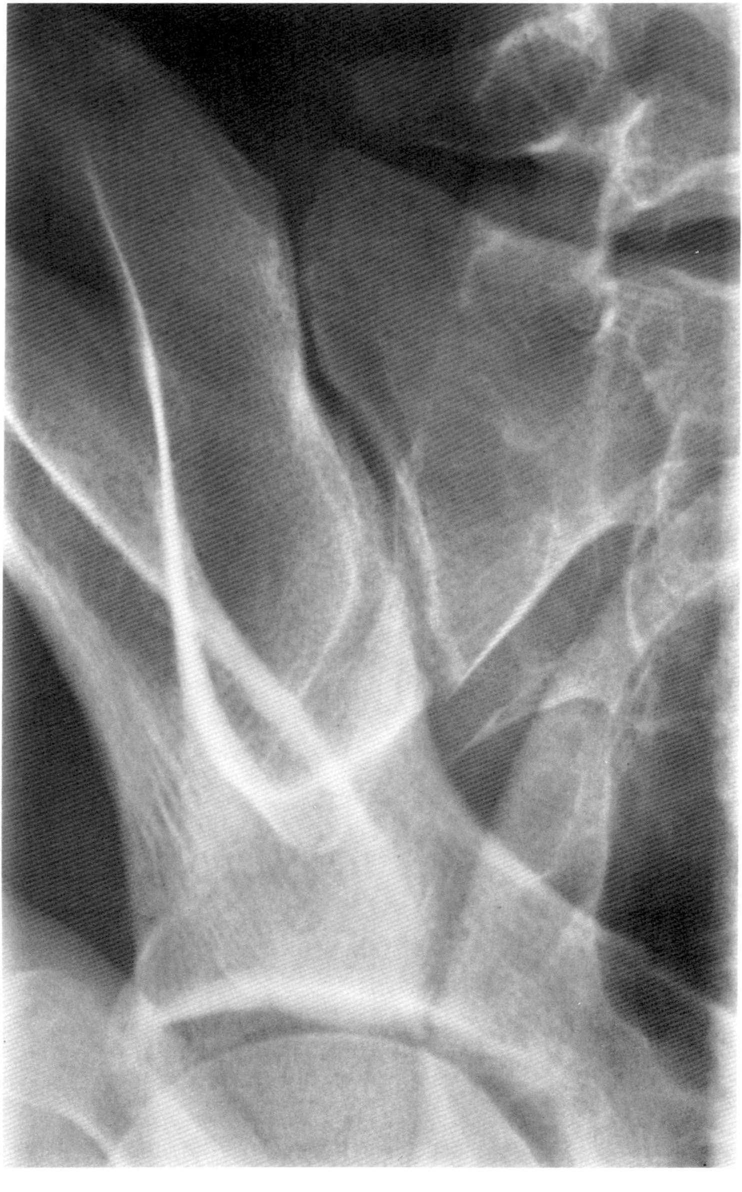

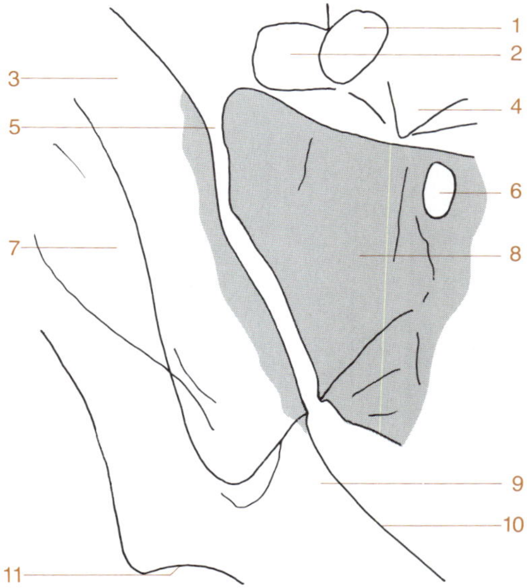

1 Pedicle, L5
2 Transverse process, L5
3 Iliac wing
4 Vertebral body, L5
5 Sacroiliac joint
6 Sacral foramen
7 Iliac wing
8 Lateral mass of the sacrum
9 Iliac bone
10 Arcuate line
11 Roof of the acetabulum

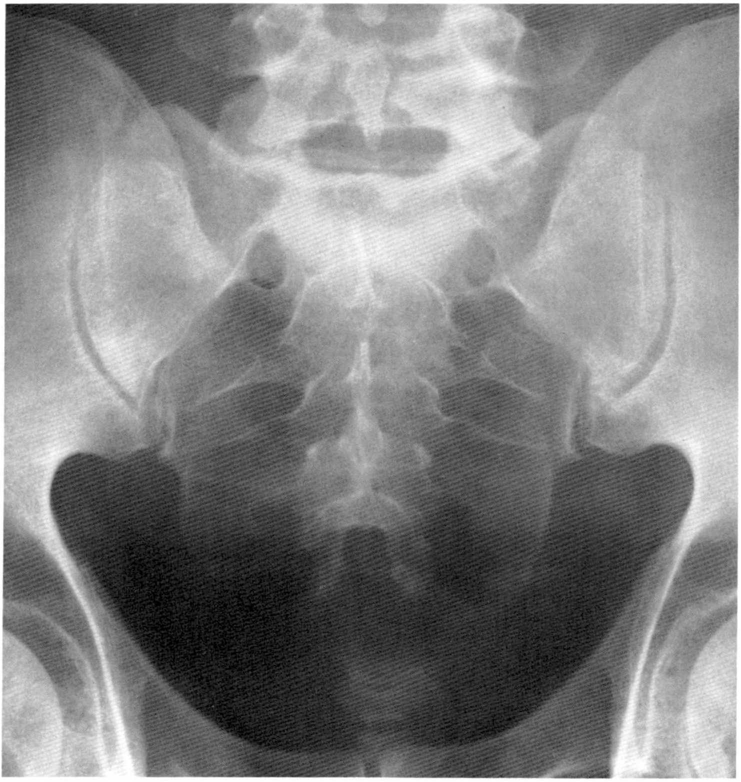

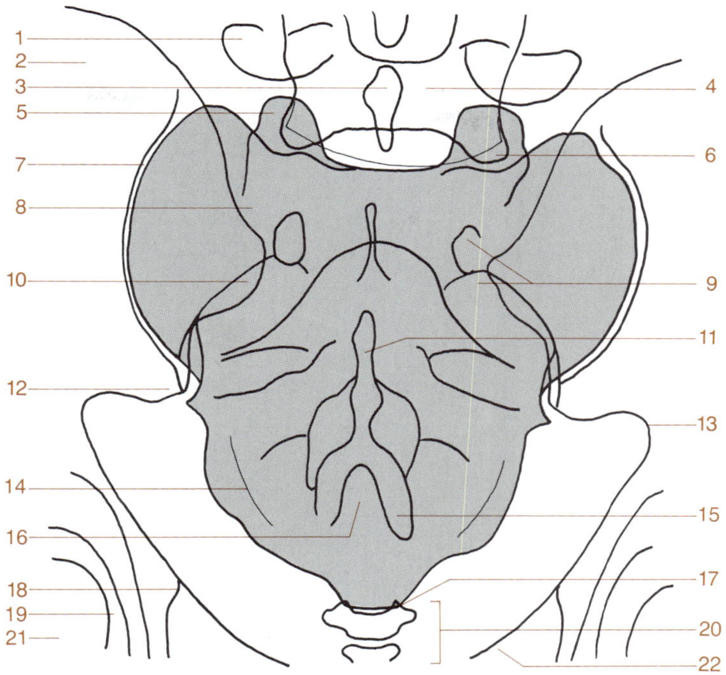

1 Transverse process
2 Iliac wing
3 Spinous process
4 L5
5 Superior articular process
6 Inferior articular process (L5)
7 Sacroiliac joint
8 Sacral wing
9 Sacral foramina
10 Posterior superior iliac spine
11 Median sacral crest
12 Posterior inferior iliac spine
13 Sciatic notch
14 Lateral sacral crest
15 Bifid spinous process
16 Sacral hiatus
17 Sacrococcygeal synchondrosis
18 Ischial spine
19 Hip joint
20 Coccygeal bone
21 Femoral head
22 Superior pubic ramus

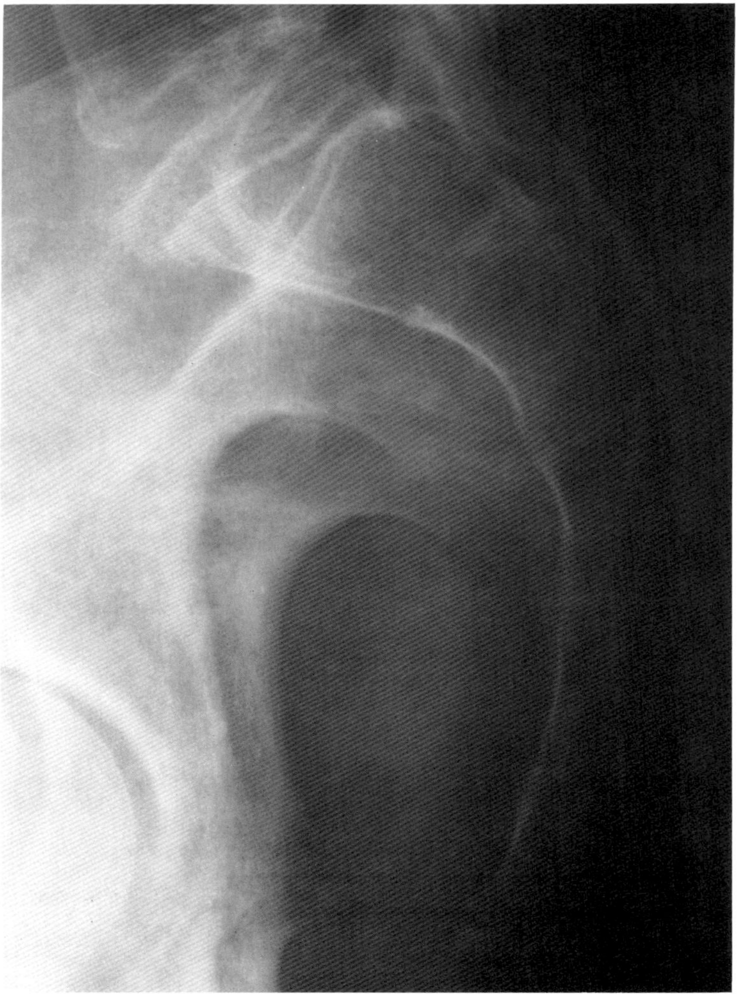

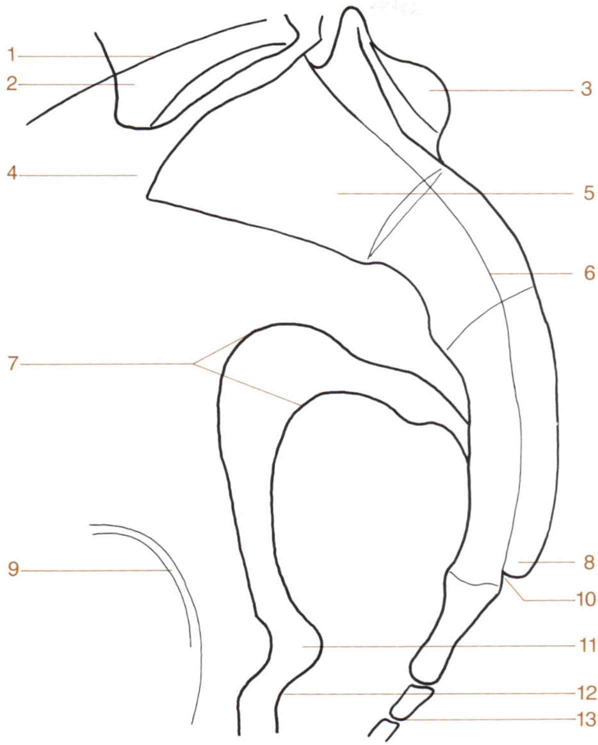

1 Iliac crest
2 L5
3 Median sacral crest
4 Promontory
5 Sacrum
6 Sacral canal
7 Greater sciatic notch
8 Fused sacral spinous processes
9 Hip joint
10 Sacral canal
11 Ischial spine
12 Lesser sciatic notch
13 Coccygeal bone

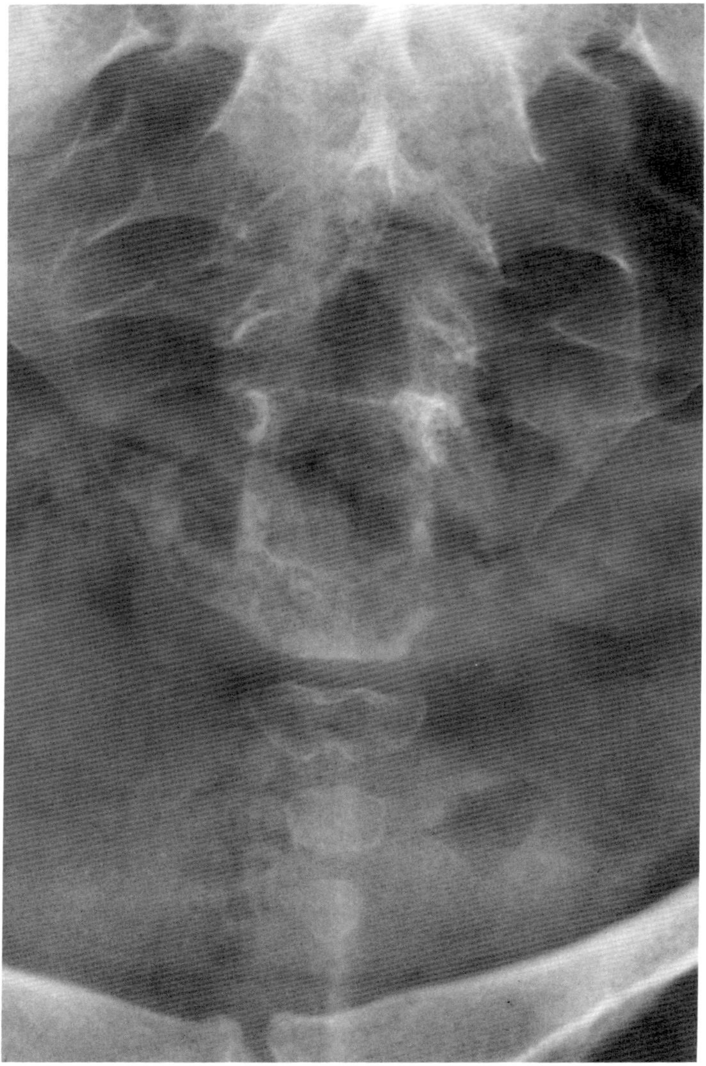

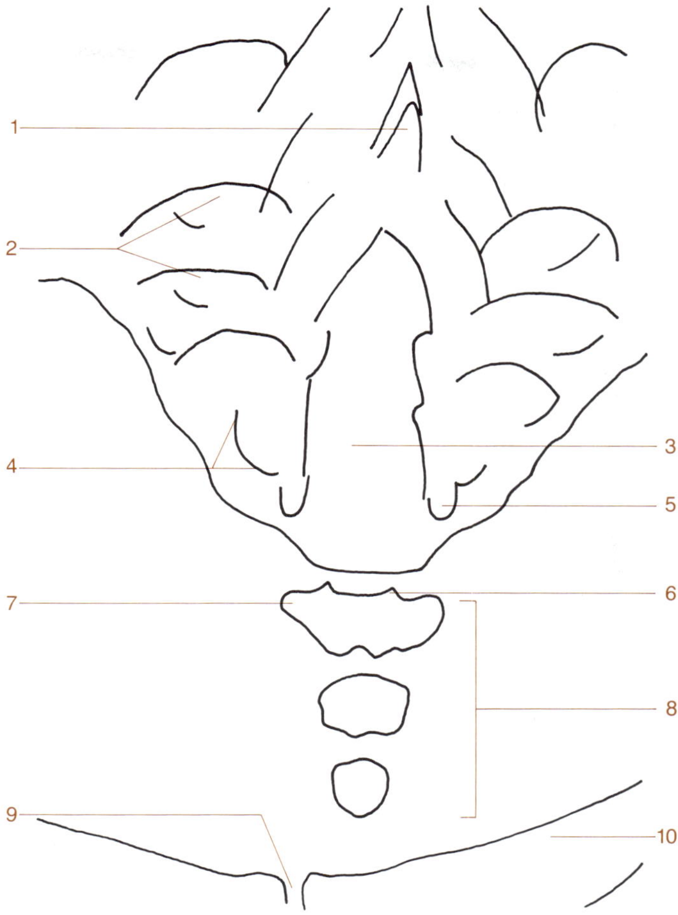

1 Median sacral crest
2 Sacral foramina
3 Sacral canal
4 Lateral sacral crest
5 Sacral horn
6 Sacrococcygeal synchondrosis
7 Transverse process
8 Coccygeal bone
9 Symphysis pubis
10 Superior pubic ramus

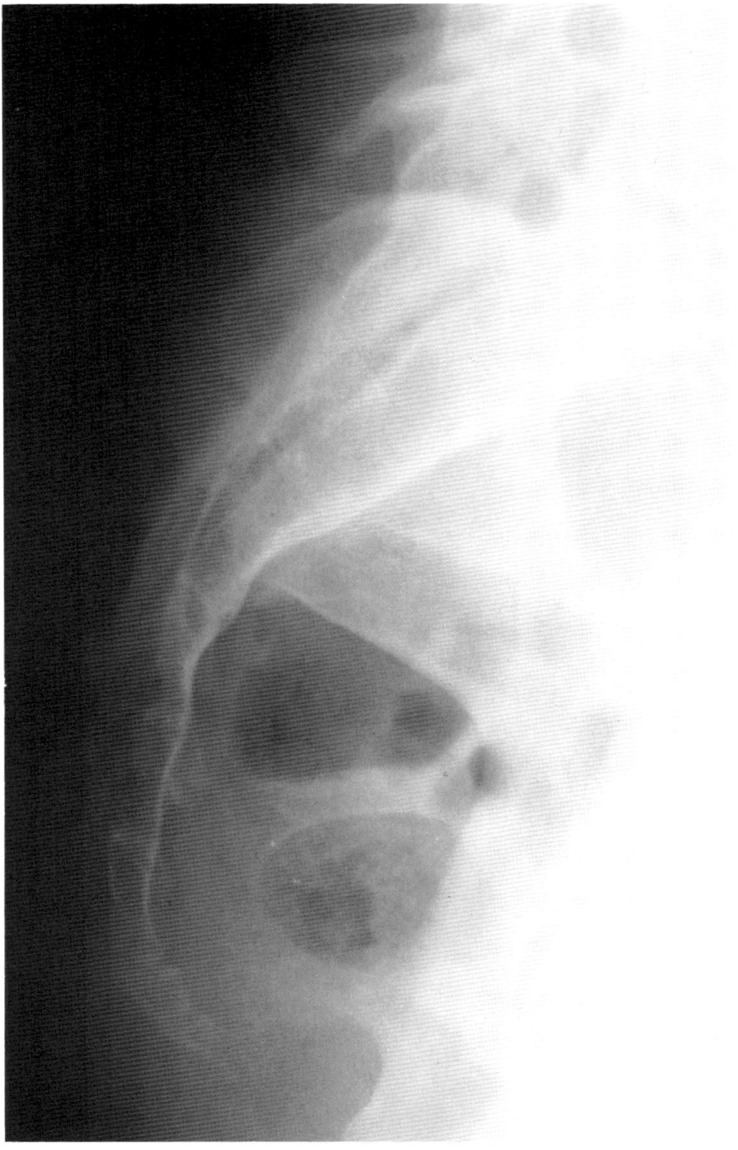

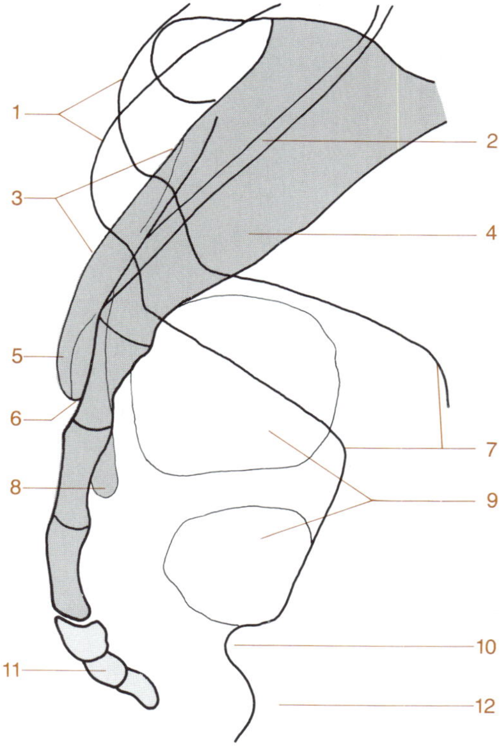

1 Iliac crest
2 Sacral canal
3 Median sacral crest
4 Sacrum
5 Sacral horn
6 Sacral canal
7 Greater sciatic notch
8 Lateral sacral crest
9 Rectal gas
10 Ischial spine
11 Coccygeal bone
12 Ischial bone

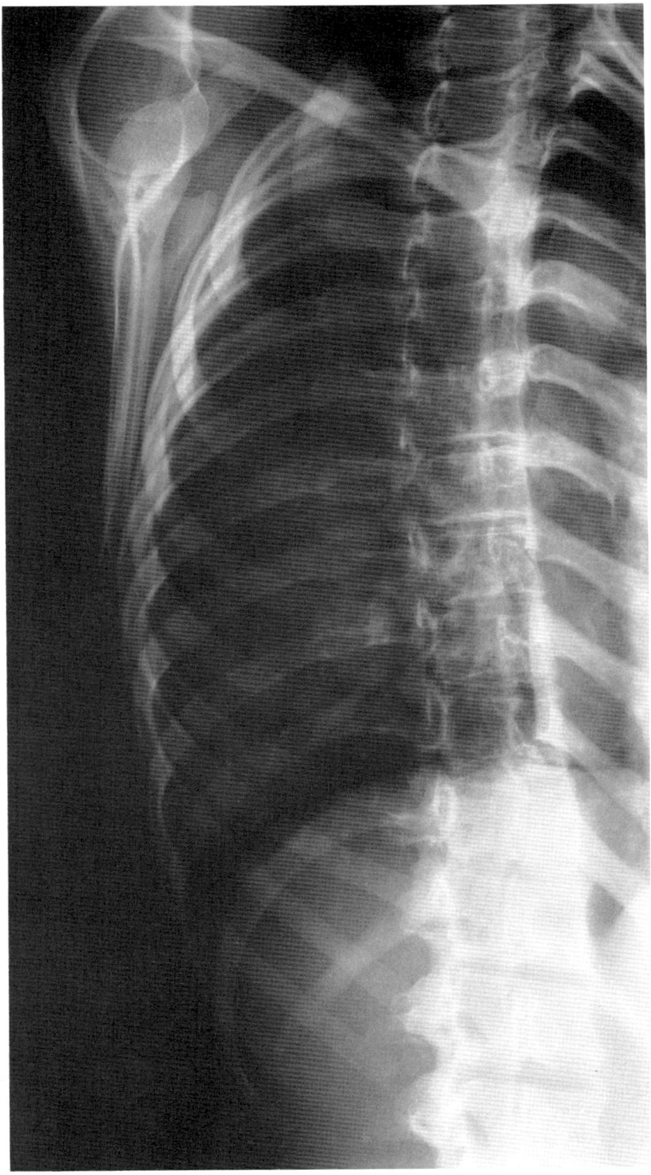

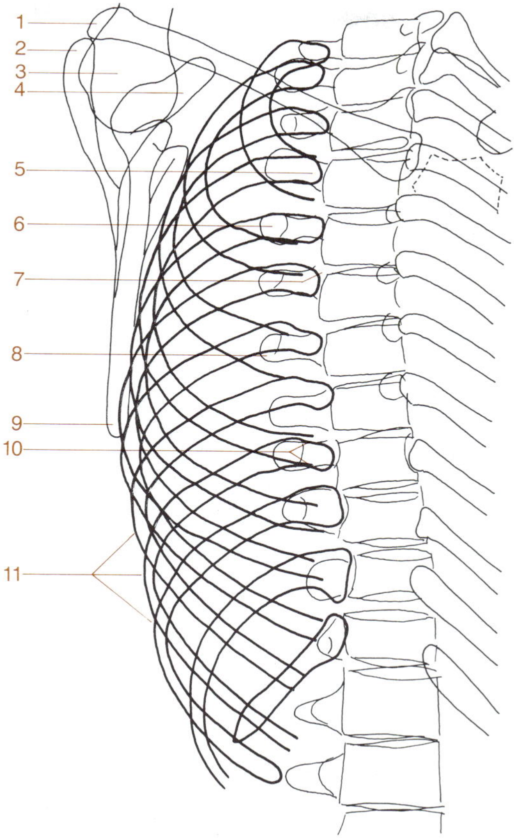

1 Clavicle (distal end)
2 Akromion
3 Humeral head
4 Coracoid process
5 Head of the rib
6 Costotransversal articulation
7 Costovertebral articulation
8 Transverse process
9 Inferior angle of the scapula
10 Rib neck
11 Costal arch

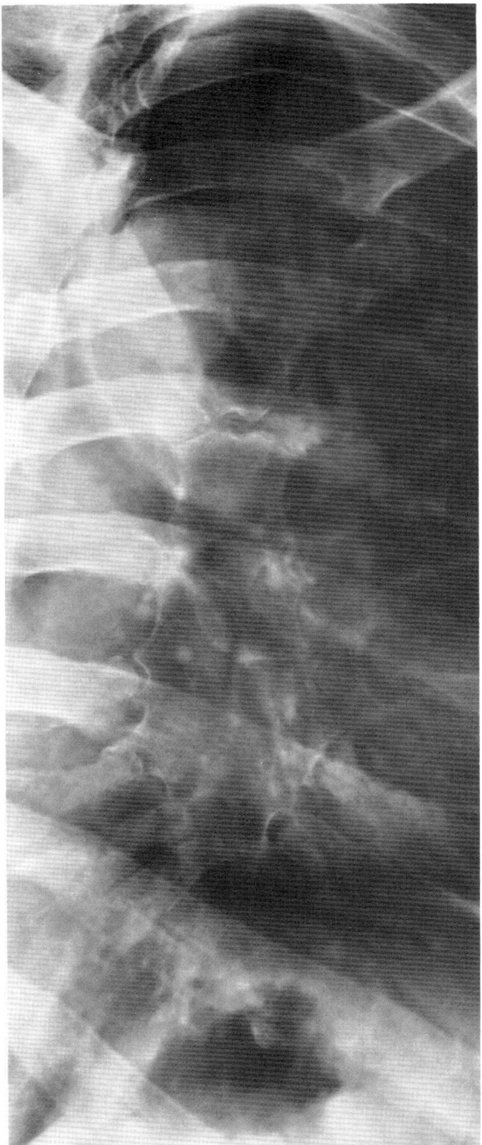

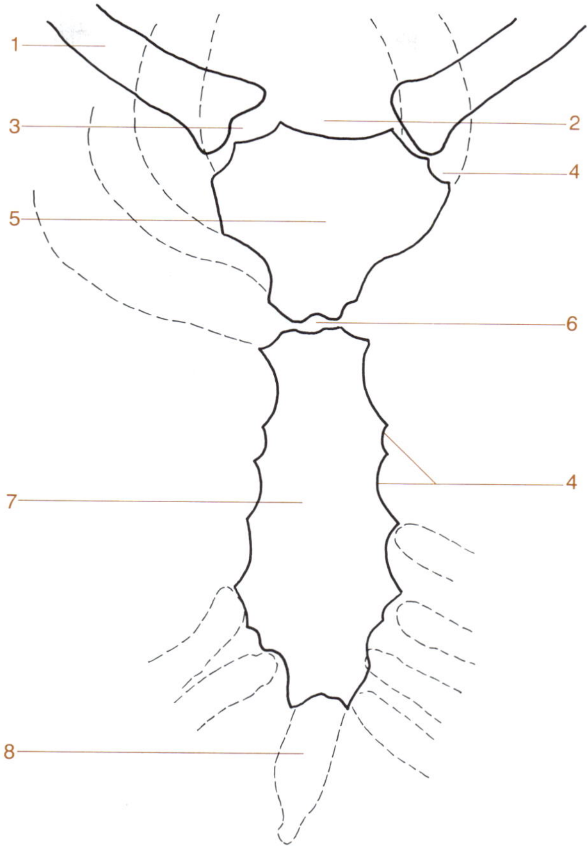

1 Clavicle
2 Sternal notch
3 Sternoclavicular joint
4 Costal incisura
5 Manubrium sterni
6 Angle of Louis
7 Sternal body
8 Xiphoid process

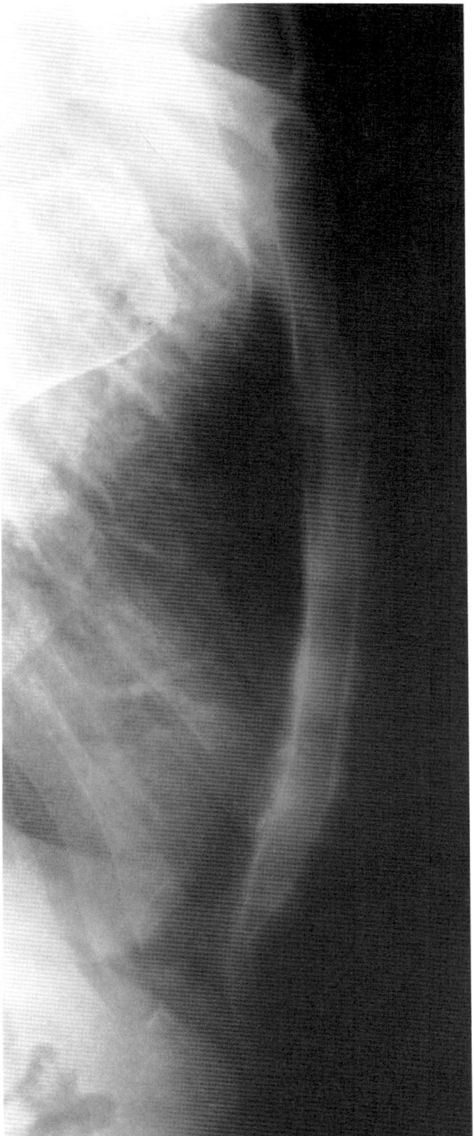

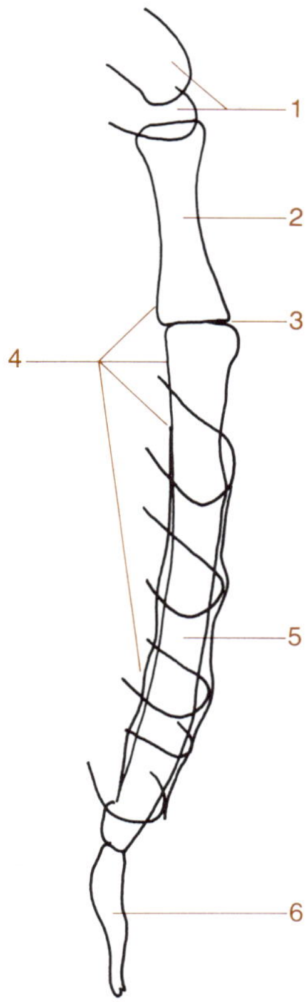

1 Clavicles
2 Manubrium sterni
3 Angle of Louis
4 Retrosternal space
5 Sternal body
6 Xiphoid process

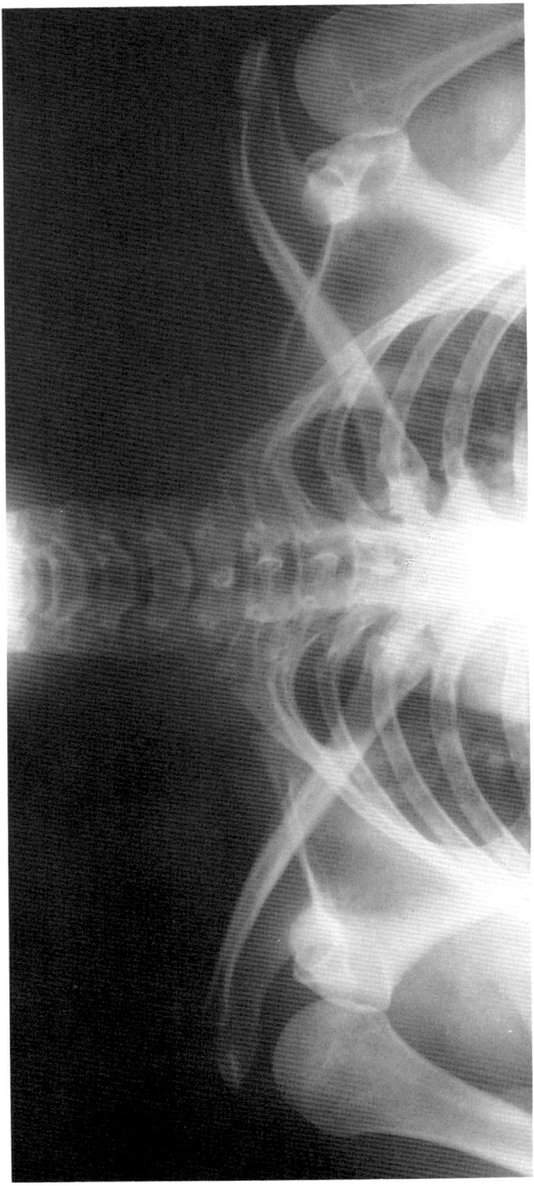

1 Cervical spine
2 Superior angle of the scapula
3 Acromioclavicular joint
4 Acromion
5 Spine of the scapula
6 Clavicle
7 Coracoid
8 Lesser tuberosity
9 Greater tuberosity
10 Humeral head
11 Glenoid fossa (articular surface)
12 Glenoid process of the scapula
13 Medial margin of the scapula
14 Proximal clavicle
15 Lateral margin of the scapula
16 Humerus

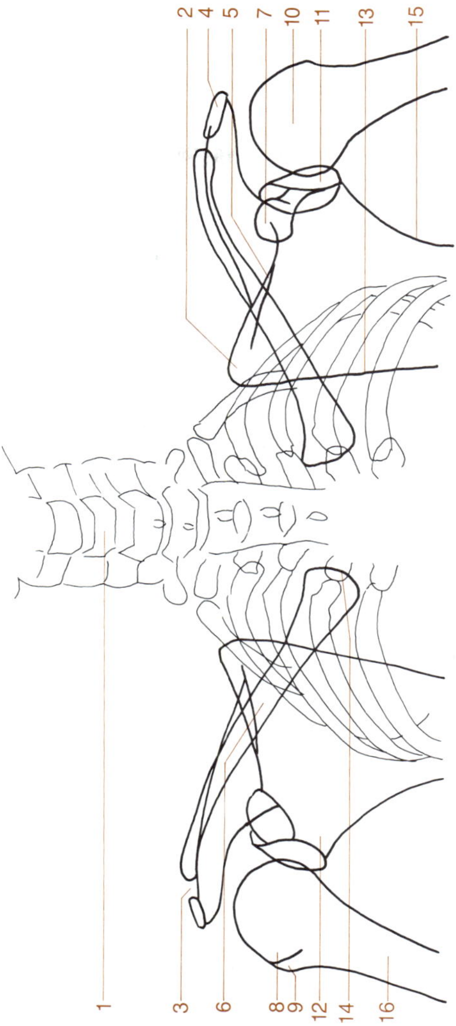

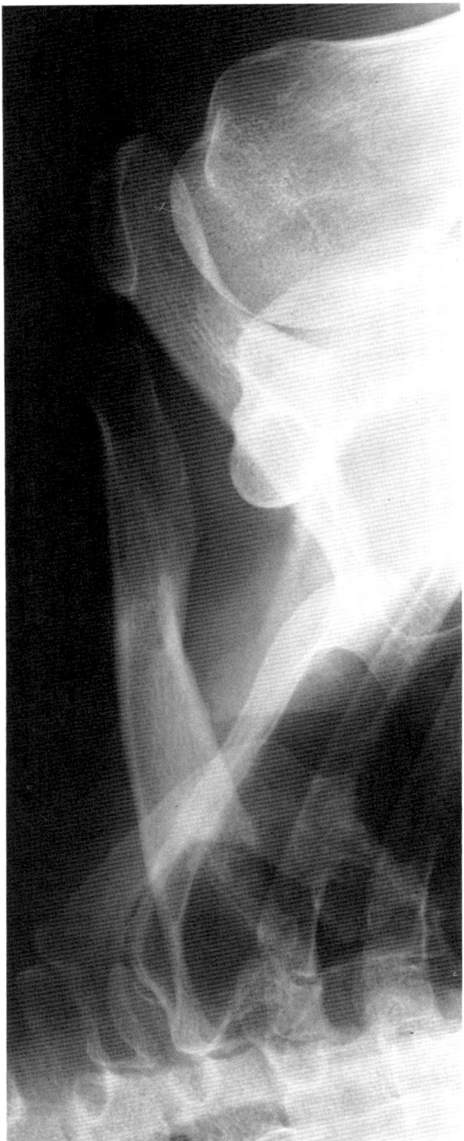

1 Conoid tubercle of the clavicle
2 Acromioclavicular joint
3 Acromion
4 Clavicle
5 Superior angle of the scapula
6 Proximal clavicle
7 Coracoid process
8 Humeral head
9 Spine of the scapula
10 Costotransversal articulation
11 Glenoid fossa

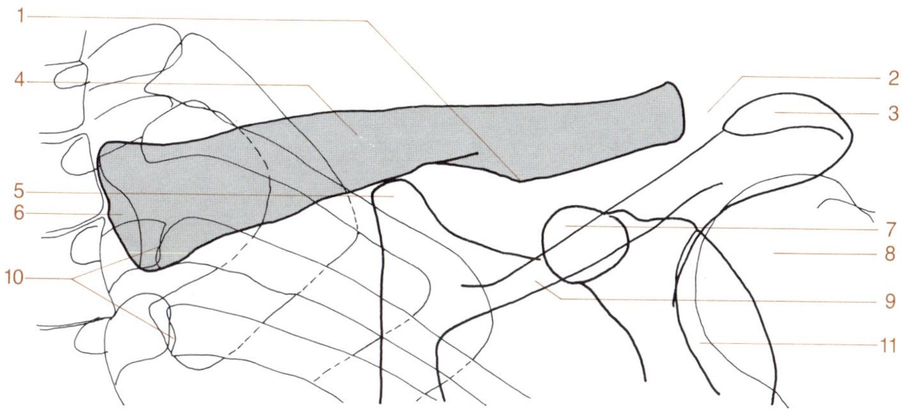

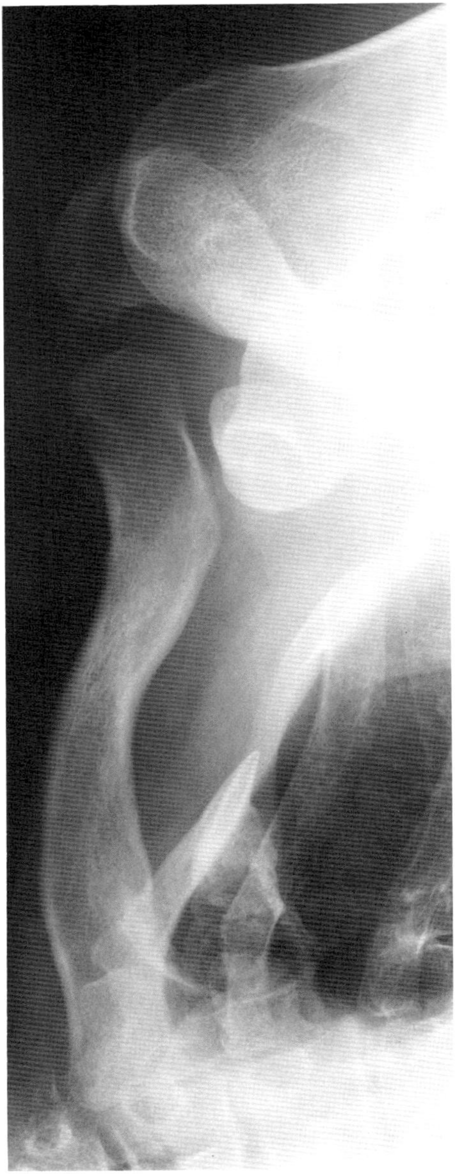

1 Sternoclavicular joint
2 Clavicle
3 Acromion
4 Acromioclavicular joint
5 Sternum (manubrium)

6 Coracoid process
7 Greater tuberosity
8 Intertubercular groove
9 Lesser tuberosity
10 Humeral head

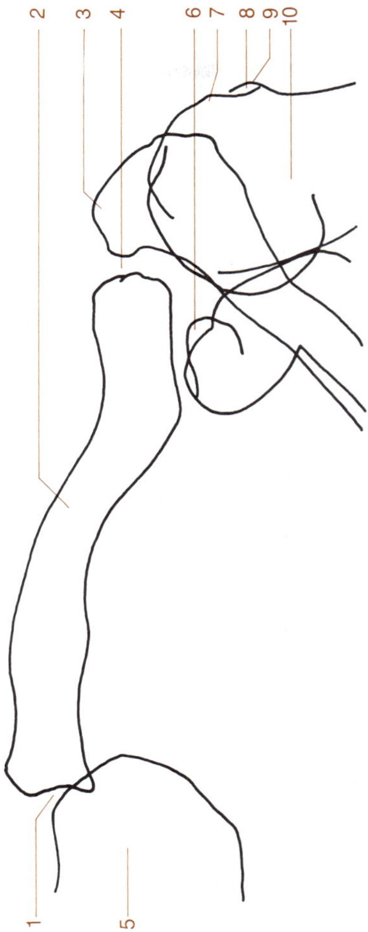

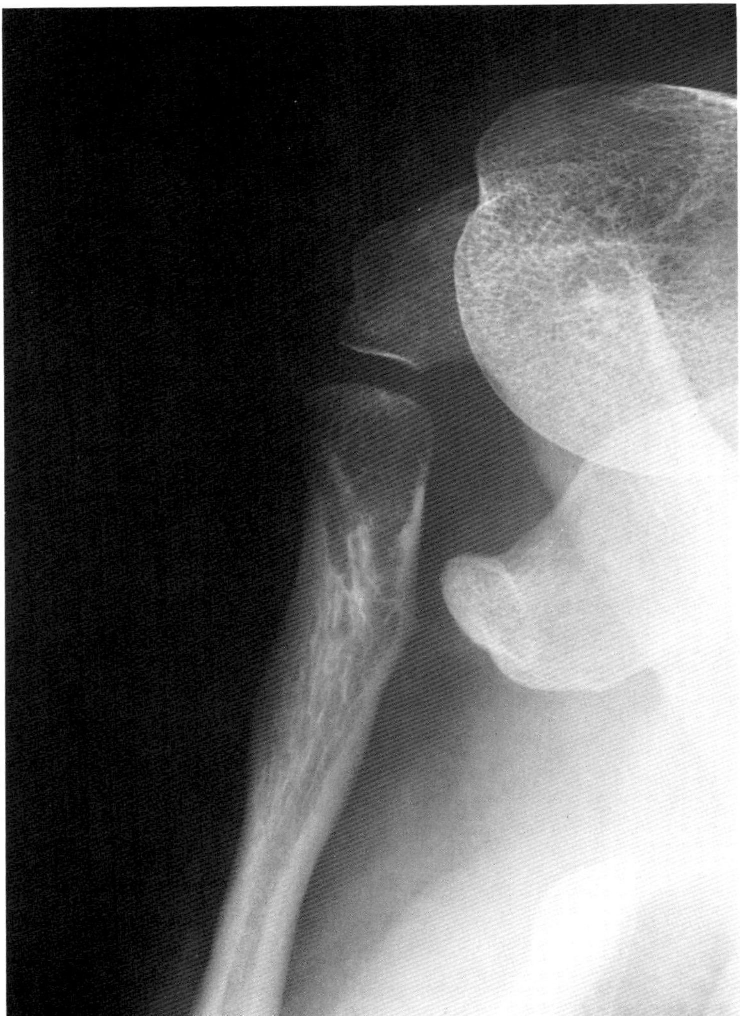

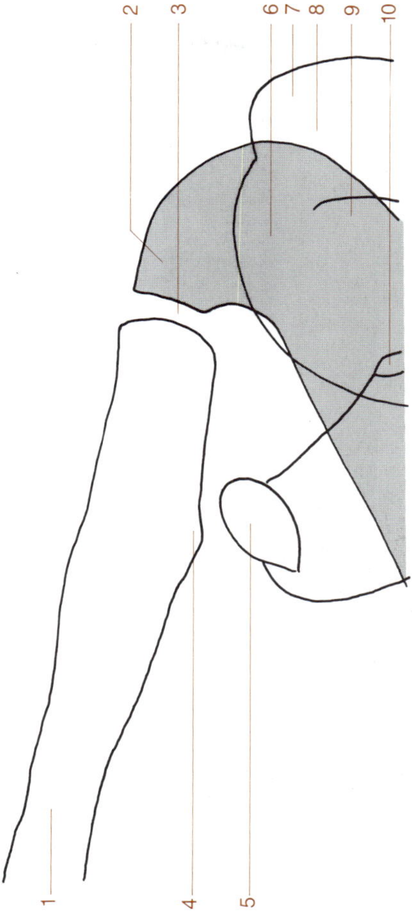

1 Clavicle
2 Acromion
3 Acromioclavicular joint
4 Conoid tubercle of the clavicle
5 Coracoid process
6 Humeral head
7 Greater tuberosity
8 Intertubercular groove
9 Lesser tuberosity
10 Glenoid fossa

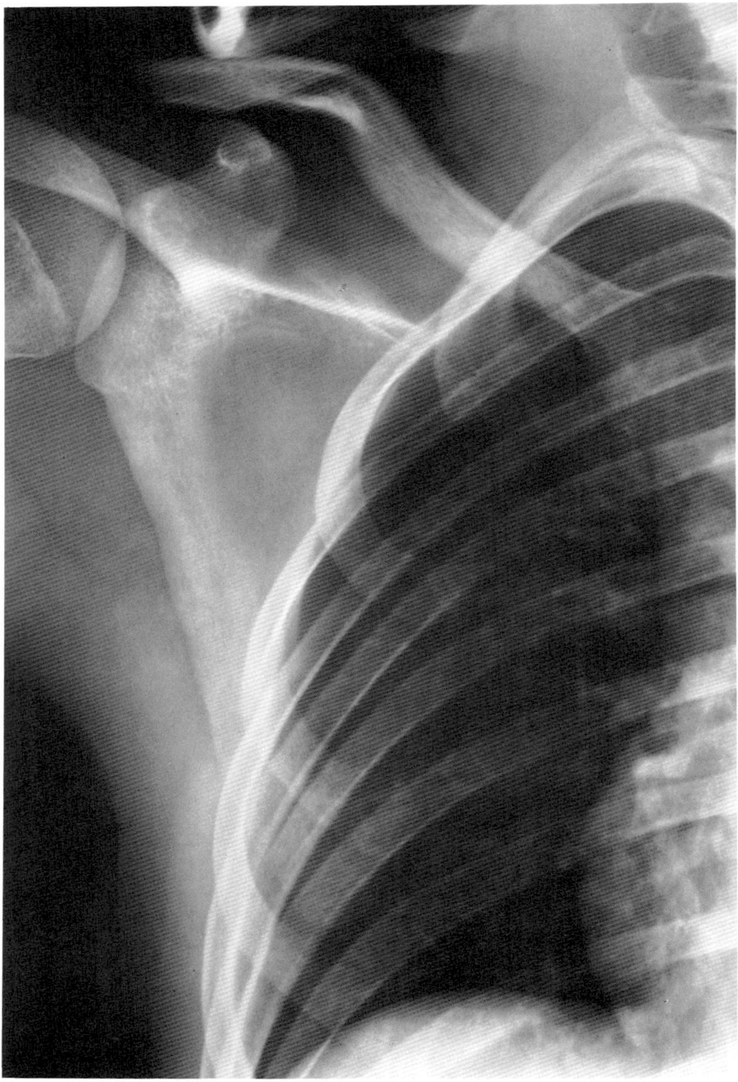

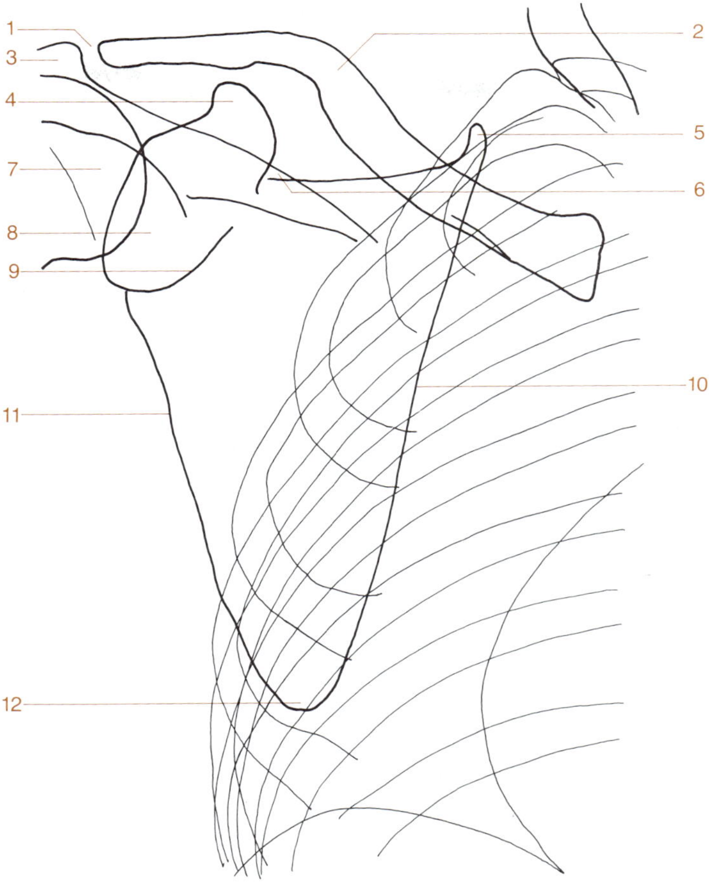

1 Acromioclavicular joint
2 Clavicle
3 Acromion
4 Coracoid process
5 Superior angle
6 Spine of the scapula
7 Humeral head
8 Articular surface
9 Glenoid process of the scapula
10 Medial margin
11 Lateral margin
12 Inferior angle

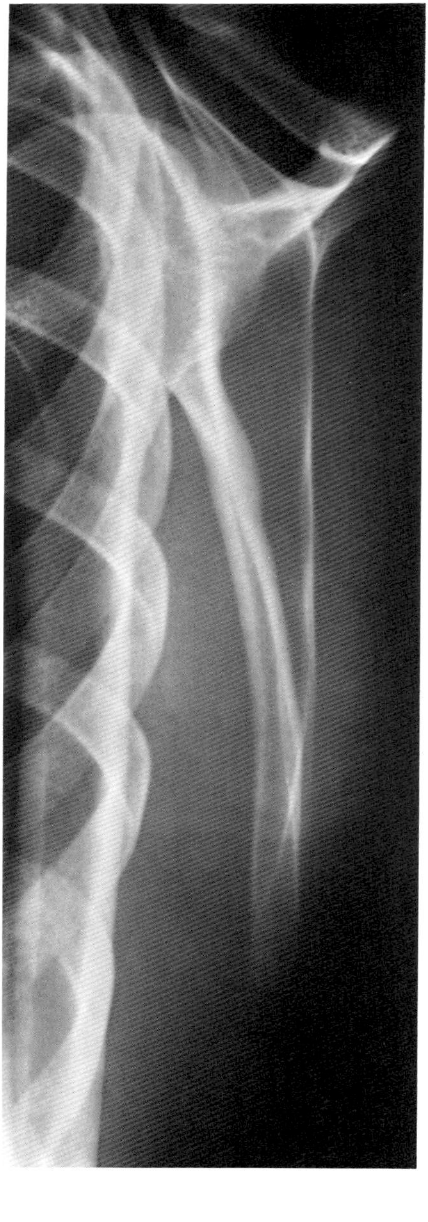

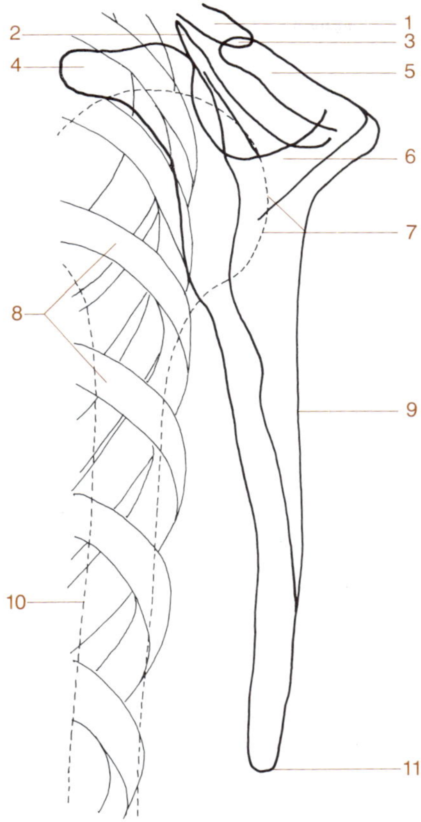

1 Distal clavicle
2 Superior angle of the scapula
3 Acromioclavicular joint
4 Coracoid process
5 Acromion
6 Spine of the scapula
7 Humeral head
8 Ribs
9 Lateral margin of the scapula
10 Humeral shaft
11 Inferior angle of the scapula

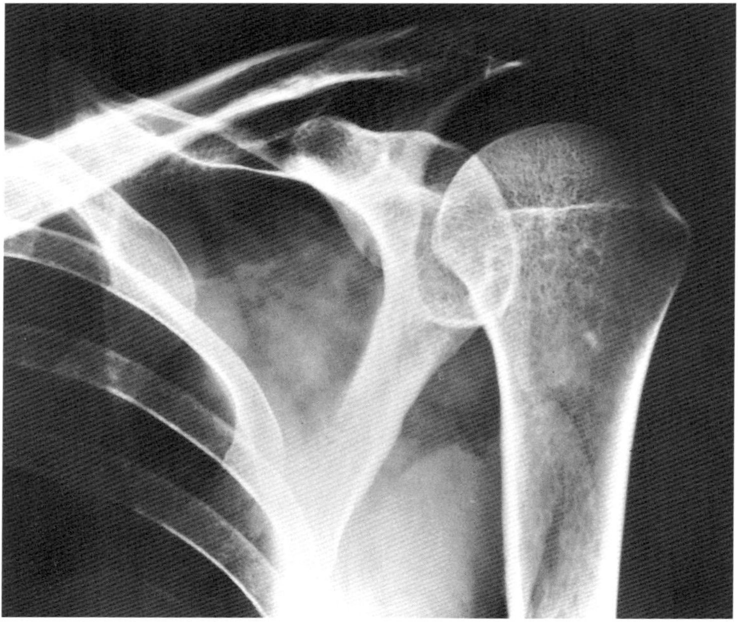

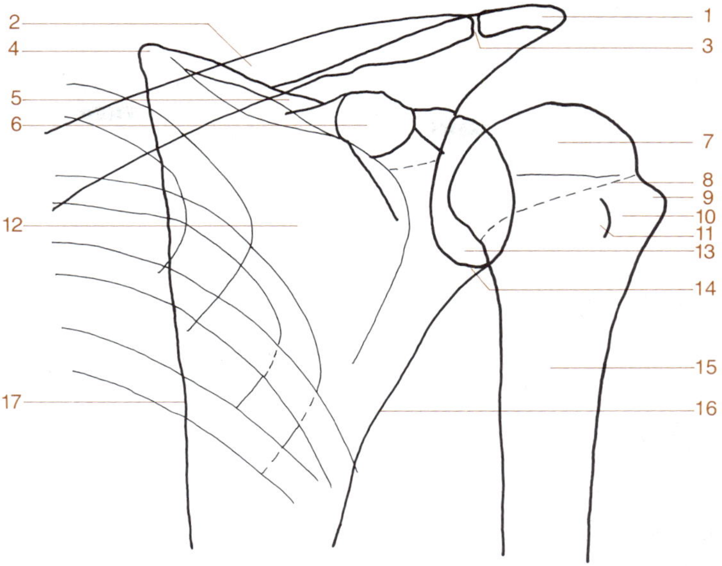

1 Acromion
2 Clavicle
3 Acromioclavicular joint
4 Superior angle of the scapula
5 Spine of the scapula
6 Coracoid process
7 Humeral head
8 Anatomical neck
9 Greater tuberosity
10 Intertubercular groove
11 Lesser tuberosity
12 Scapula
13 Glenoid fossa
14 Labrum glenoidale
15 Surgical neck
16 Lateral margin of the scapula
17 Medial margin of the scapula

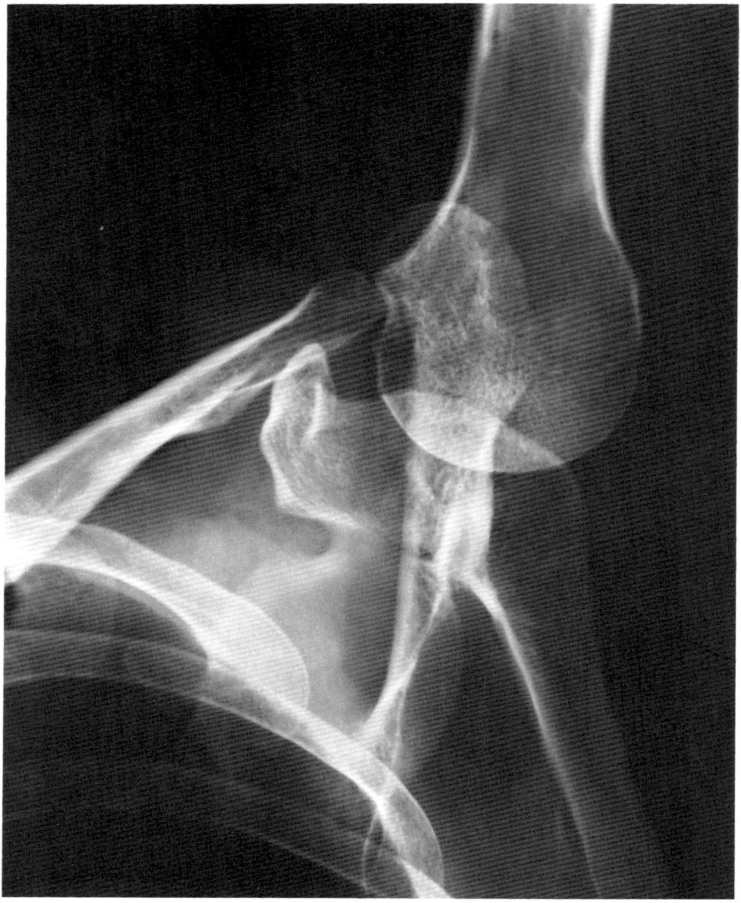

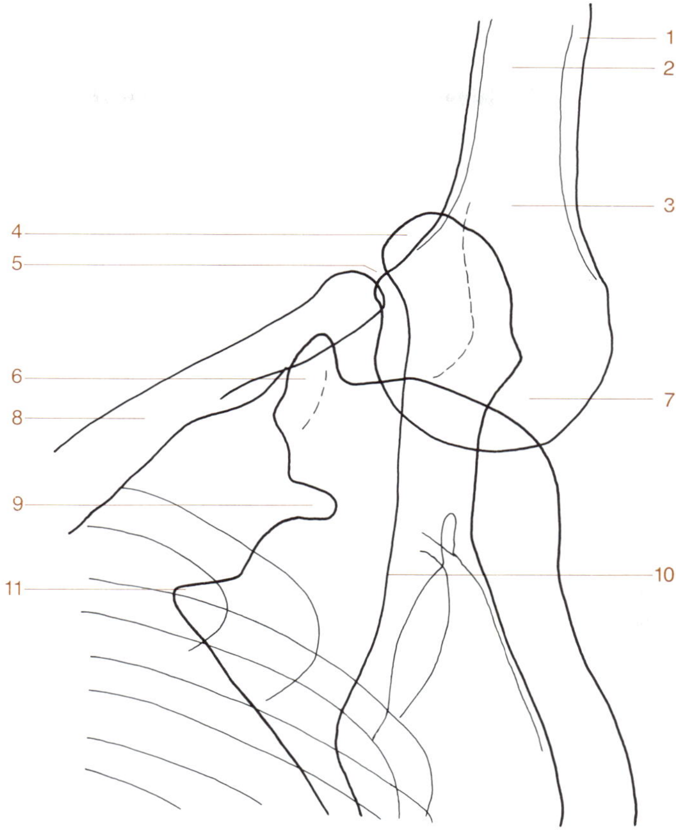

1 Cortex
2 Metaphysis
3 Surgical neck
4 Acromion
5 Acromioclavicular joint
6 Coracoid process
7 Humeral head
8 Clavicle
9 Scapular incisura or notch
10 Spine of the scapula
11 Superior angle of the scapula

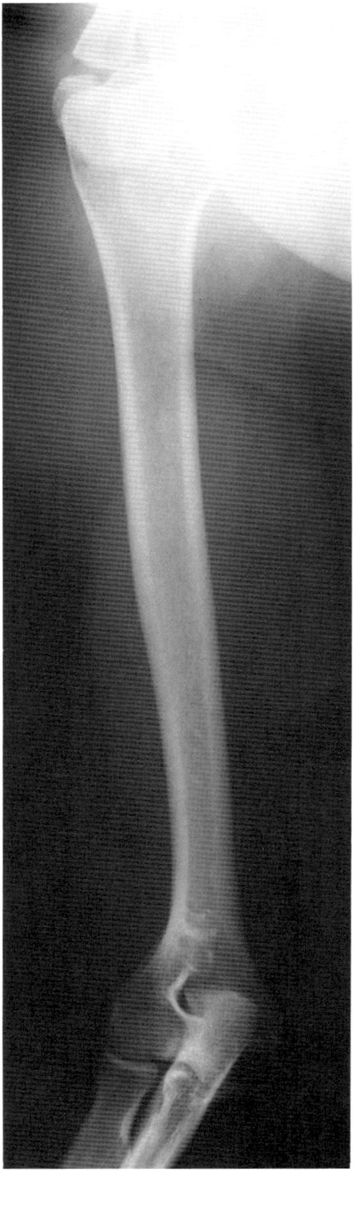

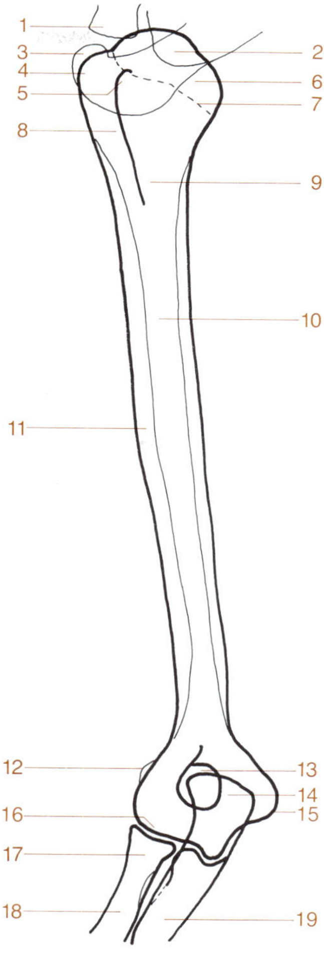

1 Clavicle
2 Glenoid process of the scapula
3 Acromion
4 Greater tuberosity
5 Lesser tuberosity
6 Humeral head
7 Anatomical neck
8 Intertubercular groove
9 Surgical neck
10 Humerus
11 Deltoid tuberosity
12 Lateral epicondyle
13 Olecranon fossa
14 Olecranon
15 Medial epicondyle
16 Capitellum and trochlea
17 Radial head
18 Radius
19 Ulna

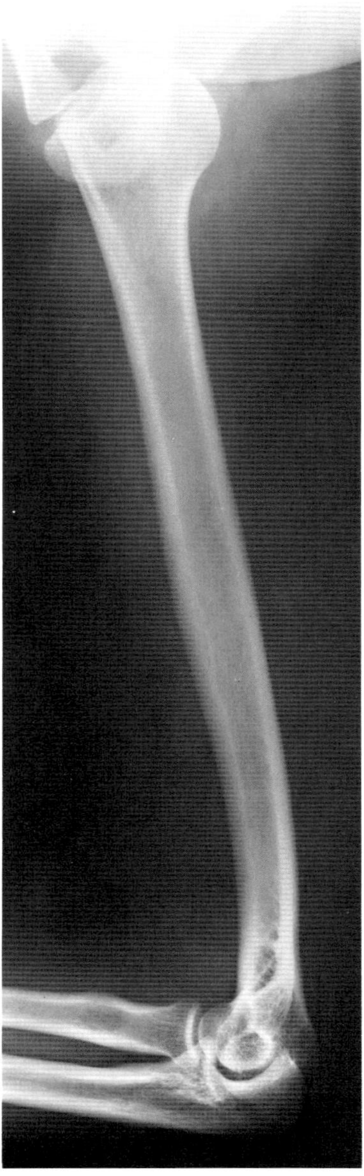

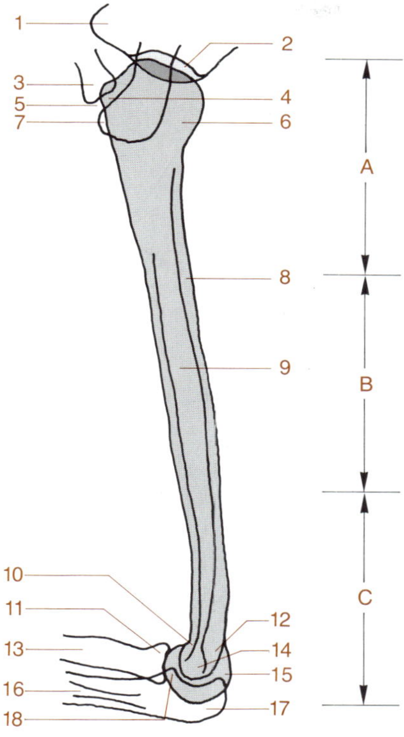

A Proximal third of the humerus
B Medial third of the humerus
C Distal third of the humerus
1 Coracoid process
2 Glenoid fossa
3 Clavicle
4 Lesser tuberosity
5 Acromioclavicular joint
6 Humeral head
7 Acromion
8 Cortex
9 Humeral shaft
10 Coronoid fossa
11 Radial shaft
12 Olecranon fossa
13 Radius
14 Trochlea of the humerus
15 Capitellum
16 Ulna
17 Olecranon
18 Coronoid process

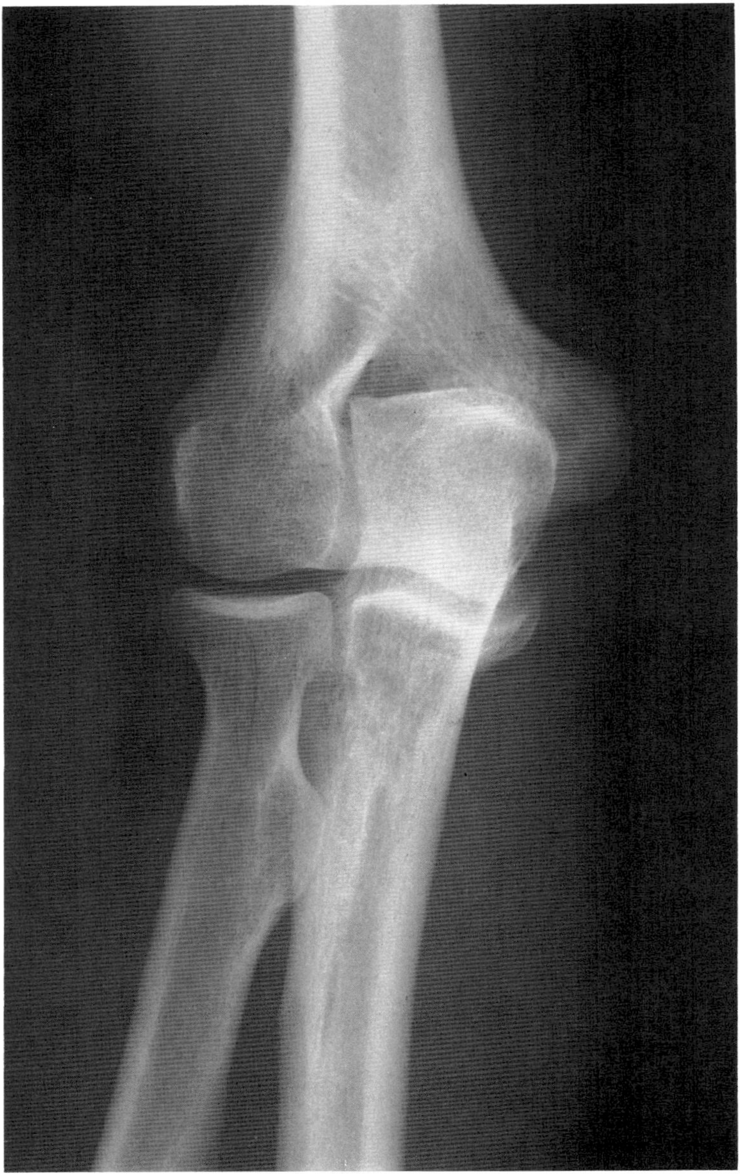

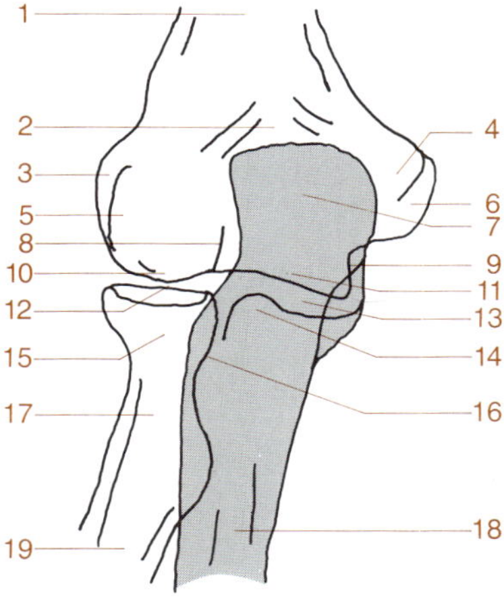

1 Humerus
2 Olecranon fossa
3 Lateral epicondyle of the humerus
4 Medial condyle of the humerus
5 Lateral condyle of the humerus
6 Medial epicondyle of the humerus
7 Olecranon
8 Lateral margin of the trochlea
9 Medial margin of the trochlea
10 Capitellum of the humerus
11 Trochlea
12 Radiohumeral articulation
13 Humeroulnar joint
14 Coronoid process
15 Radial head
16 Proximal radioulnar joint
17 Radial neck
18 Ulna
19 Radius

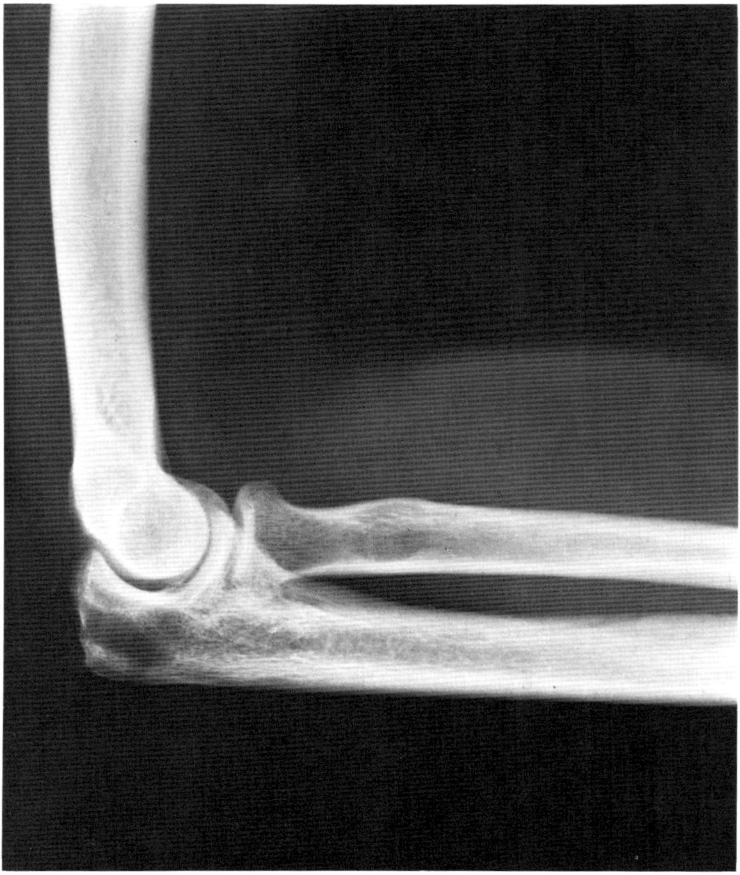

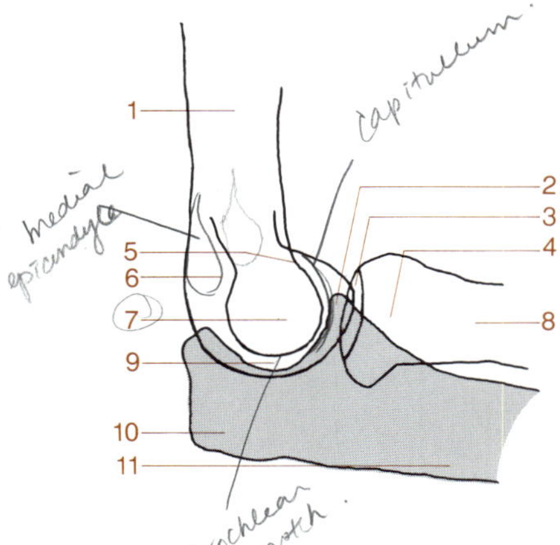

1 Humerus
2 Coronoid process
3 Radiohumeral articulation
4 Radial head
5 Coronoid fossa
6 Olecranon fossa
7 Trochlea
8 Radius
9 Humeroulnar joint
10 Olecranon
11 Ulna

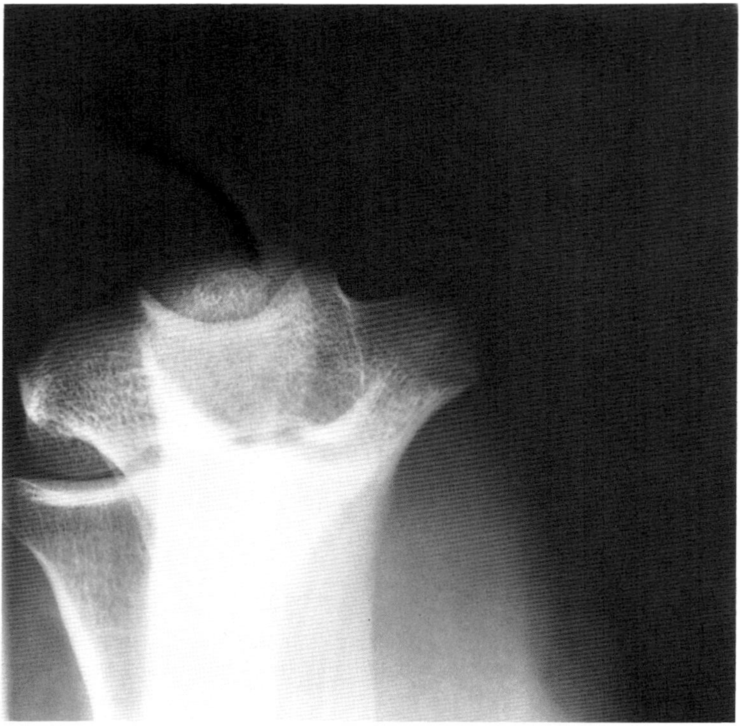

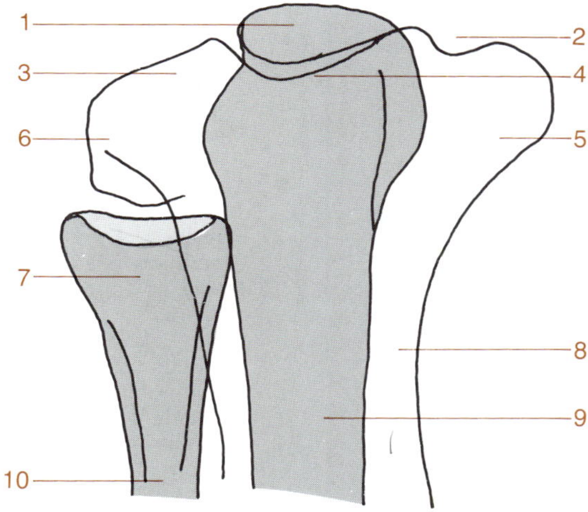

1 Olecranon
2 Cubital groove
3 Capitellum
4 Trochlea
5 Medial epicondyle
6 Lateral epicondyle
7 Radial head
8 Humerus
9 Ulna
10 Radius

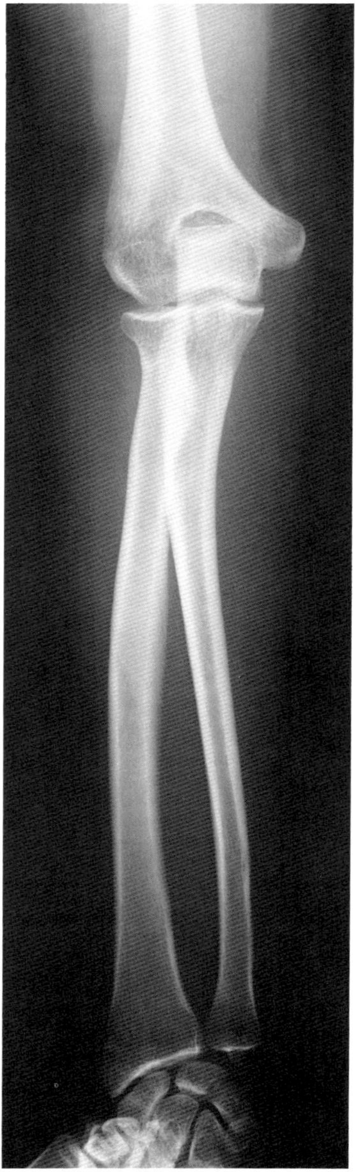

A Proximal third of the forearm
B Medial third of the forearm
C Distal third of the forearm
D Carpal bones

1 Humerus
2 Olecranon fossa
3 Medial epicondyle of the humerus
4 Lateral epicondyle of the humerus
5 Olecranon
6 Capitellum
7 Trochlea
8 Radiohumeral articulation
9 Humeroulnar joint
10 Radial head
11 Coronoid process
12 Proximal radioulnar joint
13 Radial tuberosity
14 Radial neck
15 Ulna
16 Interosseous membrane
17 Radius
18 Distal radioulnar joint
19 Radiocarpal joint
20 Ulnar styloid process
21 Radial styloid process of the radius
22 Lunate bone
23 Triquetrum
24 Navicular bone
25 Pisiform bone
22–25 Proximal carpal row

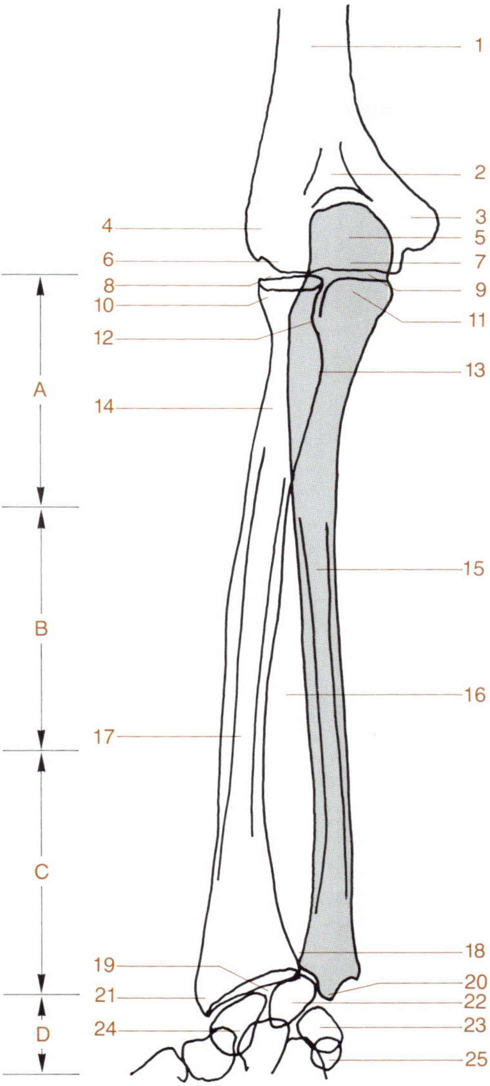
1
2
3
4
5
6
7
8
9
10
11
12
13
14
A
15
B
16
17
C
18
19
20
21
22
23
24
D
25

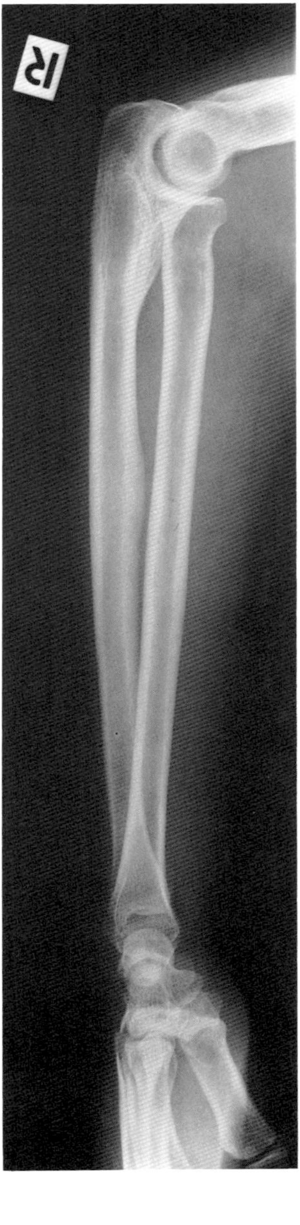

A Proximal third of the forearm
B Medial third of the forearm
C Distal third of the forearm
D Carpal bones (wrist bones)

1 Olecranon fossa
2 Olecranon
3 Humerus
4 Trochlea of the humerus
5 Coronoid fossa
6 Coronoid process
7 Radial head
8 Radial neck
9 Interosseous membrane
10 Radius
11 Ulna
12 Ulnar styloid process
13 Radiocarpal joint
14 Lunate bone
15 Pisiform bone
16 Navicular bone
17 Triquetrum
14–17 Proximal carpal row

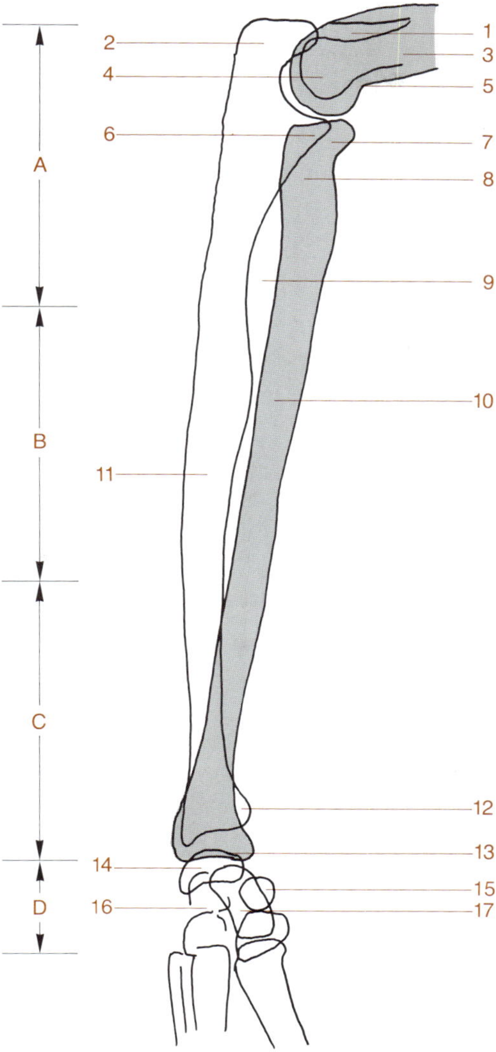
1
2
3
4
5
6
7
8
9
10
11
12
13
14
15
16
17
A
B
C
D

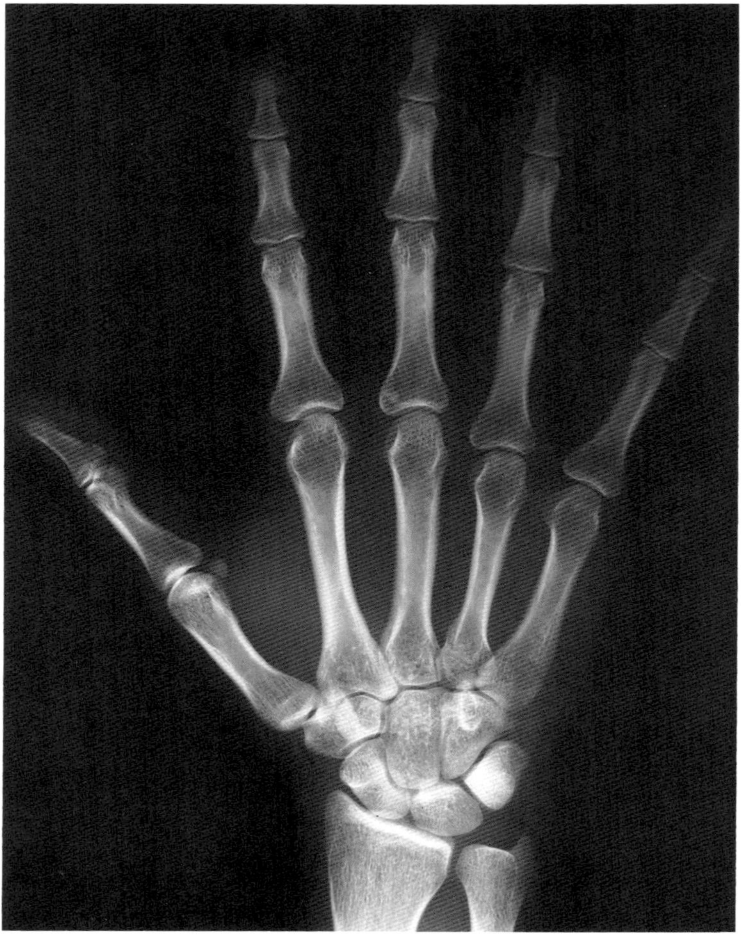

1 Distal tuft of the finger
2 Distal phalanx
3 Distal interphalangeal joint
4 Proximal interphalangeal joint
5 Middle phalanx
6 Head of the proximal phalanx
7 Proximal phalanx
8 Metacarpophalangeal joint
9 Base of the proximal phalanx
10 Head of the metacarpal bone
11 Sesamoid bone
12 Metacarpal bone
13 Base of the metacarpal bone
14 Capitate bone

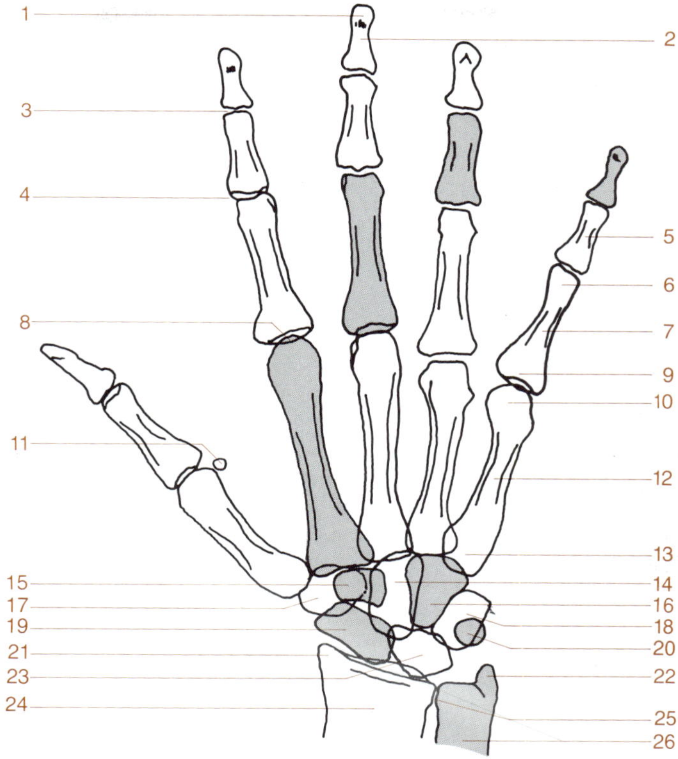

15 Trapezoid bone (lesser multangular)
16 Hamate bone
17 Trapezium bone (greater multangular)
18 Triquetrum
19 Navicular bone
20 Pisiform bone
21 Radial styloid process
22 Ulnar styloid process
23 Lunate bone
24 Distal radius
25 Distal radioulnar joint
26 Distal ulna

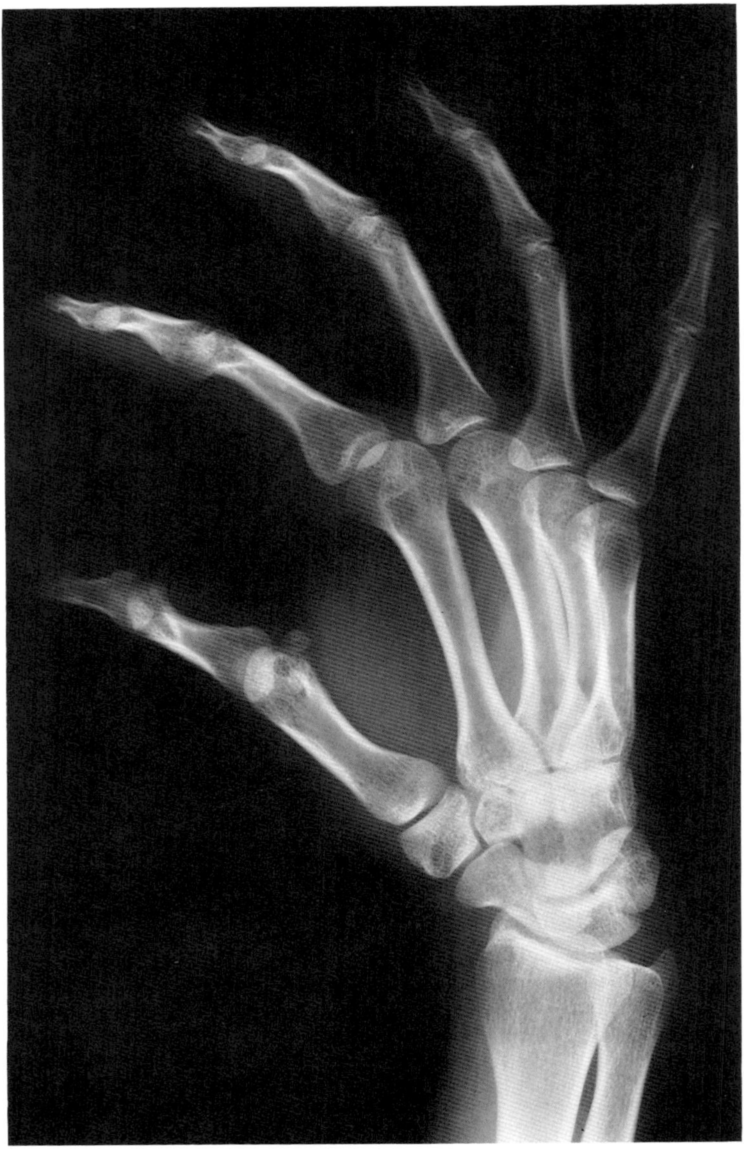

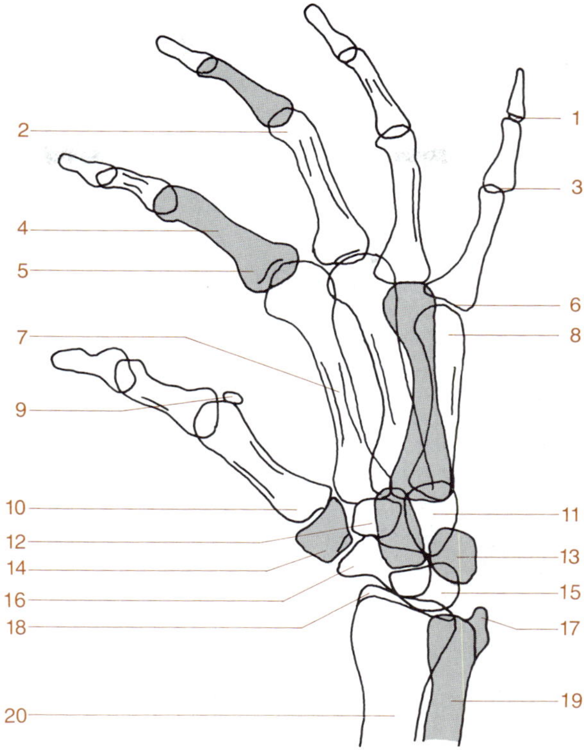

1 Distal interphalangeal joint
2 Head of the proximal phalanx
3 Proximal interphalangeal joint
4 Proximal phalanx
5 Base of the proximal phalanx
6 Metacarpophalangeal joint
7 Metacarpal bone
8 Head of the metacarpal bone
9 Sesamoid bone
10 Base of the metacarpal bone
11 Capitate bone/hamate bone
12 Trapezoid bone (lesser multangular)
13 Triquetrum
14 Trapezium bone (greater multangular)
15 Lunate bone
16 Navicular bone
17 Ulnar styloid process
18 Radial styloid process
19 Distal ulna
20 Distal radius

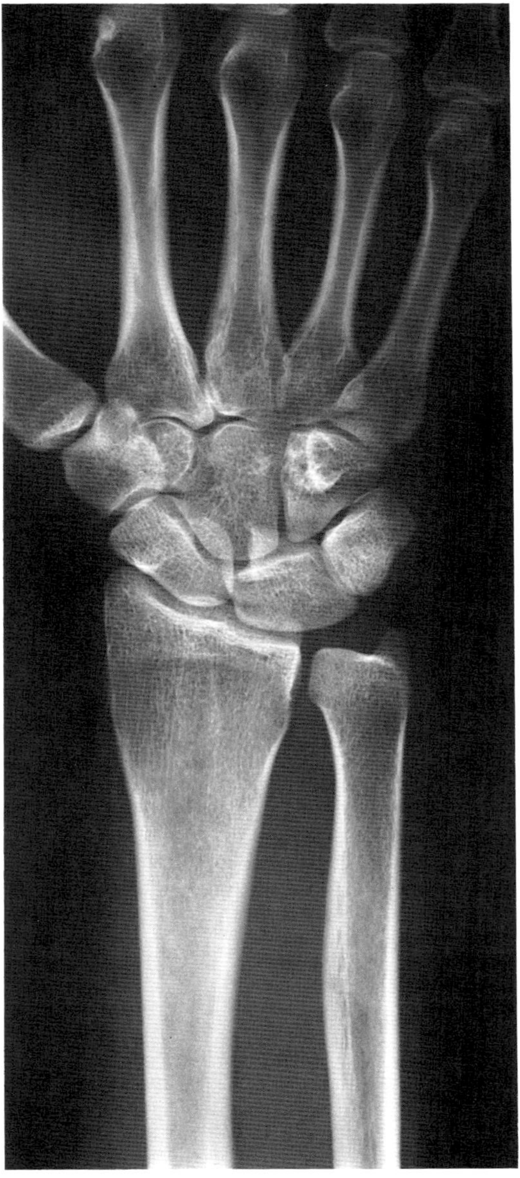

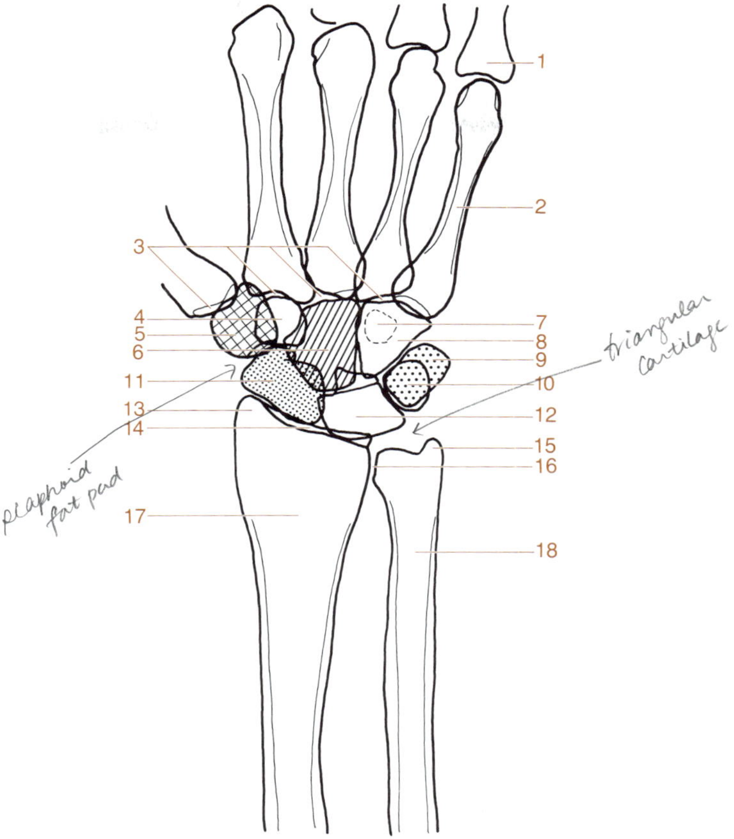

1 Proximal phalanx
2 Fifth metacarpal bone
3 Metacarpophalangeal joint
4 Trapezoid bone (lesser multangular)
5 Trapezium bone (greater multangular)
6 Capitate bone
7 Hook of the hamate bone
8 Hamate bone
9 Triquetrum
10 Pisiform bone
11 Navicular bone
12 Lunate bone
13 Radial styloid process
14 Radiocarpal joint
15 Ulnar styloid process
16 Radioulnar joint
17 Radius
18 Ulna

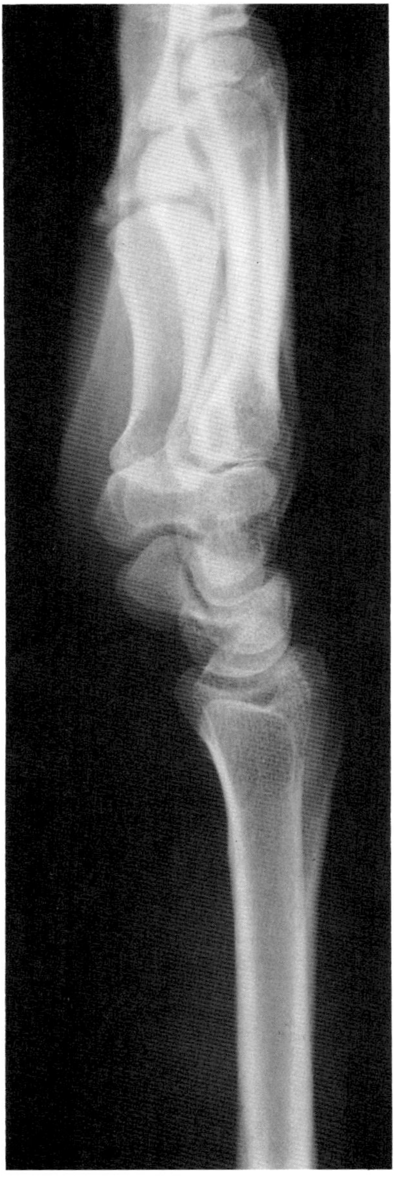

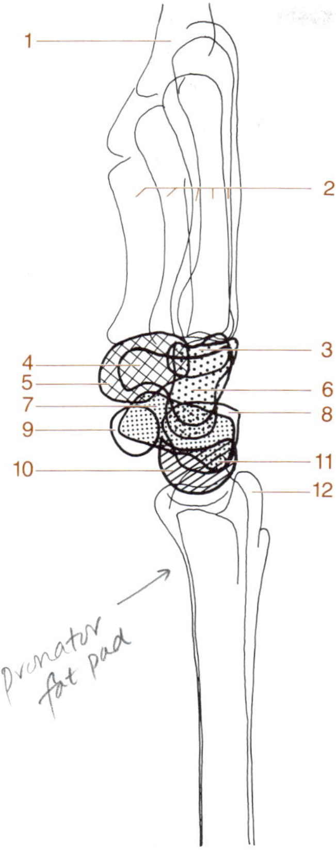

1 Proximal phalanx
2 Metacarpal bones
3 Trapezoid bone (lesser multangular)
4 Hook of the hamate bone
5 Trapezium bone (greater multangular)
6 Capitate bone
7 Navicular bone
8 Triquetrum
9 Pisiform bone
10 Lunate bone
11 Radial styloid process
12 Ulnar styloid process

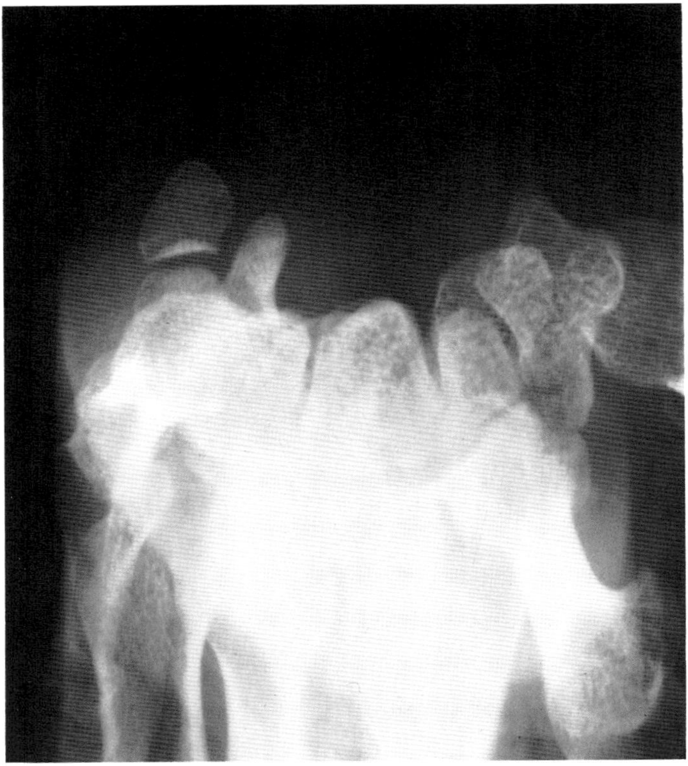

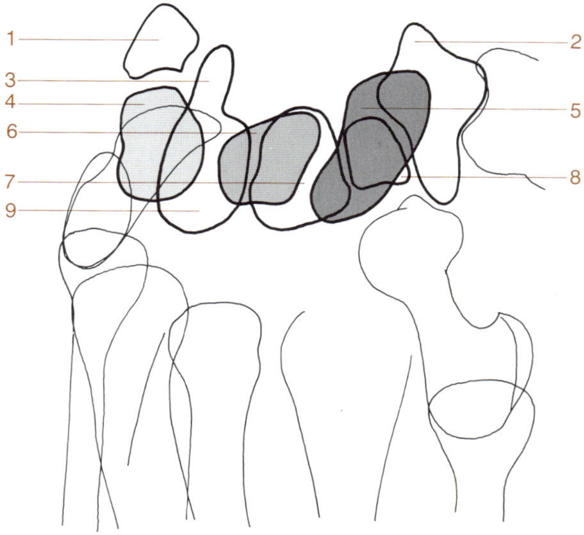

1 Pisiform bone
2 Trapezium bone (greater multangular)
3 Hook of the hamate bone
4 Triquetrum
5 Navicular bone
6 Lunate bone
7 Capitate bone
8 Trapezoid bone (lesser multangular)
9 Hamate bone

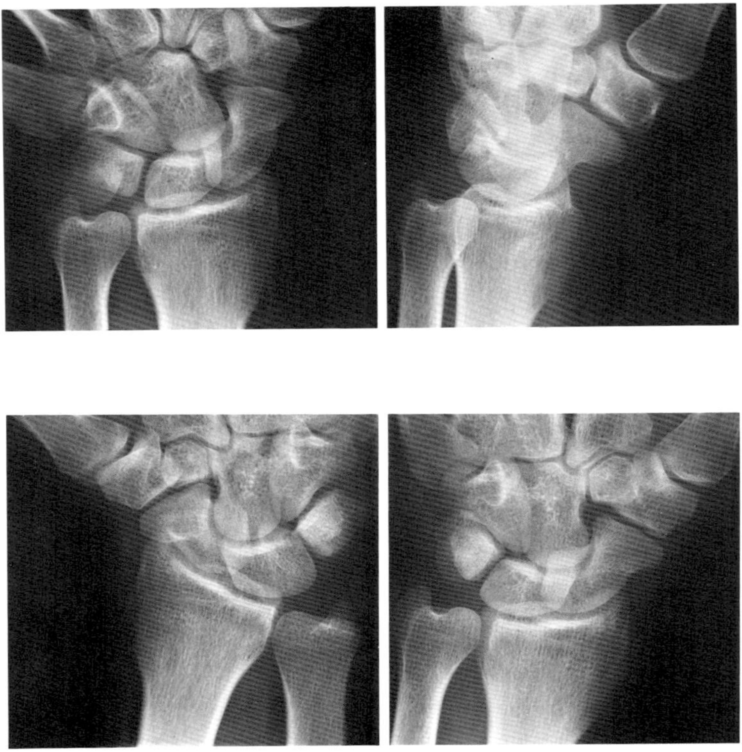

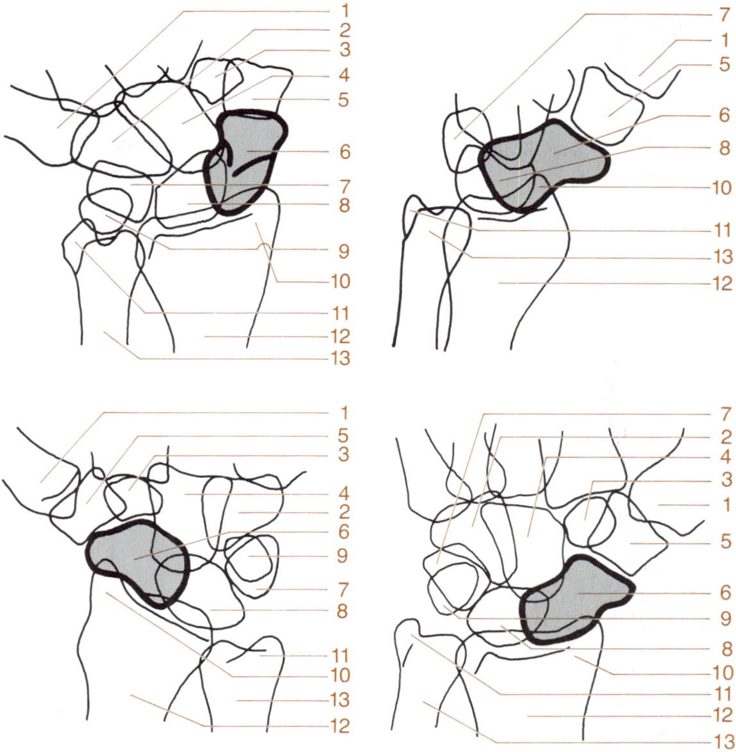

1 Metacarpal bone
2 Hamate bone
3 Trapezoid bone (lesser multangular)
4 Capitate bone
5 Trapezium bone (greater multangular)
6 Navicular bone
7 Triquetrum
8 Lunate bone
9 Pisiform bone
10 Radial styloid process
11 Ulnar styloid process
12 Radius
13 Ulna

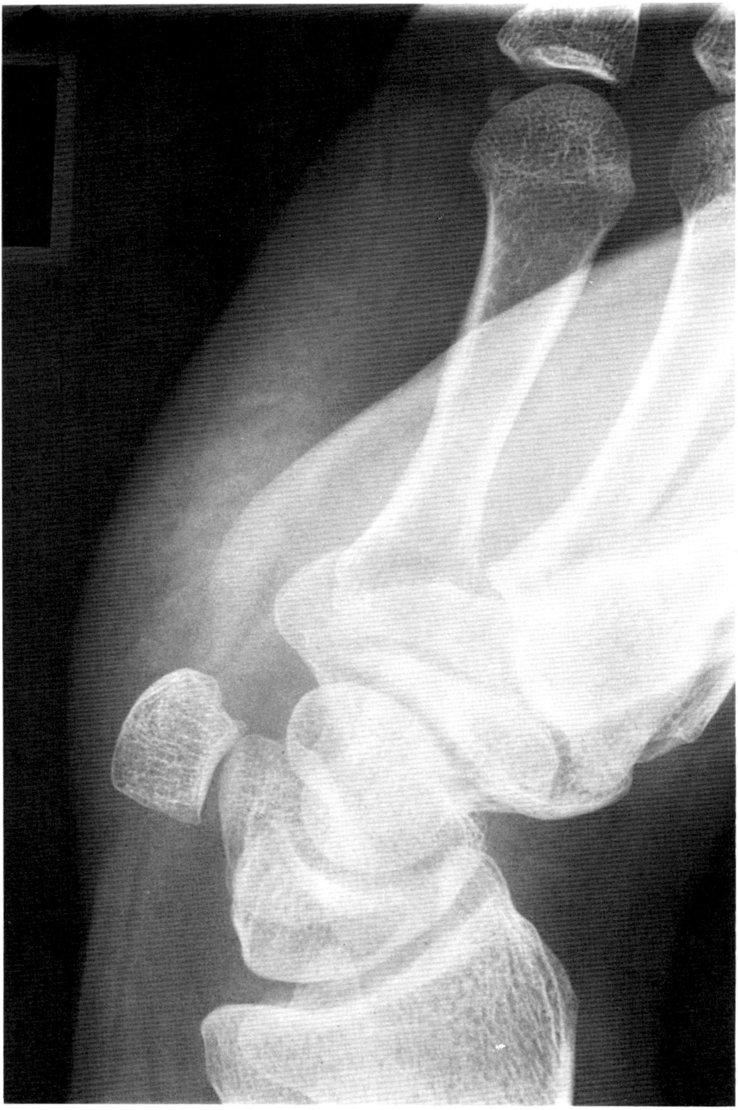

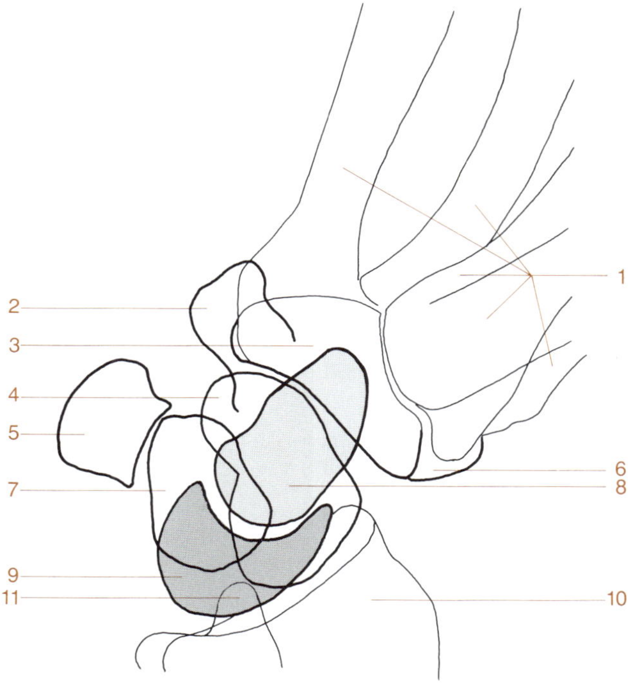

1 Metacarpal bones
2 Hamate bone
3 Trapezoid bone (lesser multangular)
4 Navicular bone
5 Pisiform bone
6 Trapezium bone (greater multangular)
7 Triquetrum
8 Capitate bone
9 Lunate bone
10 Radius
11 Ulnar styloid process

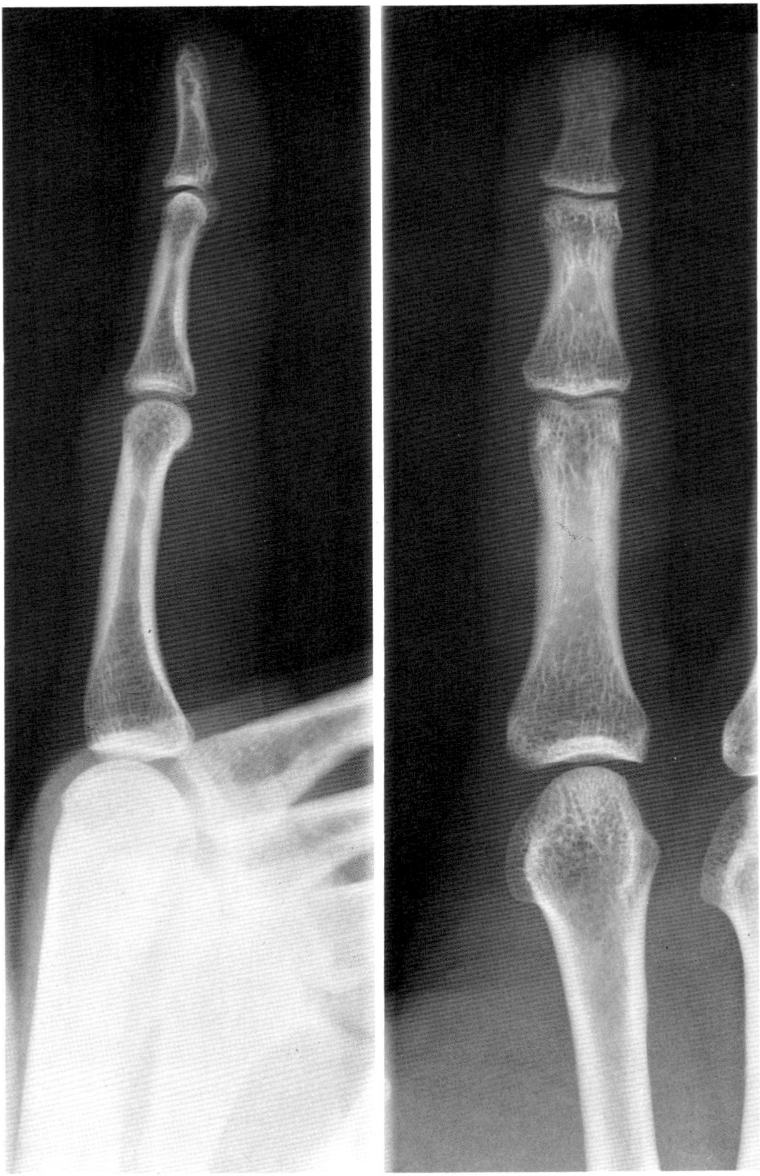

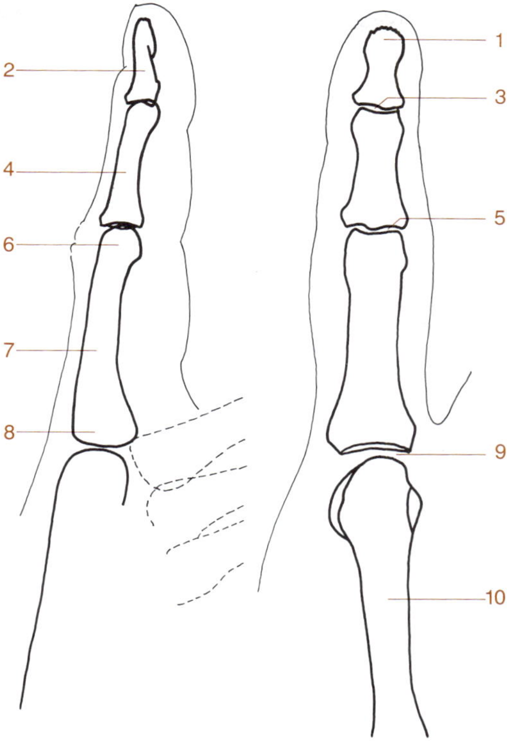

1 Distal phalangeal tuft
2 Distal phalanx
3 Distal interphalangeal joint
4 Middle phalanx
5 Proximal interphalangeal joint
6 Head of the proximal phalanx
7 Proximal phalanx
8 Base of the proximal phalanx
9 Metacarpophalangeal joint
10 Metacarpal bone

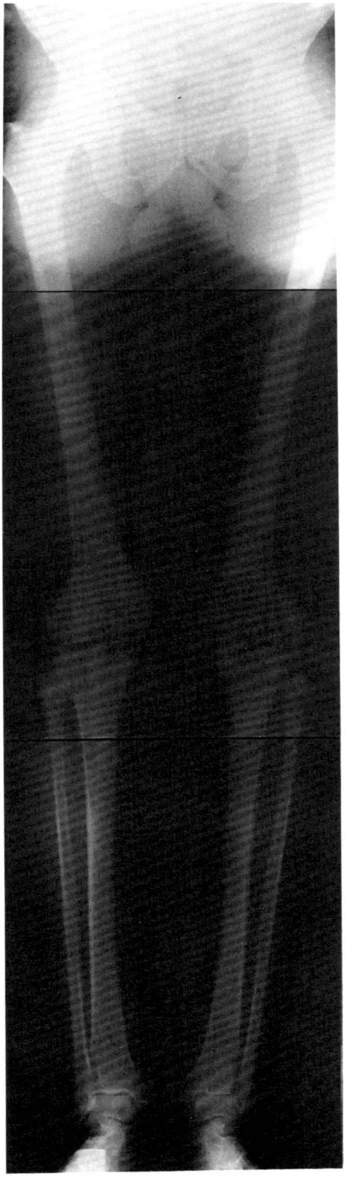

A Proximal third of the femur
B Medial third of the femur
C Distal third of the femur
D Proximal third of the lower leg
E Medial third of the lower leg
F Distal third of the lower leg

1 Hip-joint space
2 Pubic bone
3 Femoral head
4 Greater trochanter
5 Obturator foramen
6 Ischial bone
7 Ischial tuberosity
8 Femur
9 Patella
10 Medial and lateral condyles of the femur
11 Tibiofemoral joint
12 Intercondylar eminence
13 Medial and lateral condyles of the tibia
14 Tibia
15 Fibula
16 Medial malleolus
17 Lateral malleolus
18 Trochlea of the talus
19 Ankle joint

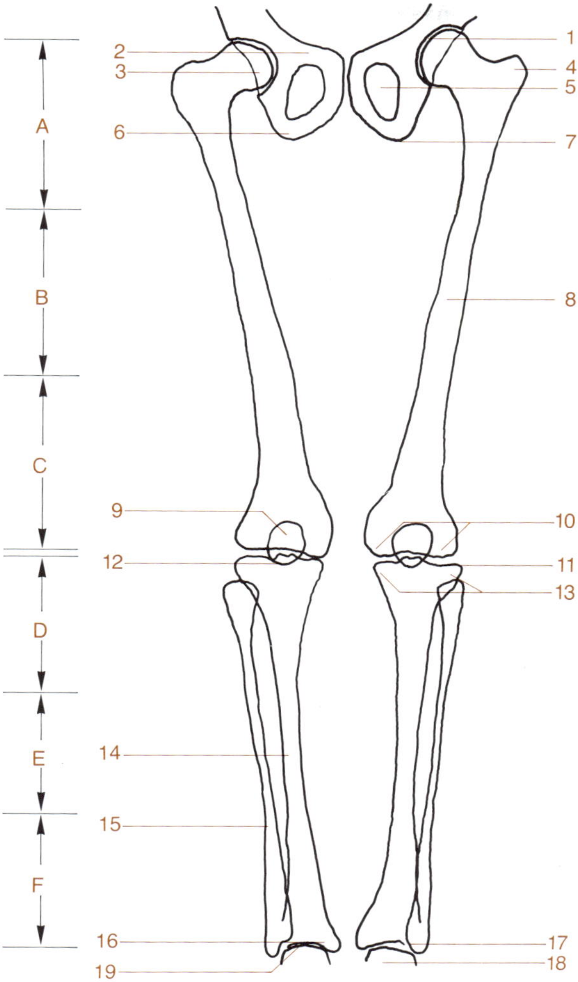
1
2
3
4
5
A
6
7
B
8
C
9
10
11
12
13
D
E
14
15
F
16
17
18
19

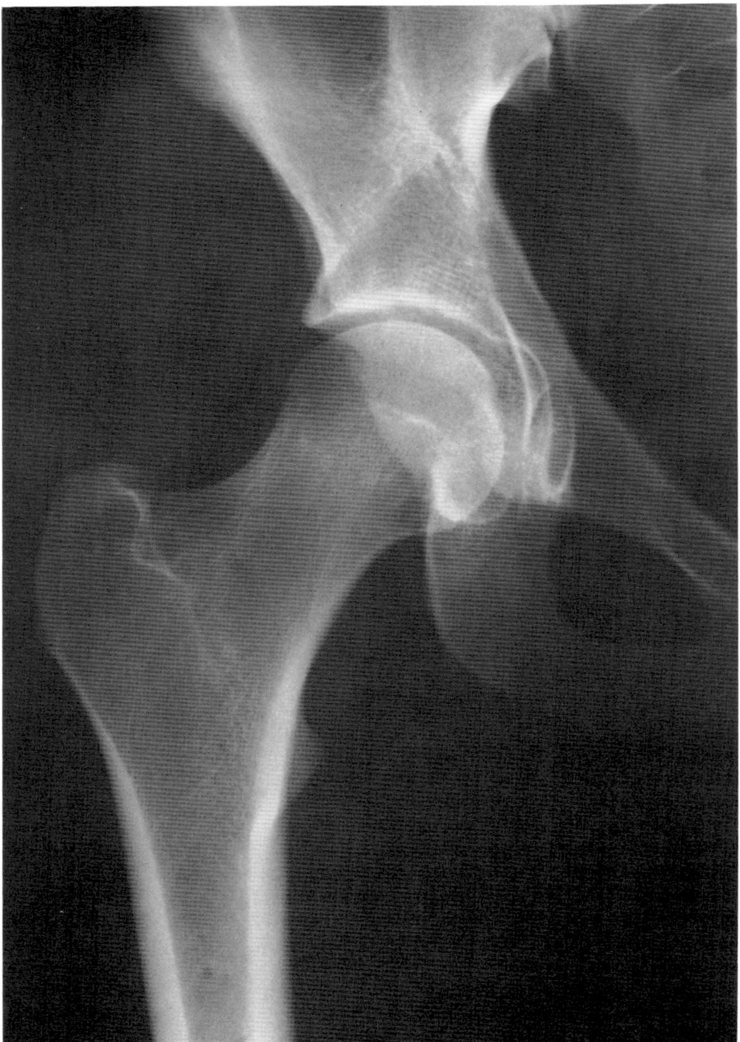

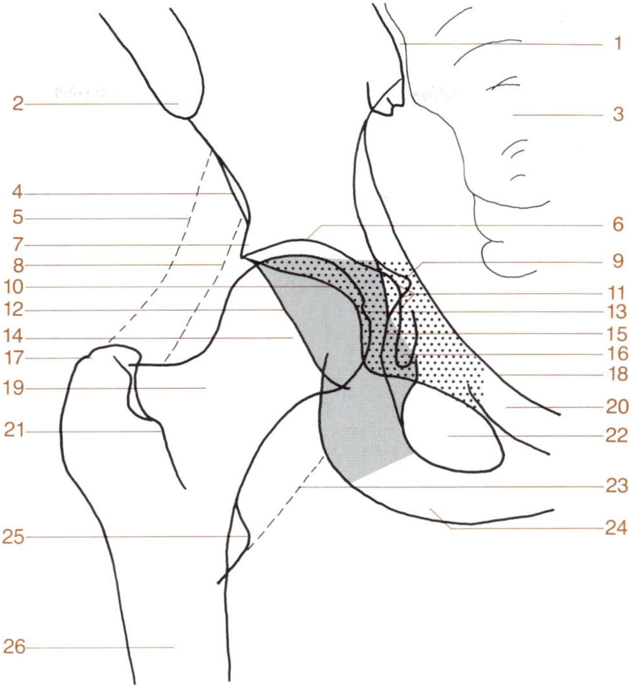

1 Sacroiliac joint
2 Anterior superior iliac spine
3 Sacrum
4 Anterior inferior iliac spine
5 Intergluteal fat plane
6 Acetabular roof
7 Superior acetabular rim
8 Fat plane medial to the gluteus minimus muscle
9 Ischial spine
10 Anterior acetabular rim
11 Acetabular floor
12 Posterior acetabular rim
13 Fovea capitis
14 Femoral head
15 Ilioischial line
16 Köhler's teardrop
17 Greater trochanter
18 Terminal line
19 Femoral neck
20 Superior pubic ramus
21 Intertrochanteric line
22 Obturator foramen
23 Iliopsoas fat plane
24 Ischial tuberosity
25 Lesser trochanter
26 Femur
Body of the ischium (posterior column)
Pubic bone, anterior column (iliopubic column)

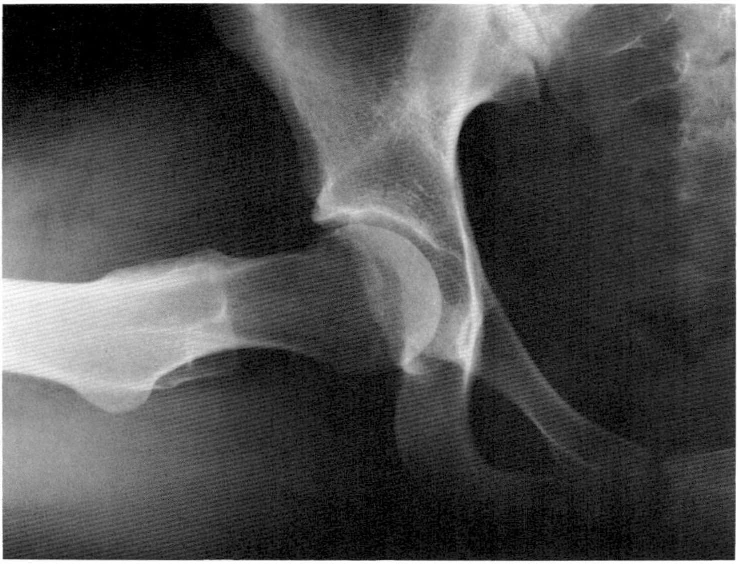

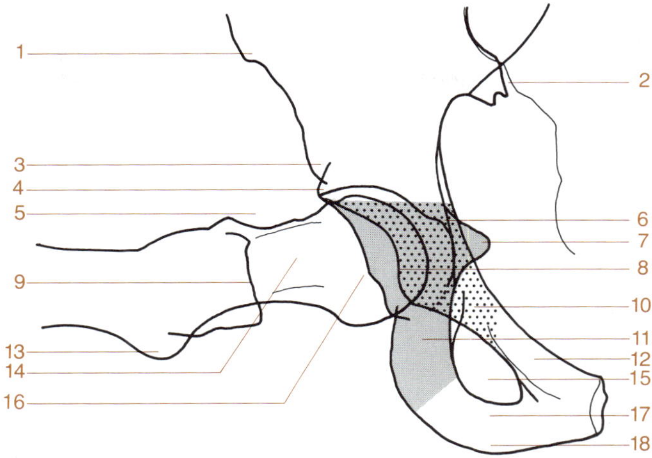

1 Anterior superior iliac spine
2 Sacroiliac joint
3 Anterior inferior iliac spine
4 Superior acetabular rim
5 Posterior acetabular rim
6 Acetabular floor
7 Ischial spine
8 Anterior acetabular rim
9 Greater trochanter
10 Pubic bone, anterior column (iliopubic column)
11 Body of the ischium (posterior column)
12 Superior pubic ramus
13 Lesser trochanter
14 Femoral neck
15 Obturator foramen
16 Femoral head
17 Inferior pubic ramus
18 Ischial tuberosity

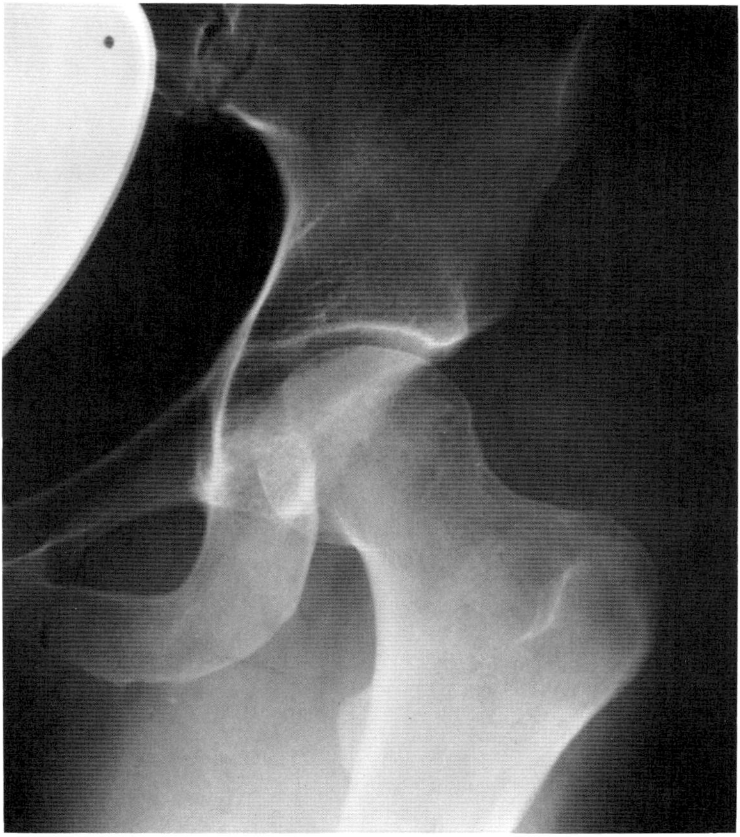

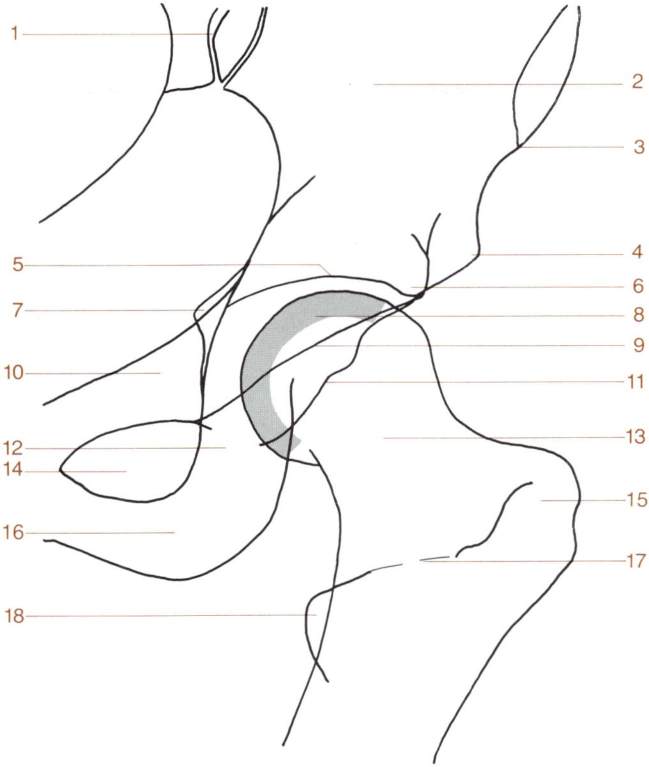

1 Sacroiliac joint
2 Iliac bone
3 Anterior superior iliac spine
4 Anterior inferior iliac spine
5 Acetabular roof
6 Superior acetabular rim
7 Ischial spine
8 Ventral articulating surface of the femoral head
9 Anterior acetabular rim
10 Body of the pubic bone (anterior column)
11 Posterior acetabular rim
12 Ischial bone
13 Femoral neck
14 Obturator foramen
15 Greater trochanter
16 Ischial tuberosity
17 Intertrochanteric line
18 Lesser trochanter

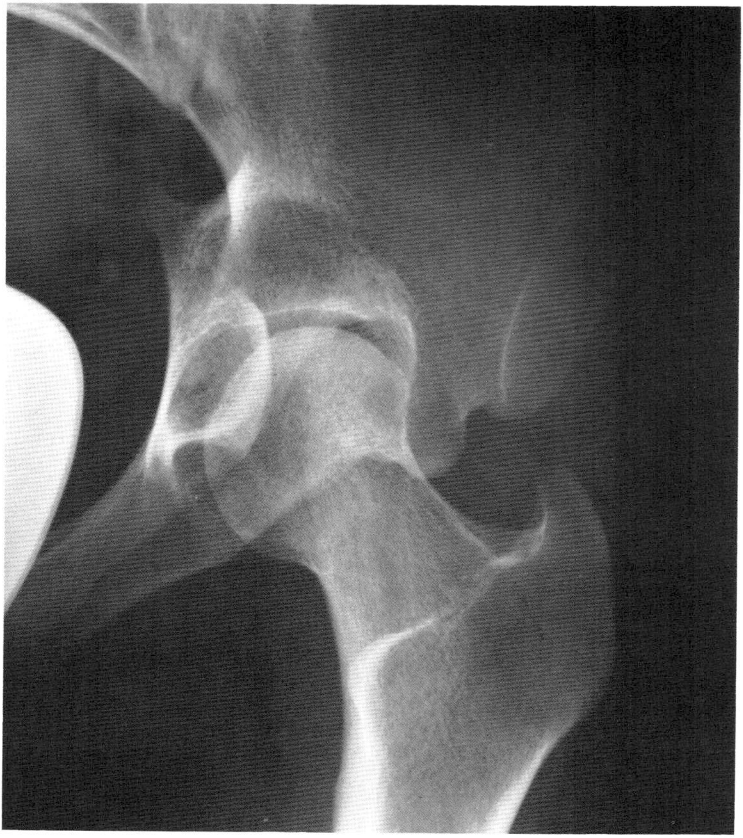

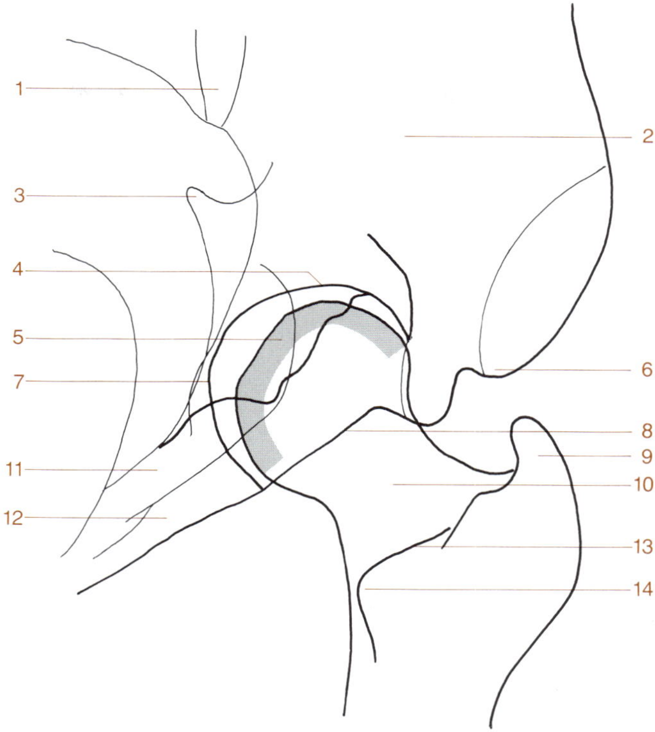

1 Sacroiliac joint
2 Iliac bone
3 Ischial spine
4 Acetabular roof
5 Dorsal articulating surface of the femoral head
6 Anterior superior iliac spine
7 Acetabular floor
8 Anterior acetabular rim
9 Greater trochanter
10 Femoral neck
11 Ischial bone
12 Pubic bone
13 Intertrochanteric line
14 Lesser trochanter

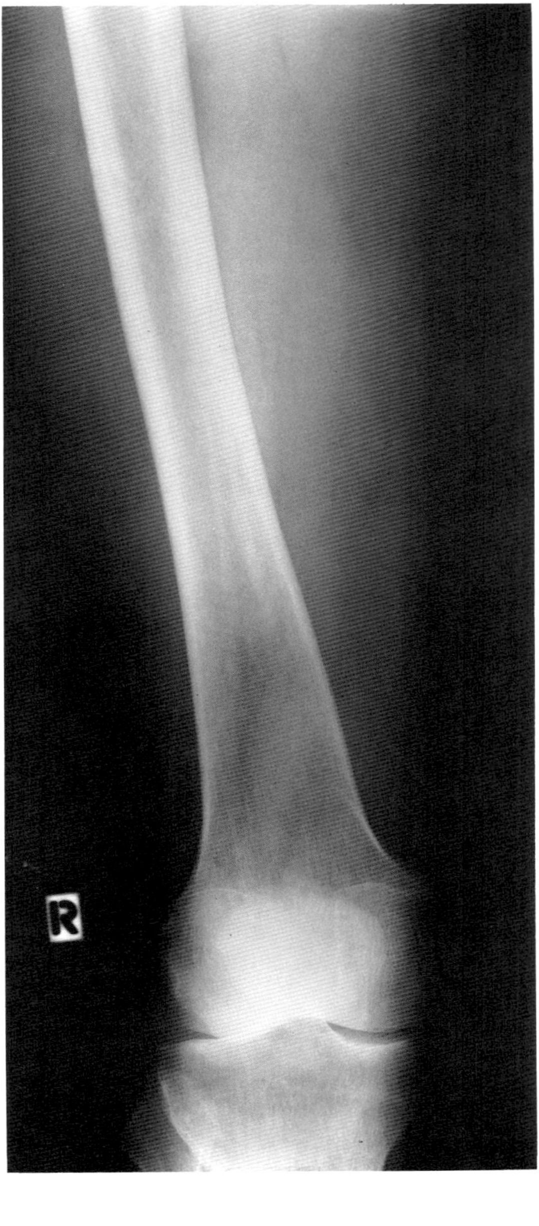
R

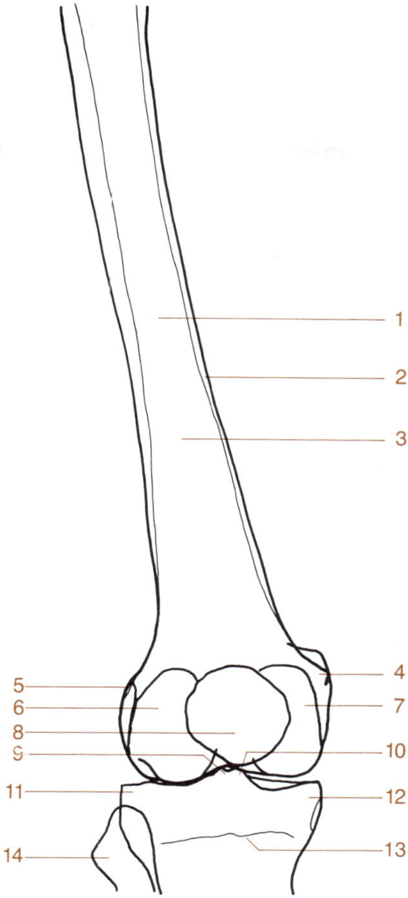

1 Femoral shaft
2 Cortex
3 Medullary space
4 Medial femoral epicondyle
5 Lateral femoral epicondyle
6 Lateral femoral condyle
7 Medial femoral condyle
8 Patella
9 Lateral intercondylar eminence
10 Medial intercondylar eminence
11 Lateral tibial condyle
12 Medial tibial condyle
13 Epiphyseal line
14 Fibular head

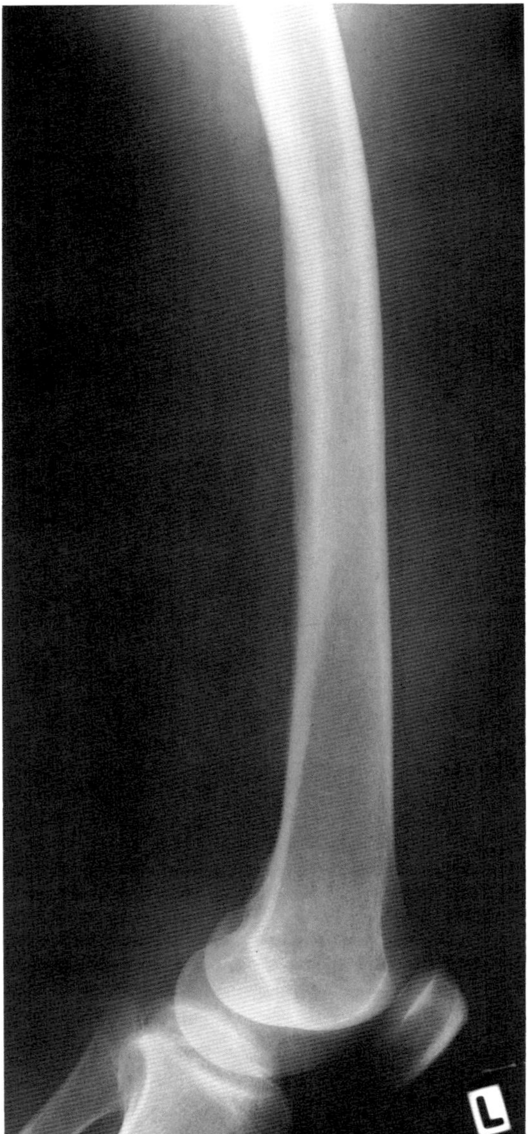
L

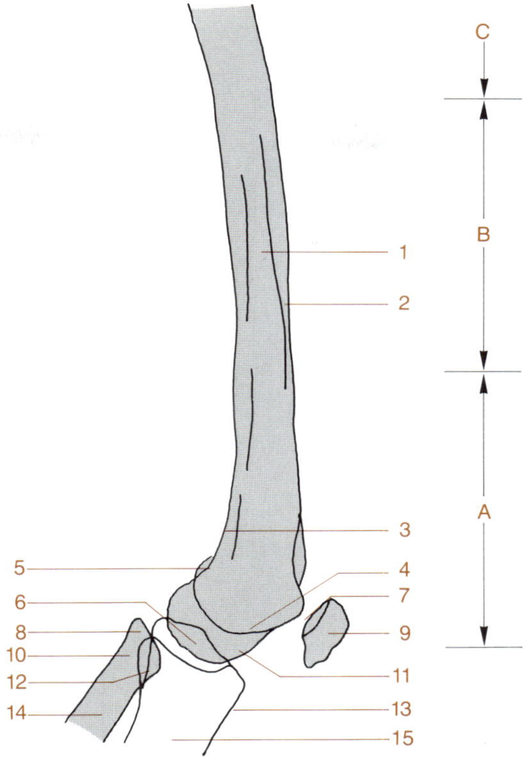

A Distal third of the femur
B Middle third of the femur
C Proximal third of the femur

1 Femur
2 Cortex
3 Popliteal fossa
4 Lateral femoral condyle
5 Intercondylar fossa
6 Intercondylar eminence
7 Patellofemoral articulation
8 Tip of fibular head
9 Patella
10 Head of the fibula
11 Medial femoral condyle
12 Tibiofibular joint
13 Tibial tuberosity
14 Fibula
15 Tibia

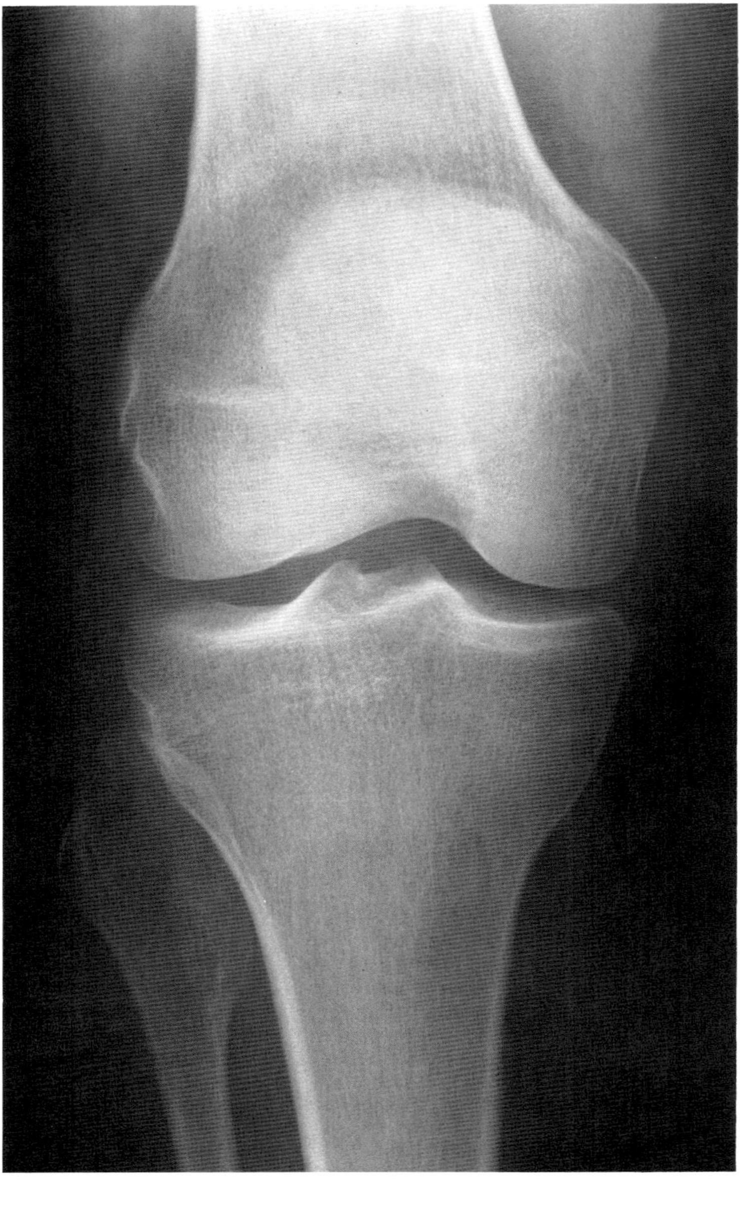

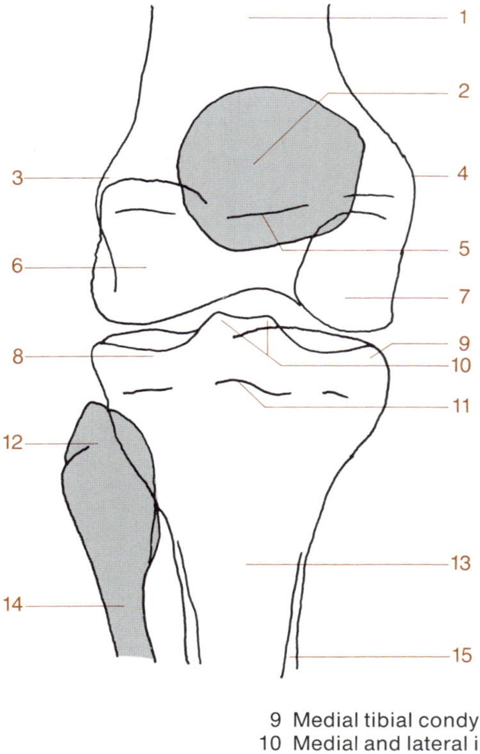

1 Femur
2 Patella
3 Lateral femoral epicondyle
4 Medial femoral epicondyle
5 Epiphyseal plate
6 Lateral femoral condyle
7 Medial femoral condyle
8 Lateral tibial condyle
9 Medial tibial condyle
10 Medial and lateral intercondylar tubercles
11 Epiphyseal plate
12 Head of the fibula
13 Tibia
14 Fibula
15 Cortical bone

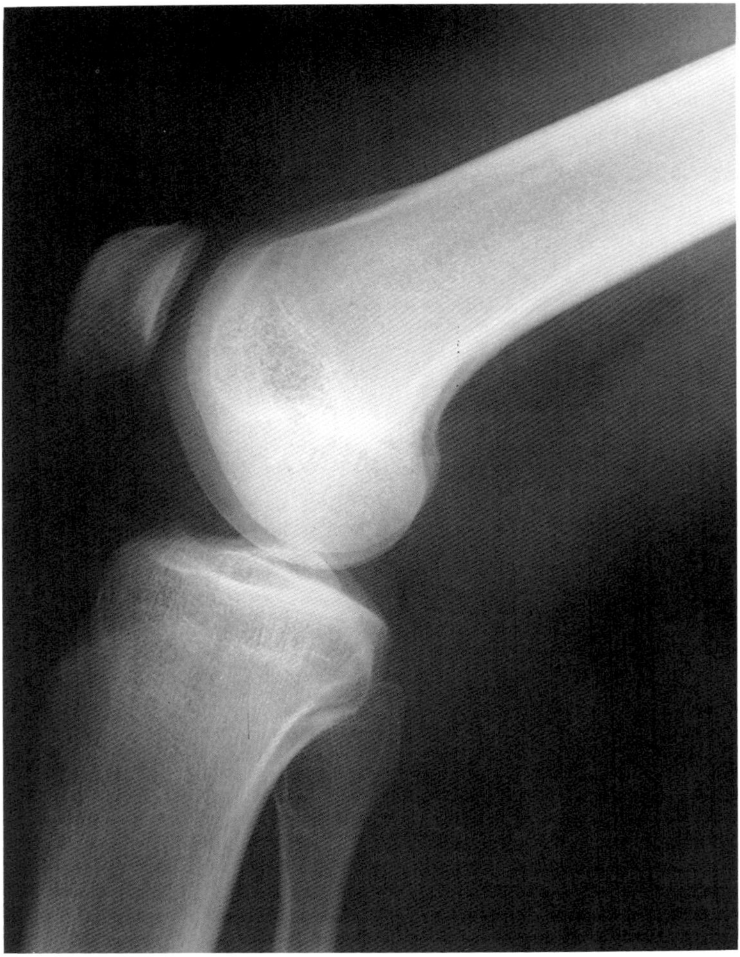

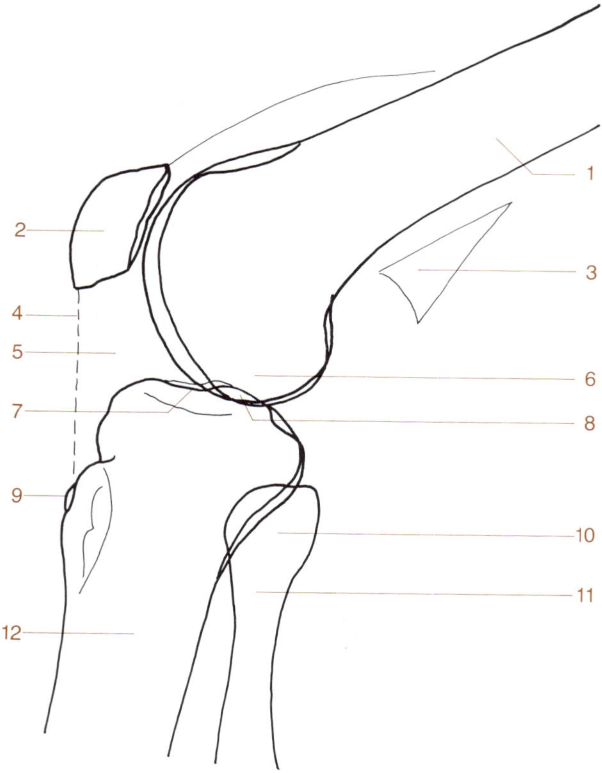

1 Femur
2 Patella
3 Fat plane
4 Ligamentum patellae
5 Infrapatellar fat pad (Hoffa)
6 Lateral femoral condyle
7 Tibial plateau
8 Intercondylar eminence
9 Tibial tuberosity
10 Fibula
11 Fibular neck
12 Tibia

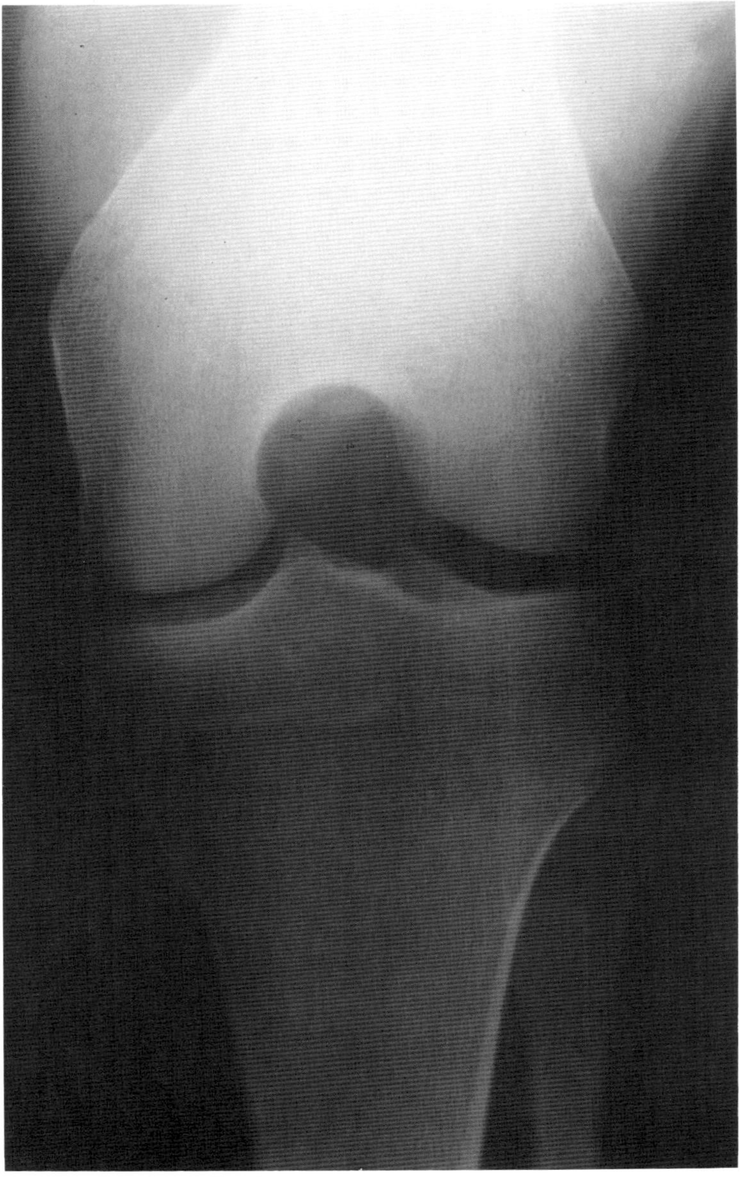

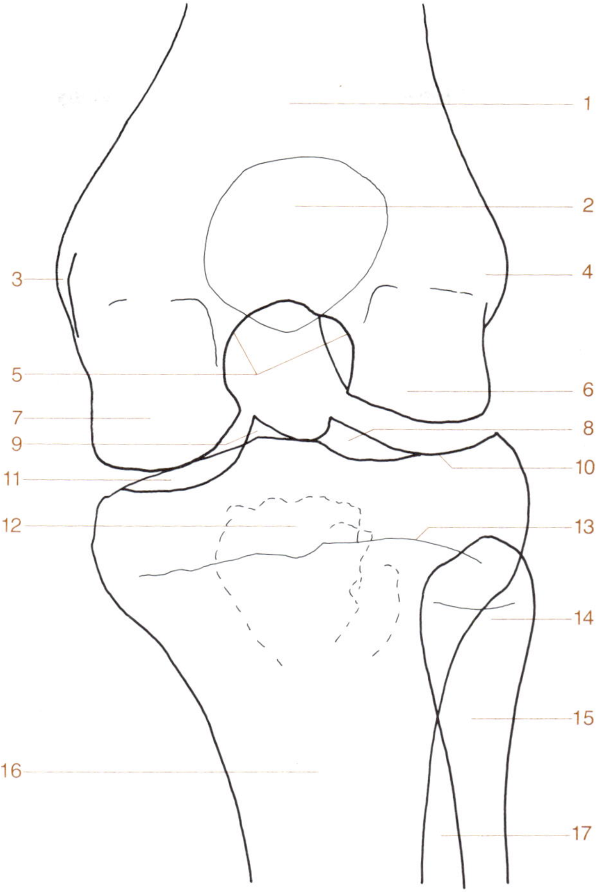

1 Femur
2 Patella
3 Medial femoral epicondyle
4 Lateral femoral epicondyle
5 Intercondylar fossa
6 Lateral femoral condyle
7 Medial femoral condyle
8 Lateral intercondylar eminence
9 Medial intercondylar eminence
10 Lateral articulating surface of the tibial plateau
11 Medial articulating surface of the tibial plateau
12 Tibial tuberosity
13 Epiphyseal plate
14 Fibular head
15 Fibular neck
16 Tibia
17 Interosseous membrane

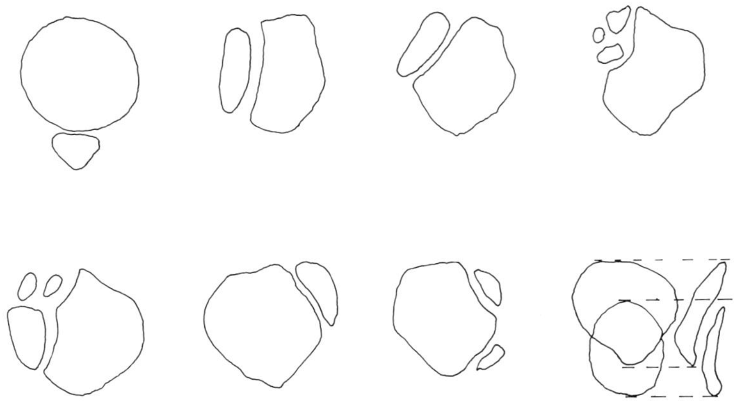

Most common forms of partate patella (after Schaer)

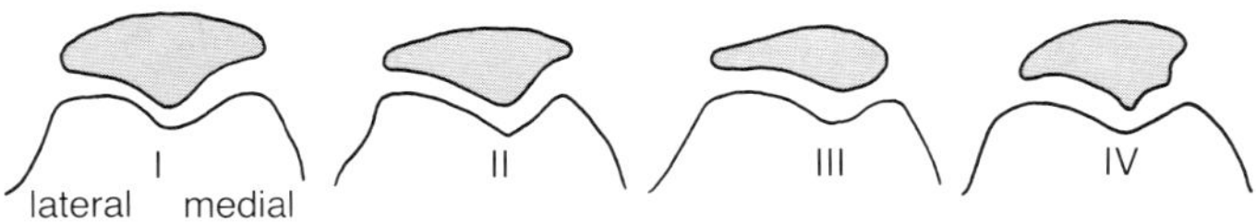

Wiberg's classification of patellar shapes (right knee)

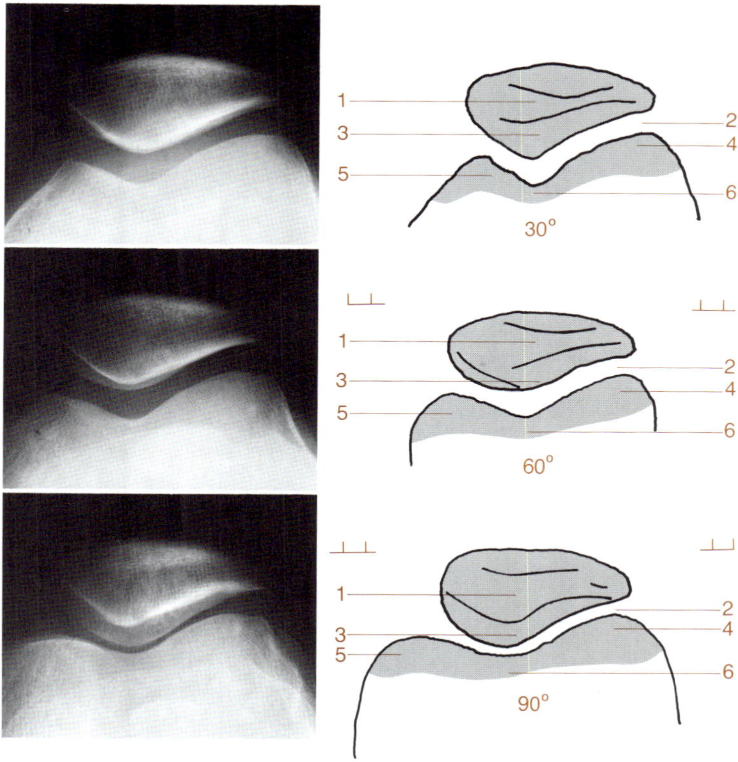

1 Patella
2 Patellofemoral articulation
3 Articular surface
4 Lateral femoral condyle
5 Medial femoral condyle
6 Intercondylar fossa

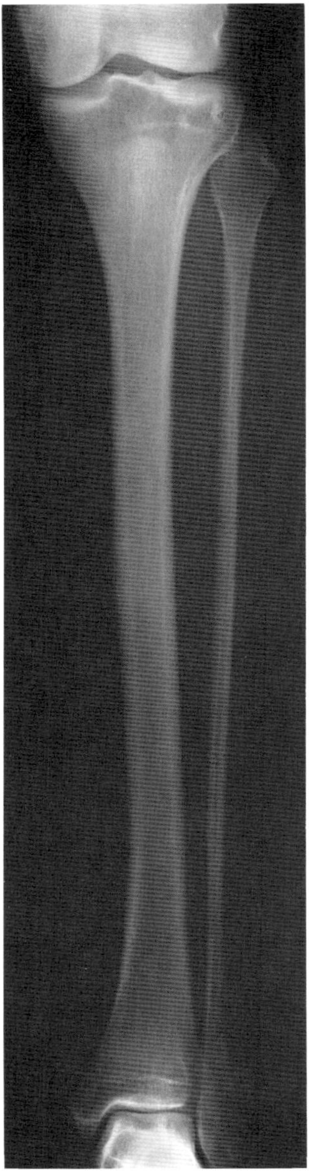

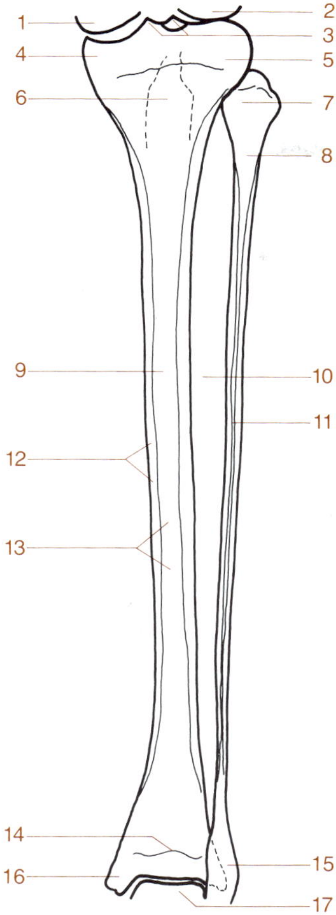

1 Medial femoral condyle
2 Lateral femoral condyle
3 Medial and lateral intercondylar eminences
4 Medial tibial condyle
5 Lateral tibial condyle
6 Tibial tuberosity
7 Fibular head
8 Fibular neck
9 Tibia
10 Interosseous membrane
11 Fibula
12 Cortex
13 Medullary space
14 Epiphyseal plate
15 Lateral malleolus
16 Medial malleolus
17 Talus

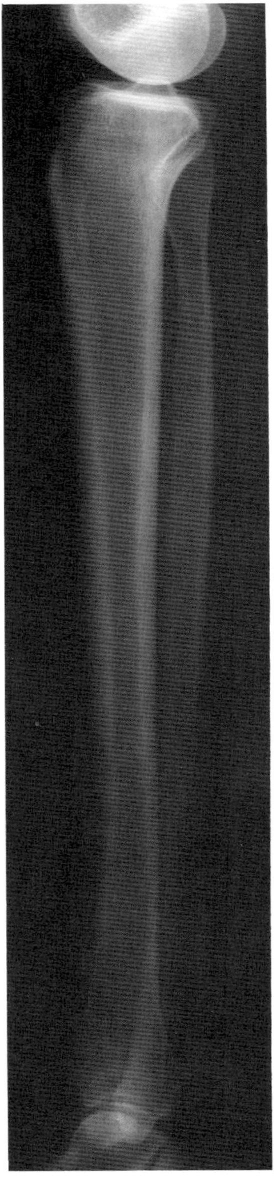

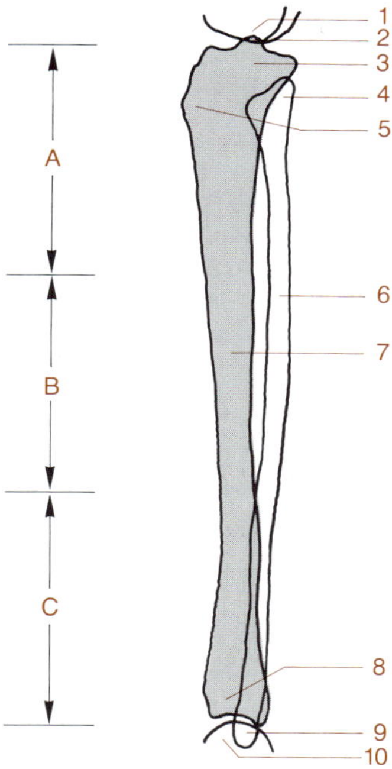

A Proximal third of the lower leg (tibia and fibula)
B Middle third of the lower leg (tibia and fibula)
C Distal third of the lower leg (tibia and fibula)

1 Medial and lateral femoral condyles
2 Intercondylar eminence
3 Medial and lateral tibial condyles
4 Fibular head
5 Tibial tuberosity (in children: proximal tibial apophysis)
6 Fibula
7 Tibia
8 Medial malleus
9 Lateral malleus
10 Trochlea of the talus

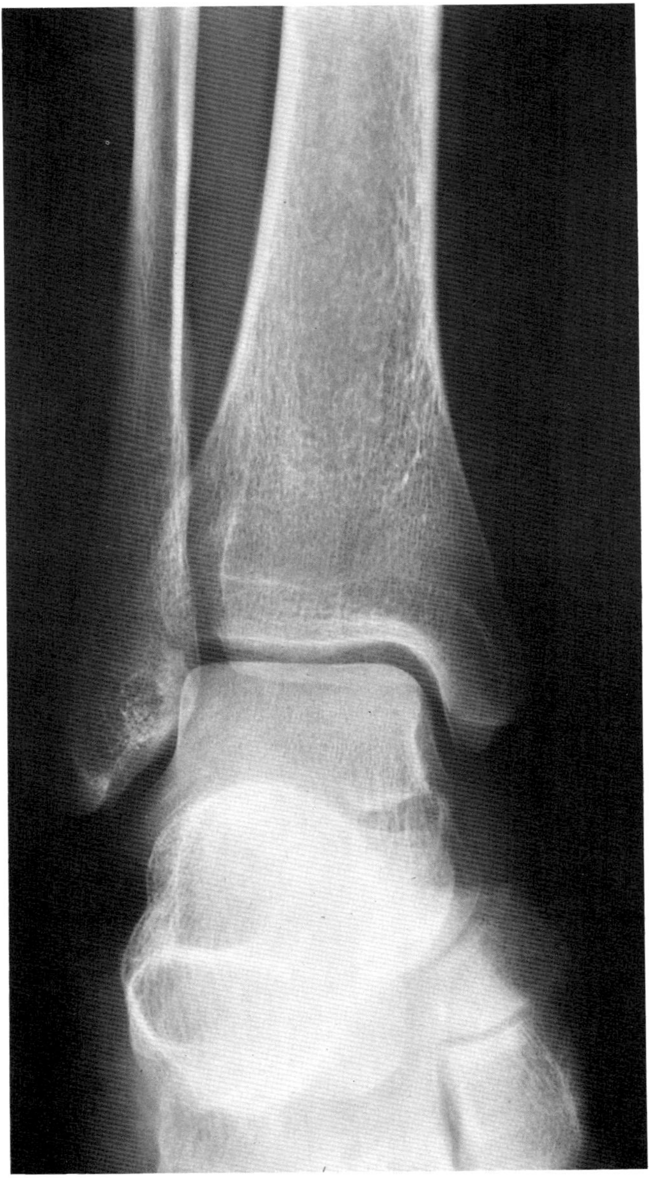

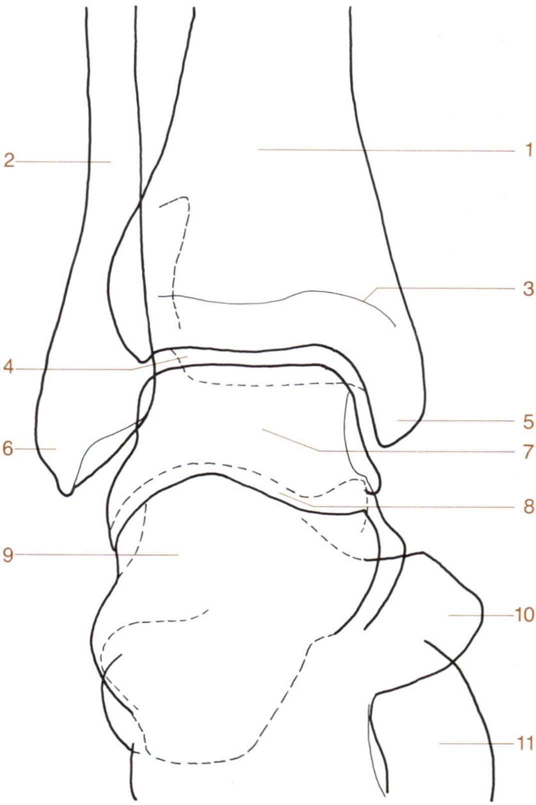

1 Tibia
2 Fibula
3 Epiphyseal plate
4 Tibiotalar joint
5 Medial malleolus
6 Lateral malleolus
7 Trochlea of the talus
8 Subtalar joint
9 Calcaneus
10 Navicular bone
11 Medial cuneiform bone

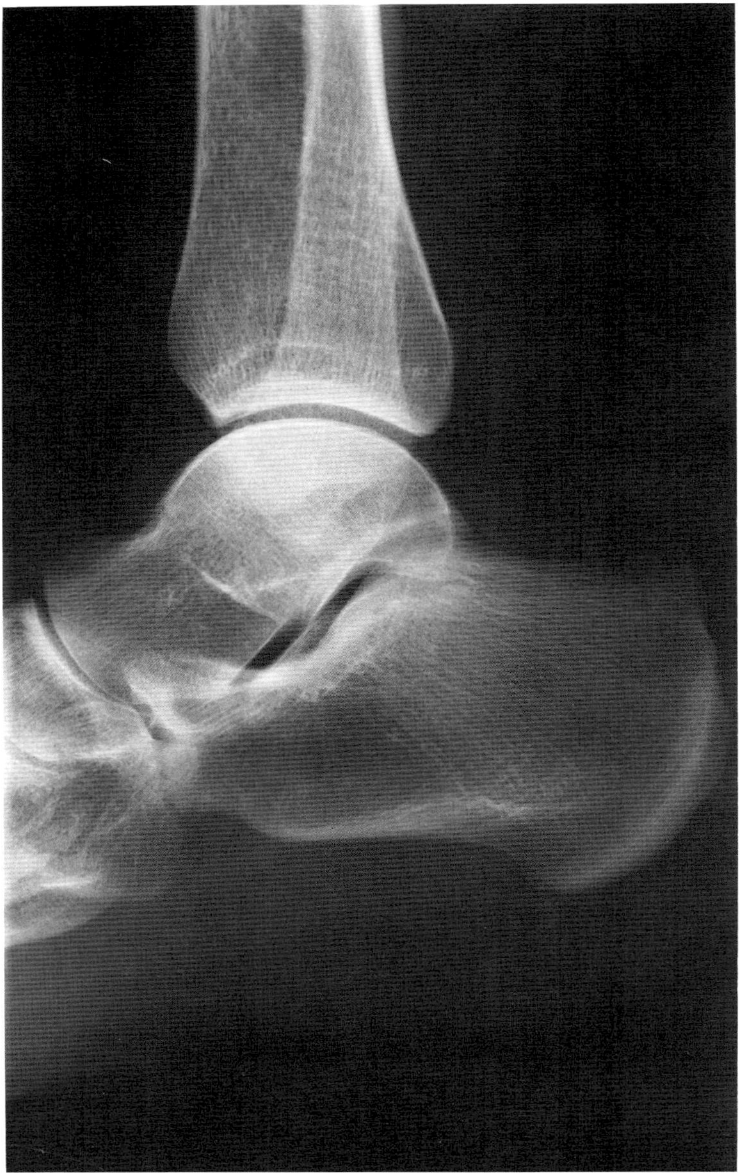

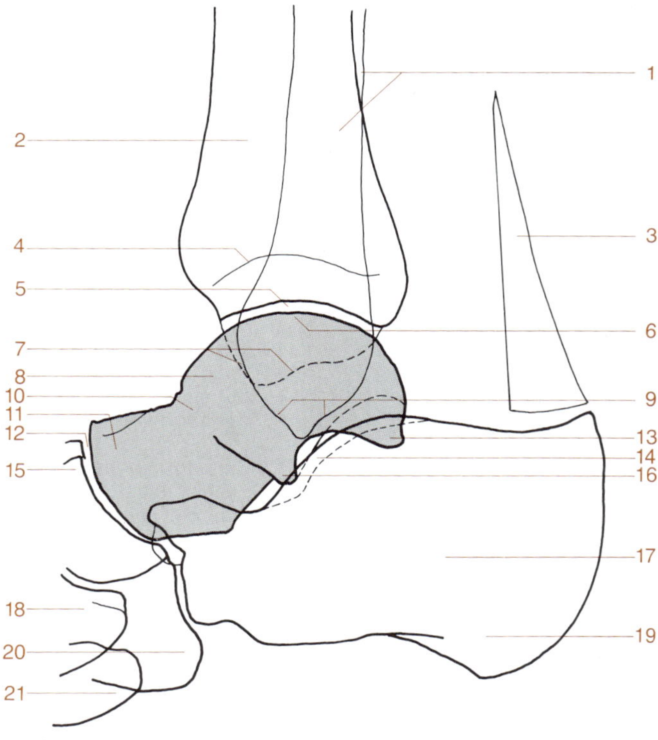

1 Fibula
2 Tibia
3 Achilles tendon
4 Epiphyseal plate
5 Tibiotalar joint
6 Trochlea of the talus
7 Medial malleolus
8 Talus
9 Lateral malleolus
10 Neck of the talus
11 Head of the talus
12 Talonavicular joint
13 Posterior process of the talus
14 Tarsal sinus
15 Navicular bone
16 Lateral process of the talus
17 Calcaneus
18 Medial cuneiform bone
19 Tuber calcanei
20 Cuboid bone
21 Base of fifth metatarsal bone

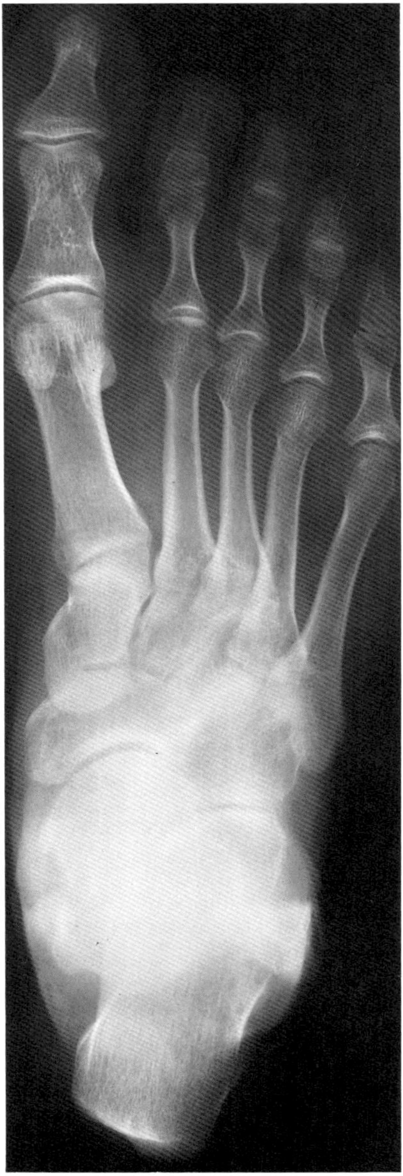

1 Distal phalangeal tuft
2 Distal phalanx of the big toe
3 Distal interphalangeal joint, big toe
4 Distal interphalangeal joint
5 Proximal interphalangeal joint
6 Distal phalanx
7 Middle phalanx
8 Head of the proximal phalanx
9 Proximal phalanx
10 Sesamoid bone
11 Base of the phalanx
12 Metatarsophalangeal joint
13 Metatarsal bone
14 Head of the metatarsal
15 Cuneiform bone I (medial)
16 Cuneiform bone II (intermediate)
17 Cuneiform bone III (lateral)
18 Base of the metatarsal bone/ tuberosity of metatarsal bone V
19 Navicular bone
20 Head of the talus
21 Cuboid bone
22 Medial malleolus
23 Lateral malleolus
24 Calcaneus
25 Tarsometatarsal joint (Lisfranc)
26 Intertarsal joint (Chopart)
27 Os intermetatarseum
28 Os vesalianum
29 Os peroneum
30 Os cuboideum secundarium
31 Os tibiale externum
32 Os supratalare

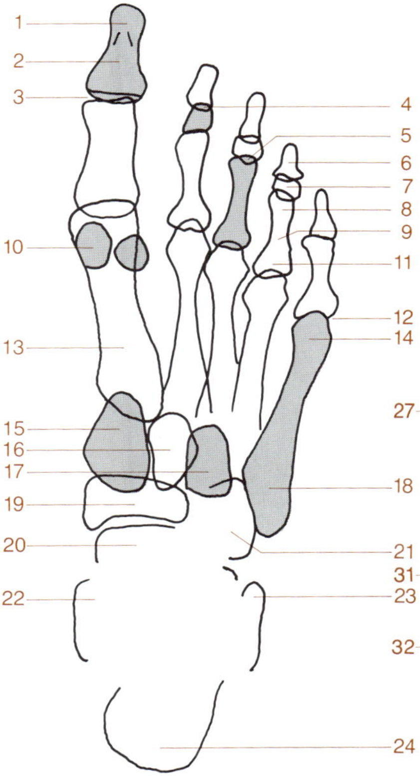

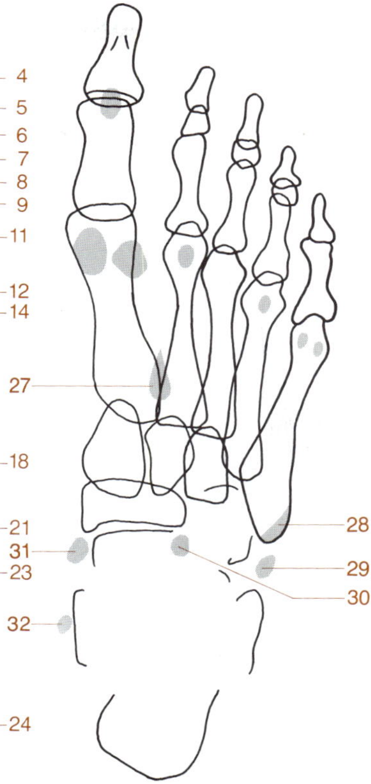

Commom sesamoid bones and accessory bones in the foot

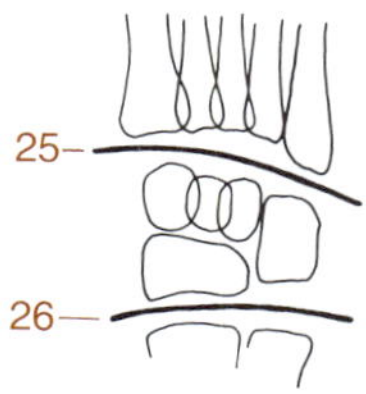

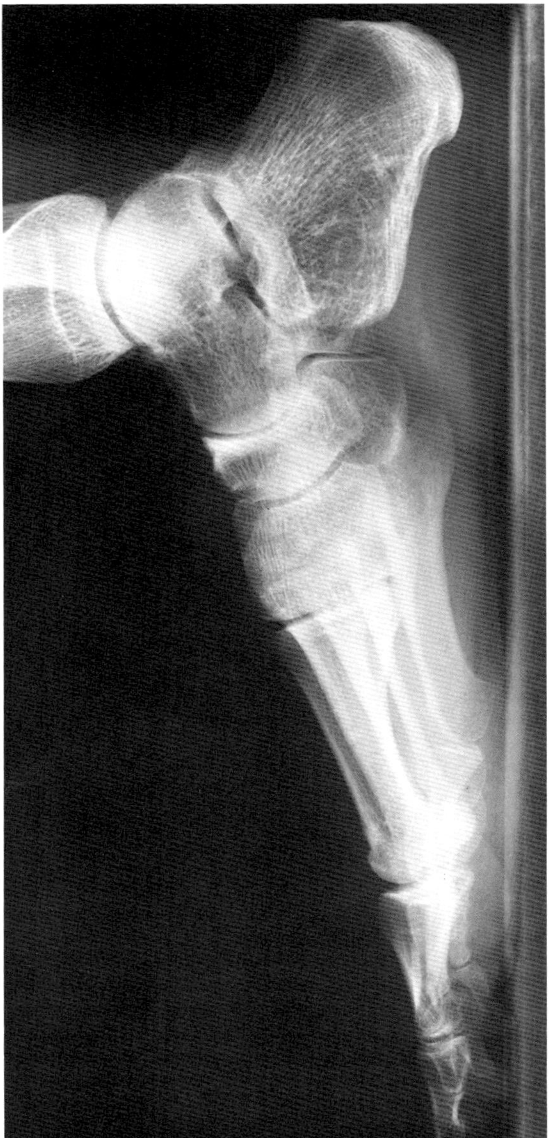

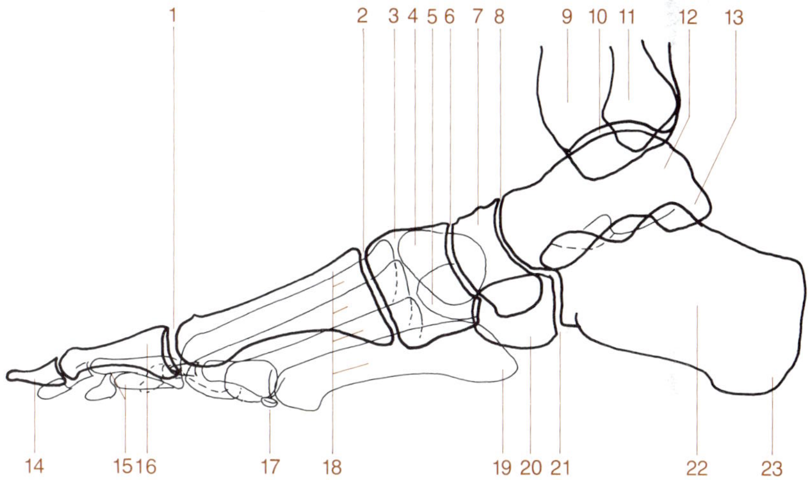

1 Metatarsophalangeal joint
2 Tarsometatarsal joint
3 Medial cuneiform bone
4 Intermediate cuneiform bone
5 Lateral cuneiform bone
6 Cuneonavicular articulation
7 Navicular bone
8 Talonavicular joint space
9 Tibia
10 Tibiotalar joint space
11 Fibula
12 Talus
13 Posterior talar process
14 Distal phalanx
15 Middle phalanx
16 Proximal phalanx
17 Sesamoid bone
18 Metatarsal bone
19 Tuberosity of metatarsal bone V
20 Cuboid bone
21 Calcaneocuboid joint
22 Calcaneus
23 Tuber calcanei

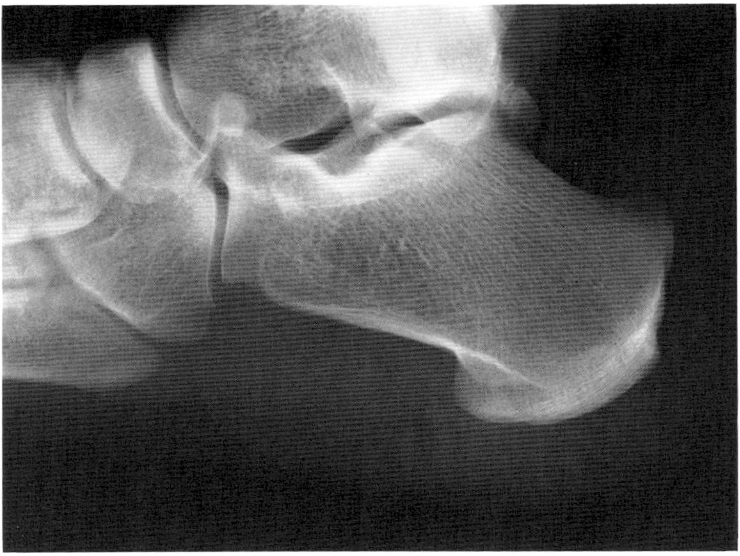

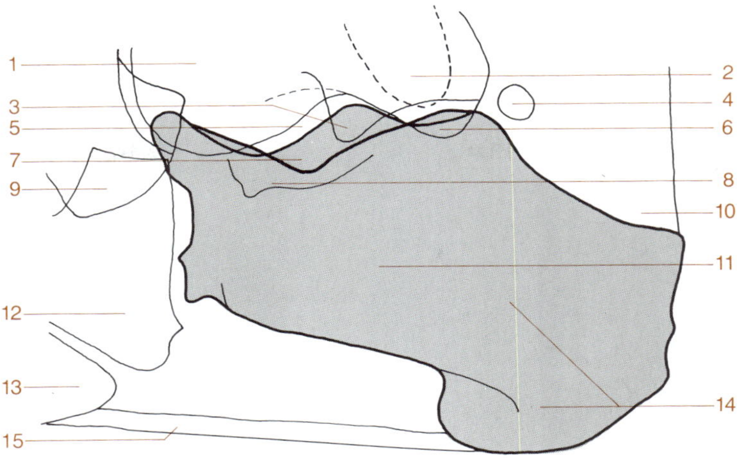

1 Talus
2 Lateral malleolus
3 Lateral process of the talus
4 Os trigonum
5 Subtalar joint
6 Posterior process of the talus
7 Tarsal sinus
8 Sustentaculum tali
9 Navicular bone
10 Achilles tendon
11 Calcaneus
12 Cuboid bone
13 Base of metatarsal bone V
14 Tuber calcanei
15 Plantar aponeurosis

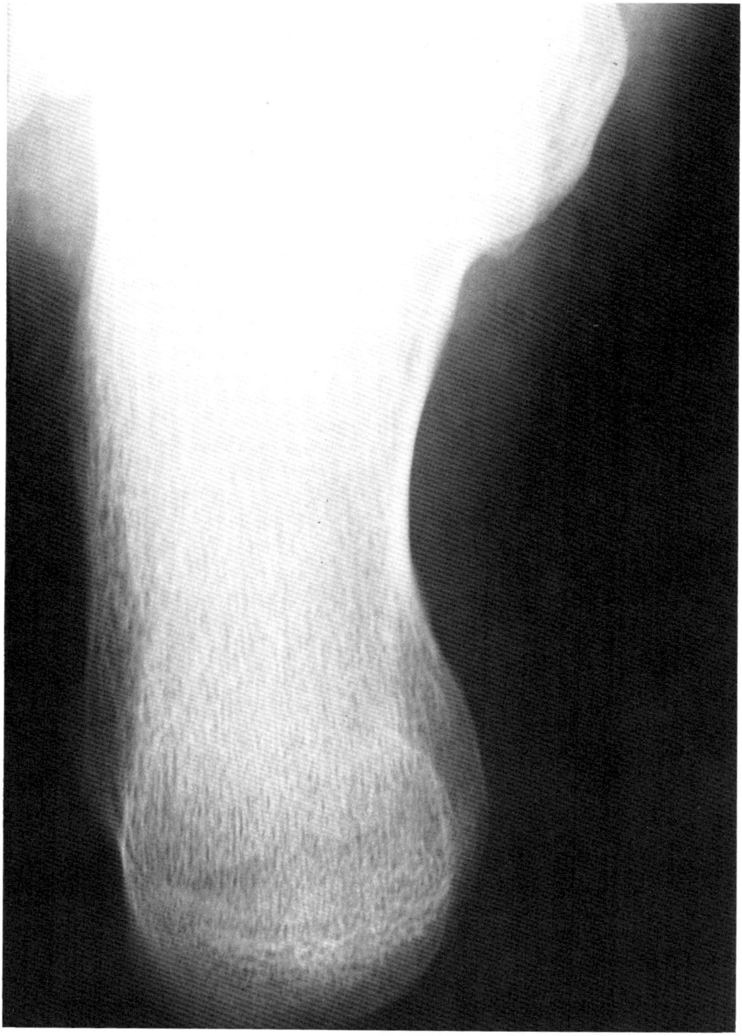

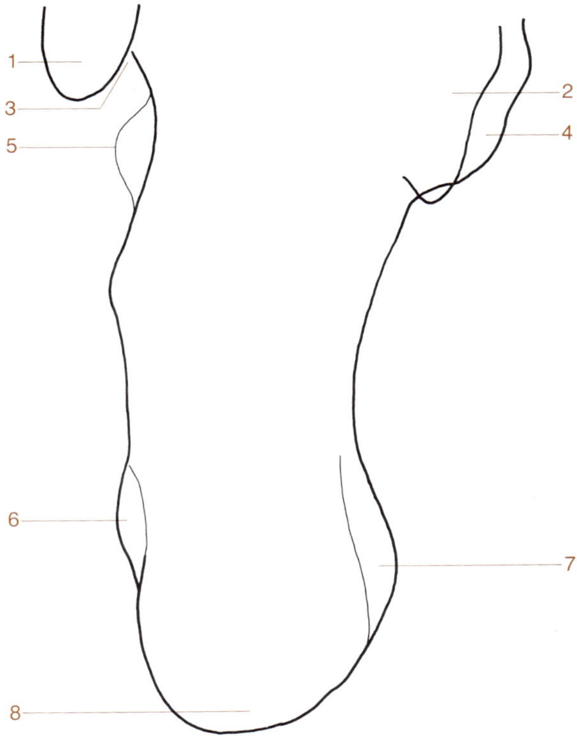

1 Lateral malleolus
2 Talus
3 Groove for the tendon of the peroneus longus muscle
4 Sustentaculum tali
5 Peroneal trochlea
6 Lateral process of the calcaneal tuberosity
7 Medial process of the calcaneal tuberosity
8 Tuber calcanei

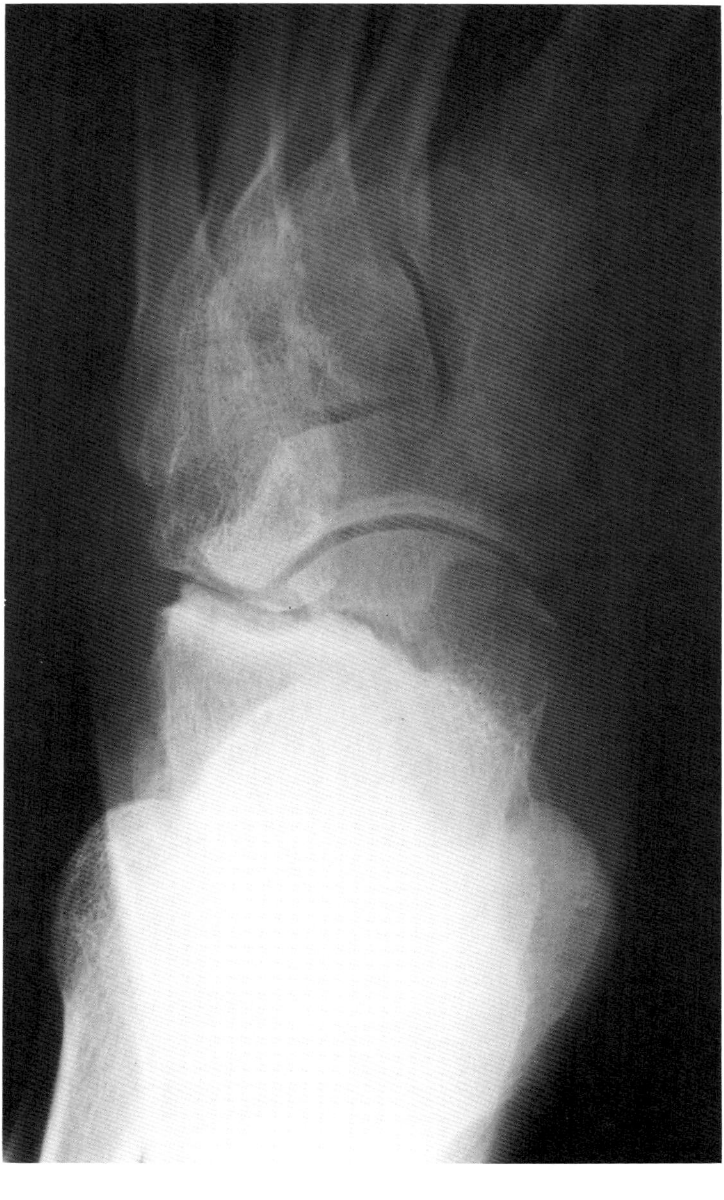

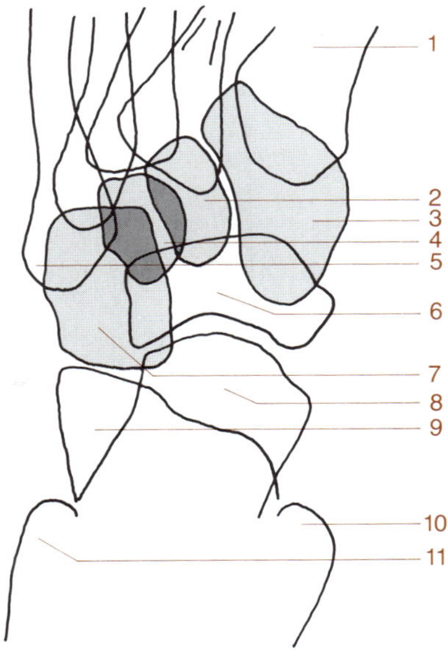

1 Metatarsal bone
2 Intermediate cuneiform bone
3 Medial cuneiform bone
4 Lateral cuneiform bone
5 Tuberosity of metatarsal bone V
6 Navicular bone
7 Cuboid bone
8 Head of the talus
9 Calcaneus
10 Medial malleolus
11 Lateral malleolus

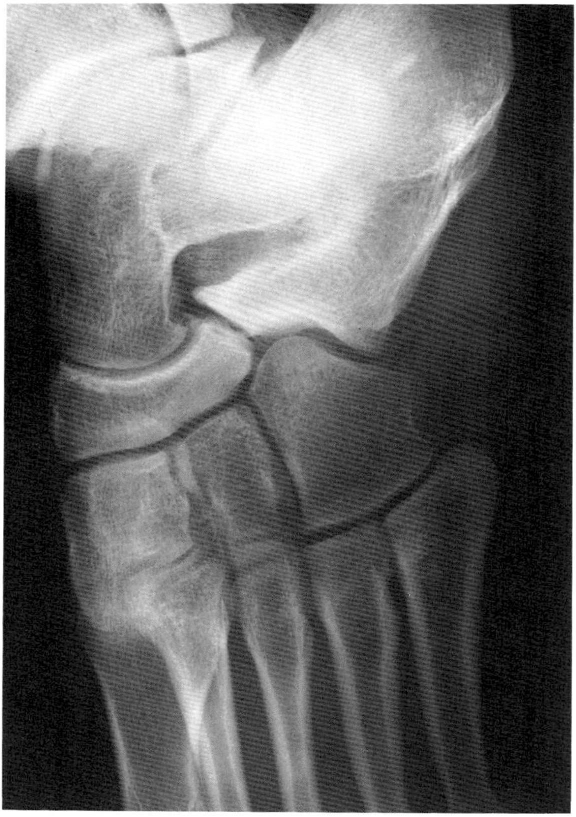

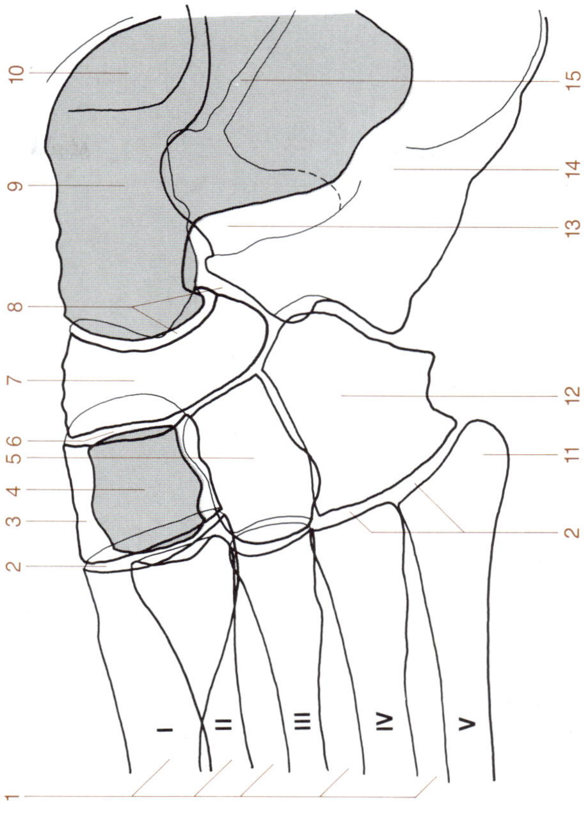

1 Metatarsal bones
2 Tarsometatarsal joint
3 Medial cuneiform bone
4 Intermediate cuneiform bone
5 Lateral cuneiform bone
6 Cuneonavicular articulation
7 Navicular bone
8 Talocalcaneonavicular joint
9 Talus
10 Medial malleolus
11 Tuberosity of metatarsal bone V
12 Cuboid bone
13 Tarsal sinus
14 Calcaneus
15 Subtalar joint

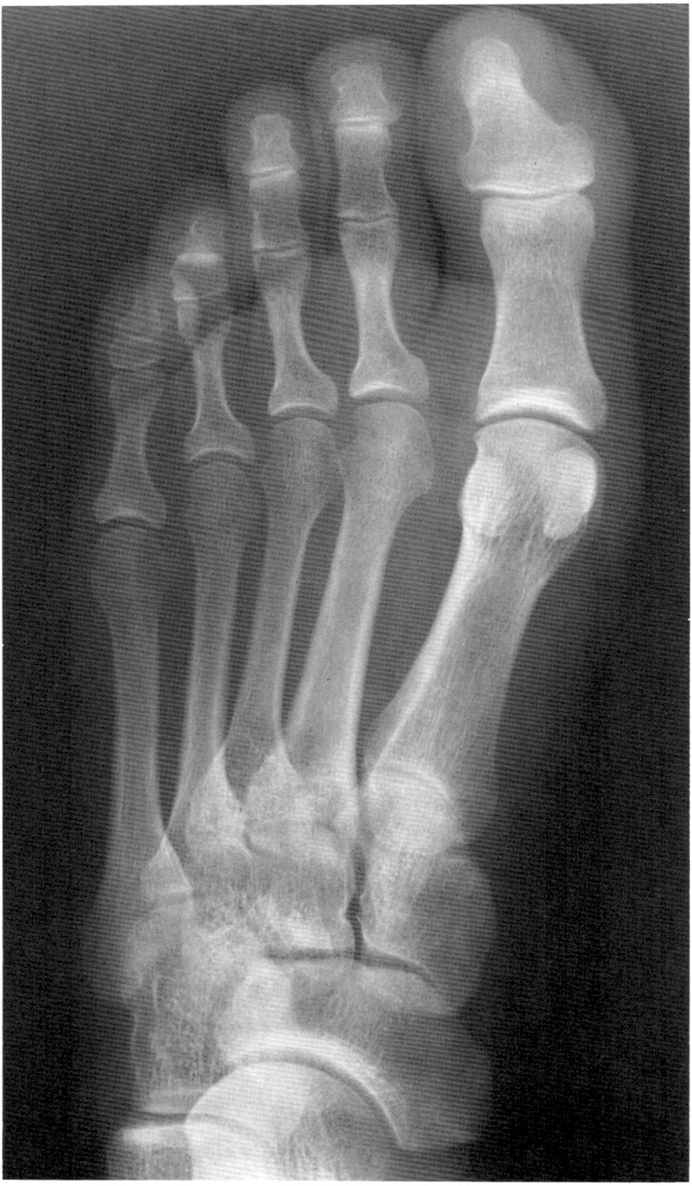

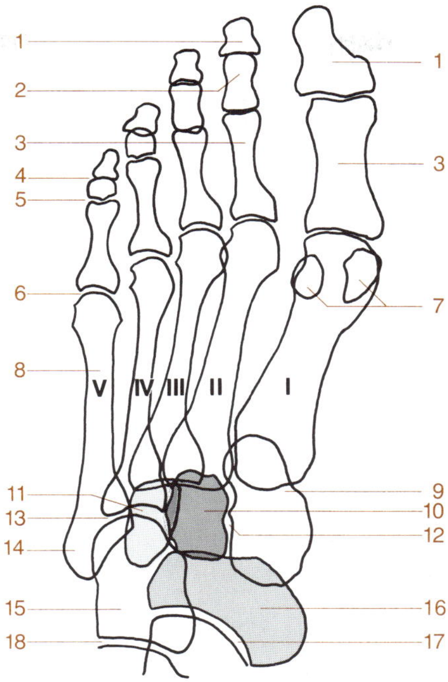

1 Distal phalanx
2 Middle phalanx
3 Proximal phalanx
4 Distal interphalangeal joint
5 Proximal interphalangeal joint
6 Metatarsophalangeal joint
7 Sesamoid bones
8 Metatarsal bones (I–V)
9 Medial cuneiform bone
10 Intermediate cuneiform bone
11 Lateral cuneiform bone
12 Intertarsal joint
13 Metatarsophalangeal joint
14 Tuberosity of metatarsal bone V
15 Cuboid bone
16 Navicular bone
17 Talonavicular joint space
18 Calcaneocuboid joint

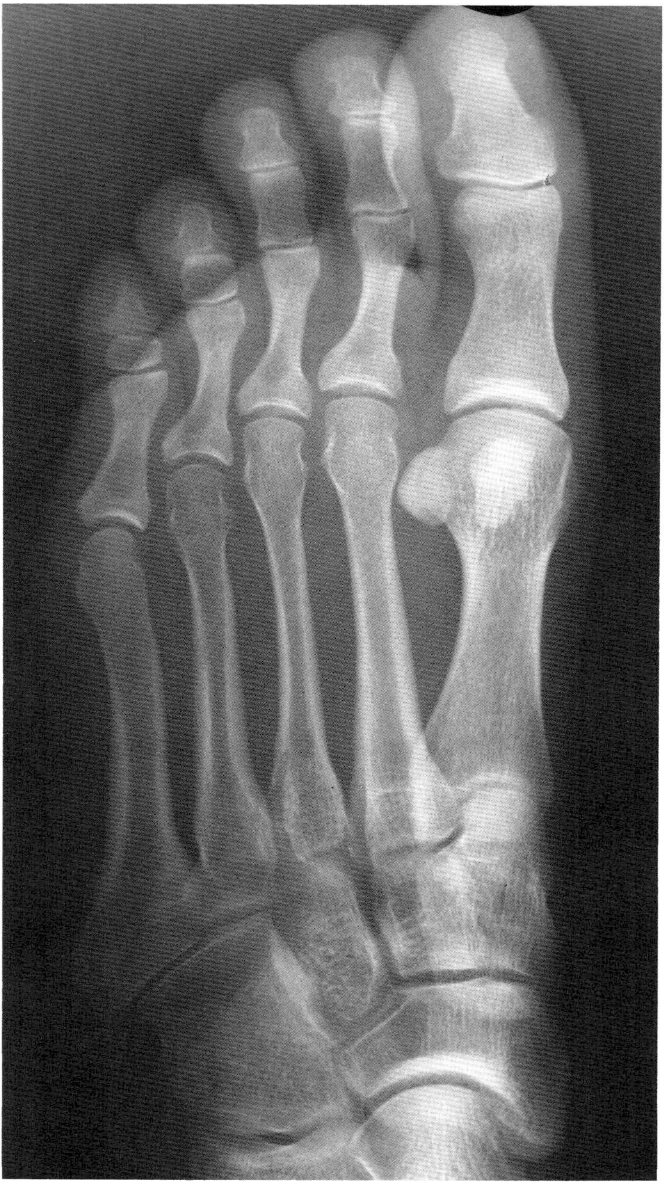

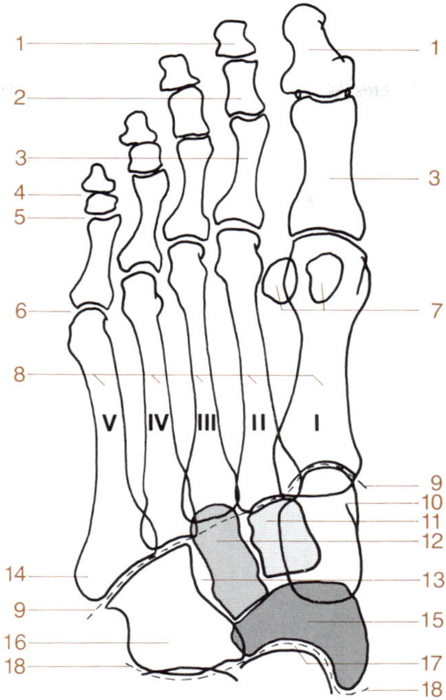

1 Distal phalanx
2 Middle phalanx
3 Proximal phalanx
4 Distal interphalangeal joint
5 Proximal interphalangeal joint
6 Metatarsophalangeal joint
7 Sesamoid bones
8 Metatarsal bones
9 Tarsometatarsal joint (Lisfranc's line)
10 Medial cuneiform bone
11 Intermediate cuneiform bone
12 Lateral cuneiform bone
13 Intertarsal joint
14 Tuberosity of metatarsal bone V
15 Navicular bone
16 Cuboid bone
17 Talonavicular joint space
18 Intertarsal joint space (Chopart's line, separating the proximal and distal tarsal bones)

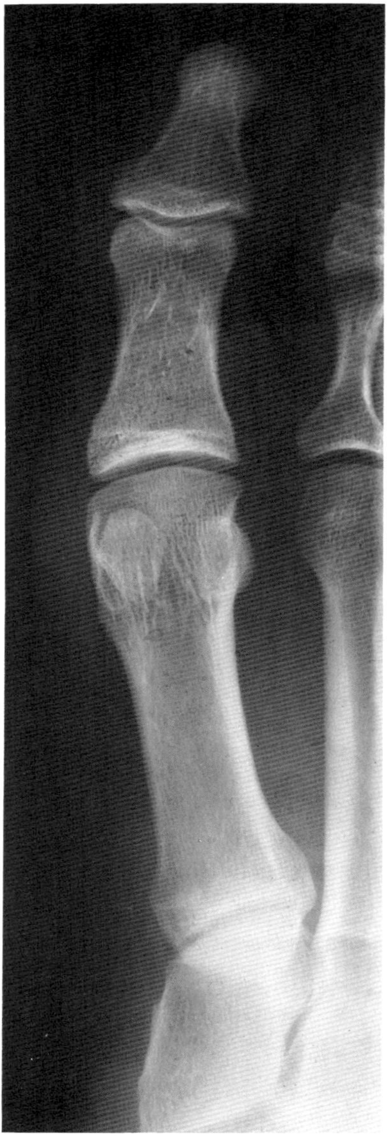

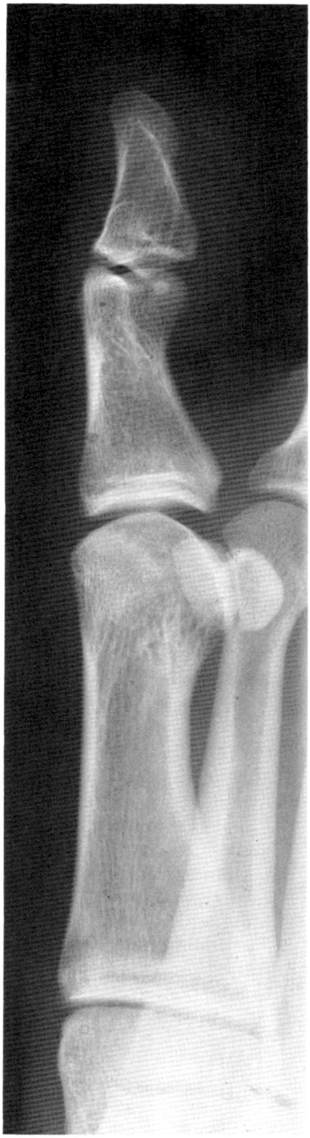

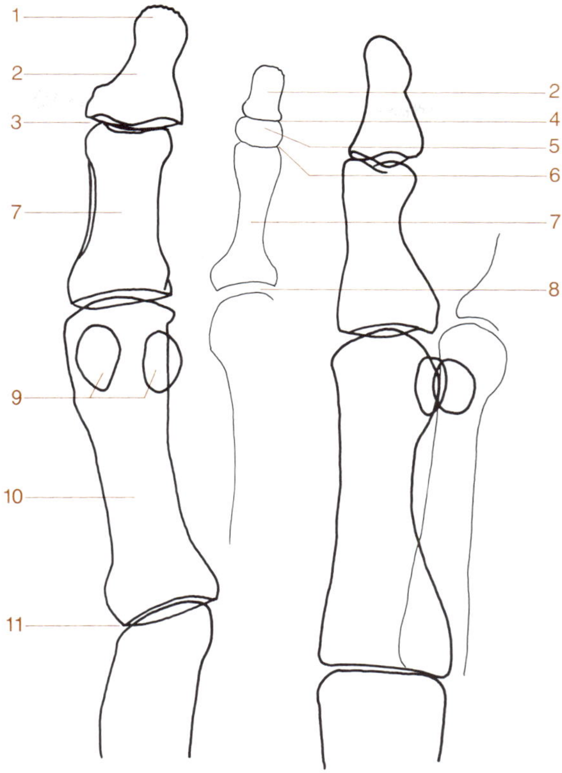

1 Distal phalangeal tuft
2 Distal phalanx
3 Interphalangeal joint I
4 Distal interphalangeal joint
5 Middle phalanx
6 Proximal interphalangeal joint
7 Proximal phalanx
8 Metatarsophalangeal joint
9 Sesamoid bone
10 Metatarsal bone I
11 Tarsometatarsal joint

Anatomy of Miscellaneous Plain Films

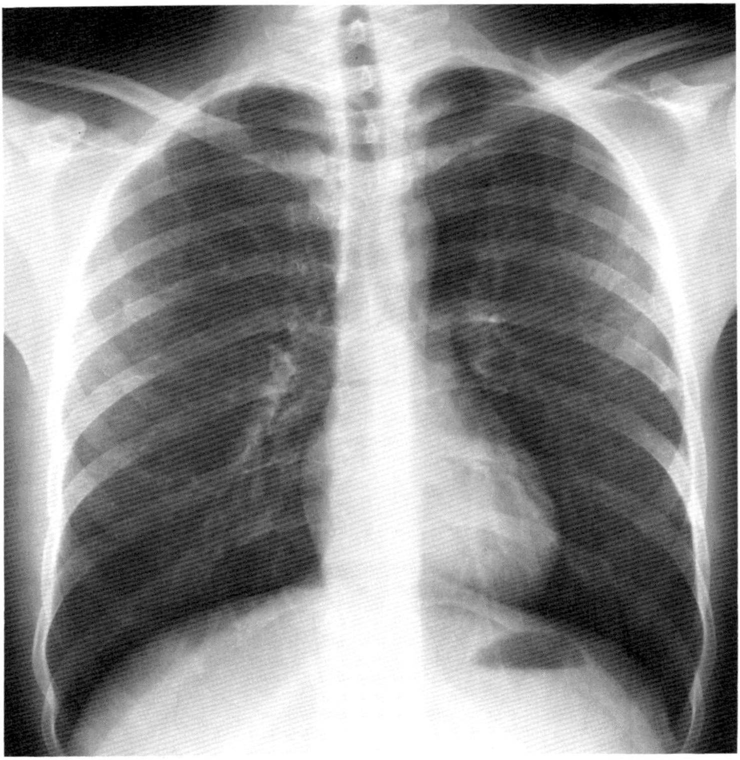

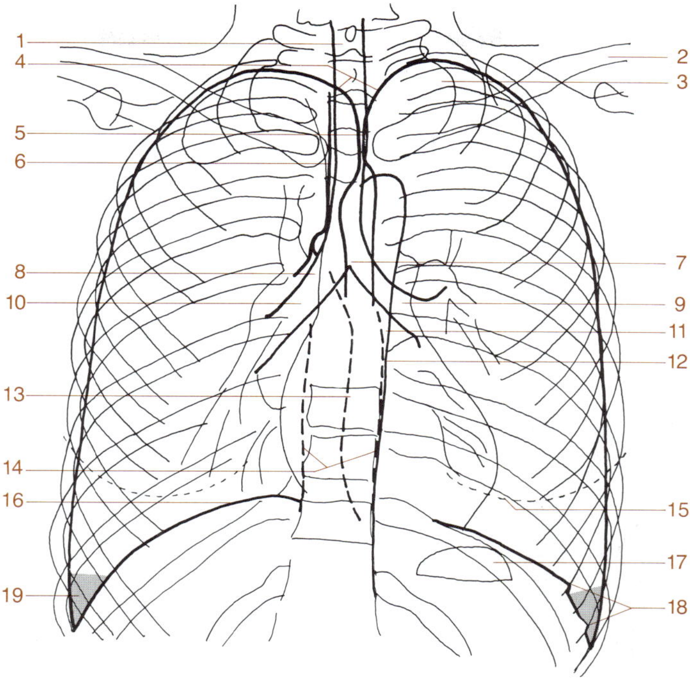

1 Trachea
2 Clavicle
3 Lung apex
4, 5 Posterior superior junction-line complex
6 Right paratracheal stripe
7 Tracheal carina
8 Right main stem bronchus
9 Left main stem bronchus
10 Bronchus intermedius
11 Preaortic stripe
12 Descending aorta
13 Azygoesophageal stripe
14 Paraspinal stripe
15 Breast contour
16 Dome of the diaphragm
17 Stomach bubble
18 Diaphragmatic muscle slips
19 Costophrenic sulcus

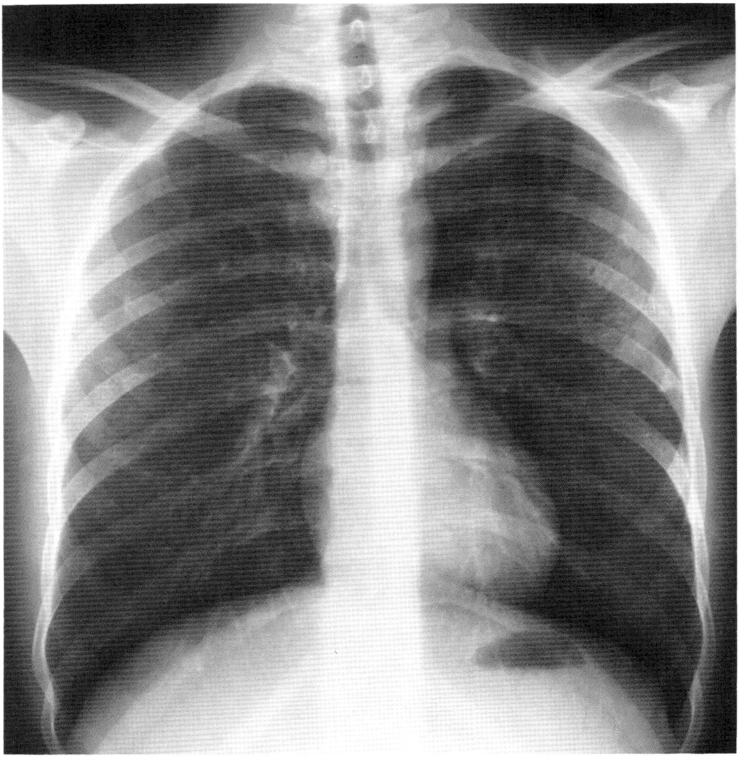

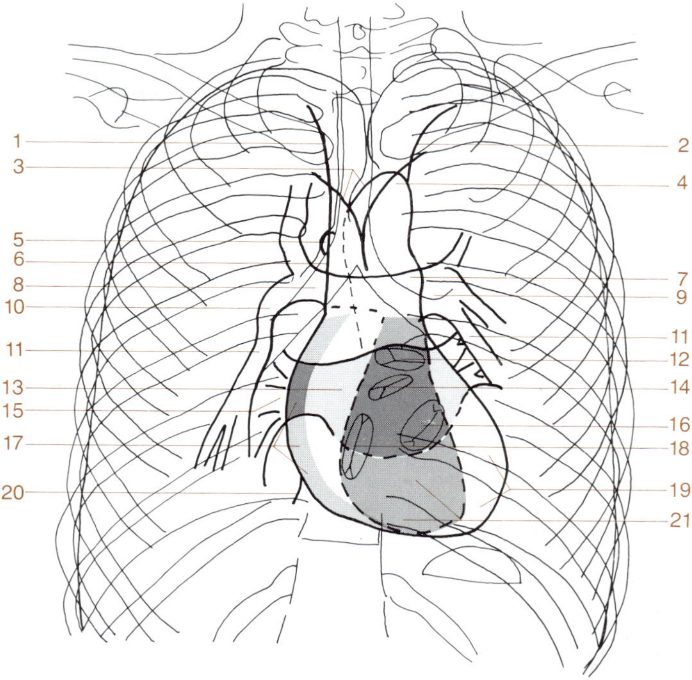

1 Contour of the right brachiocephalic vein
2 Contour of the subclavian artery
3 Anterior junction line
4 Aortic arch
5 Azygos vein
6 Superior vena cava
7 Main pulmonary artery segment
8 Right pulmonary artery
9 Left pulmonary artery
10 Interlobar pulmonary artery
11 Right lower lobe pulmonary artery
12 Pulmonic valve
13 Left atrium
14 Aortic valve
15 Confluence of pulmonary veins
16 Mitral valve
17 Right atrium
18 Tricuspid valve
19 Left ventricle
20 Inferior vena cava
21 Right ventricle

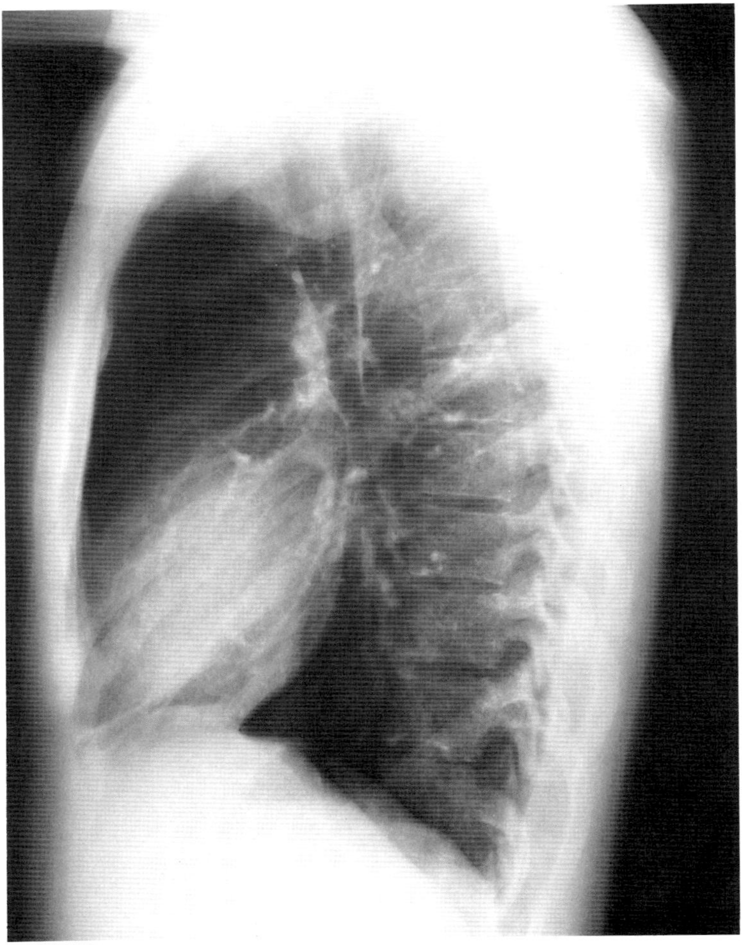

1 Shoulder soft tissues
2 Trachea
3 Scapula
4 Angle of Louis
5 Aortic arch
6 Sternal body
7 Aortopulmonary window
8 Ascending aorta
9 Right upper lobe bronchus
10 Retrosternal space
11 Left upper lobe bronchus
12 Main pulmonary artery segment
13 Descending aorta
14 Pulmonic valve
15 Right lower lobe pulmonary veins

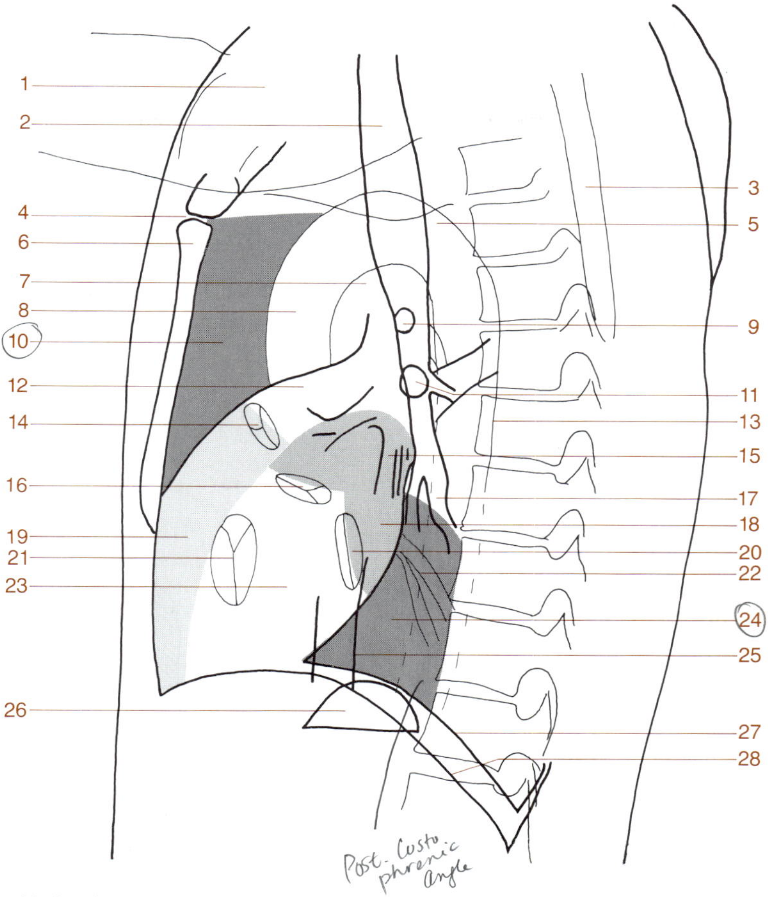

16 Aortic valve
17 Lower lobe bronchus
18 Left atrium
19 Right ventricle
20 Mitral valve
21 Tricuspid valve
22 Left lower lobe pulmonary veins
23 Left ventricle
24 Retrocardiac space
25 Inferior vena cava
26 Stomach bubble
27 Left hemidiaphragm
28 Right hemidiaphragm

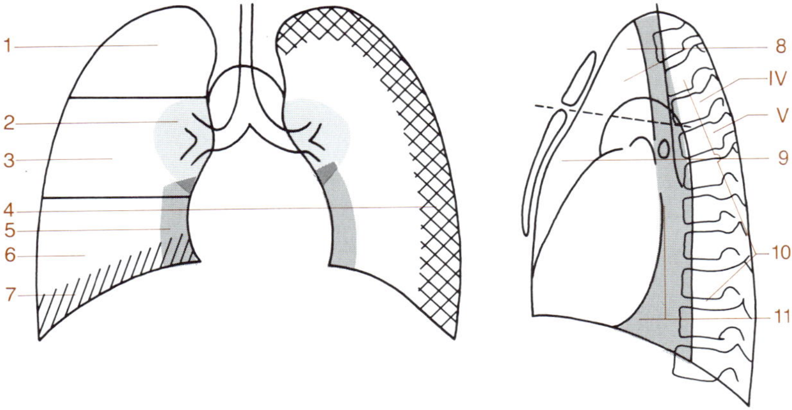

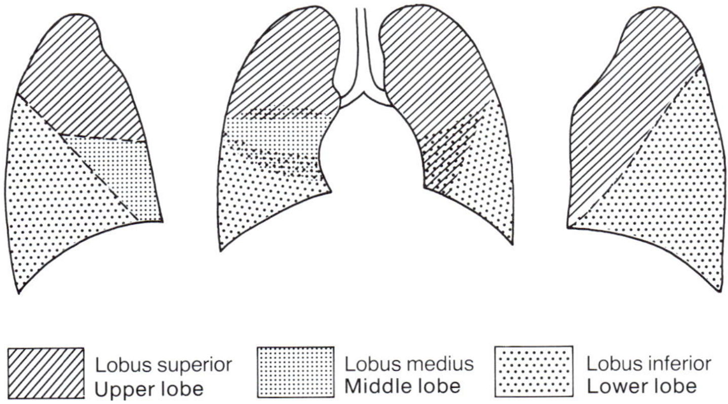

1 Upper lung zone
2 Perihilar region
3 Mid-lung zone
4 Chest wall
5 Pericardiac region
6 Lower lung zone
7 Supradiaphragmatic region
8 Superior anterior mediastinum
9 Inferior anterior mediastinum
10 Posterior mediastinum
11 Middle mediastinum
IV, V Thoracic vertebrae

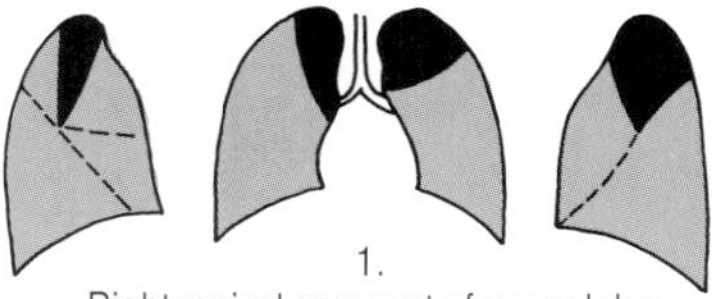

1.
Right: apical segment of upper lobe
Left: apical–posterior segment of upper lobe

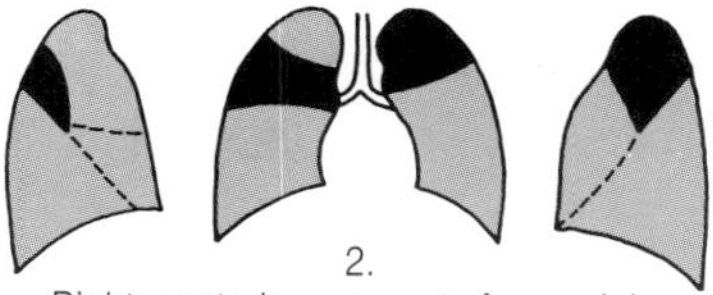

2.
Right: posterior segment of upper lobe
Left: apical–posterior segment of upper lobe

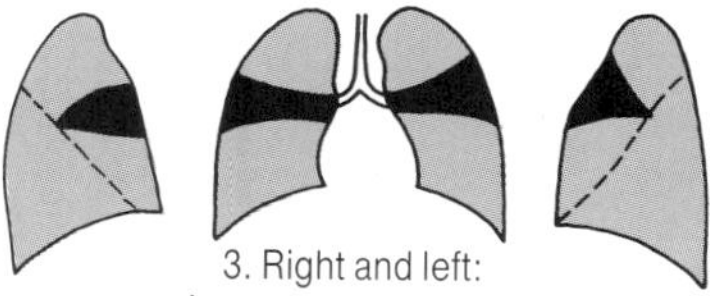

3. Right and left:
anterior segment of upper lobe

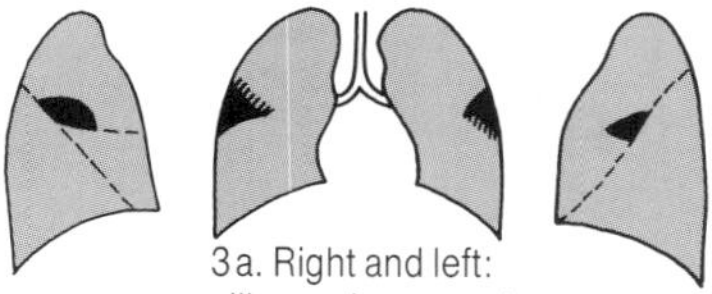

3a. Right and left:
axillary subsegment

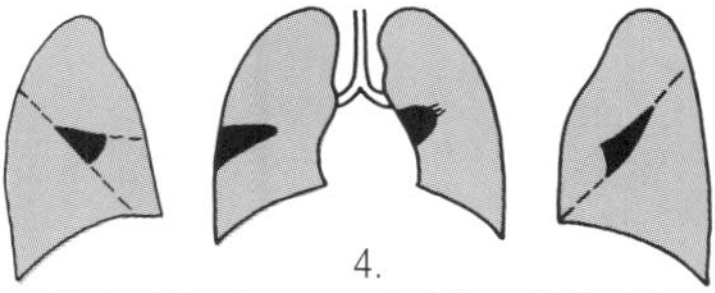

4.
Right: lateral segment of the middle lobe
Left: superior lingular segment

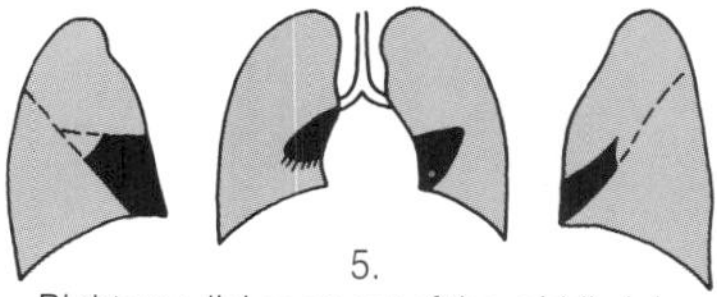

5.
Right: medial segment of the middle lobe
Left: inferior lingular segment

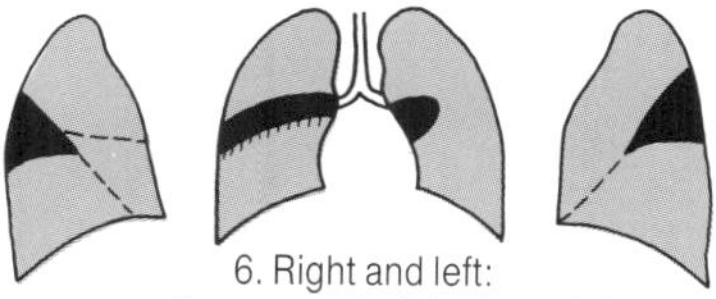

6. Right and left:
superior segment of the lower lobe

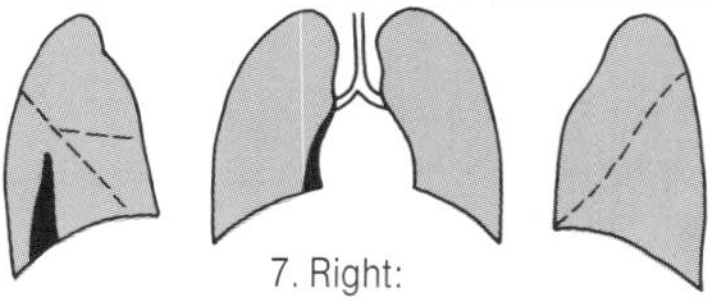

7. Right:
medial segment of the lower lobe

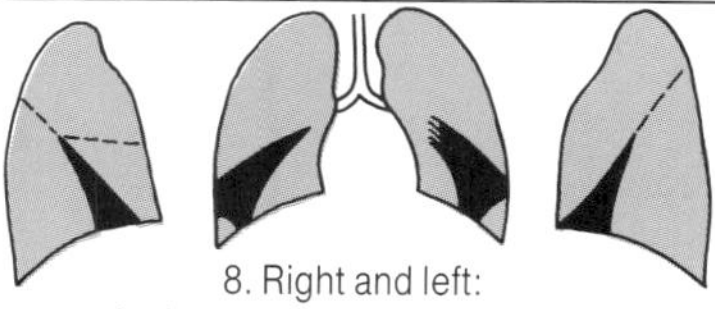

8. Right and left:
anterior basal segment of the lower lobe

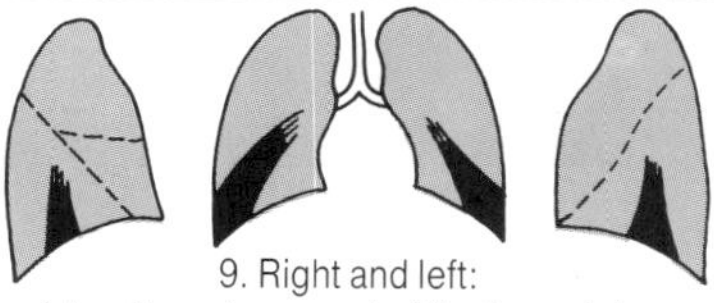

9. Right and left:
lateral basal segment of the lower lobe

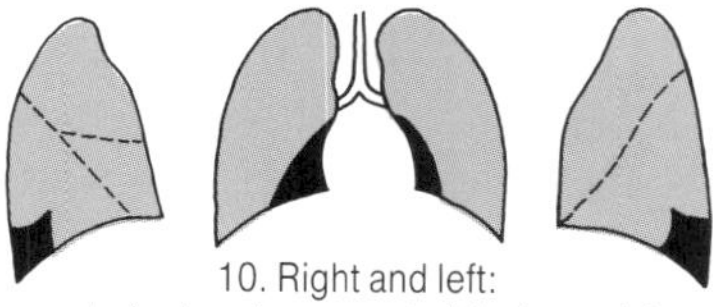

10. Right and left:
posterior basal segment of the lower lobe

Lung segments

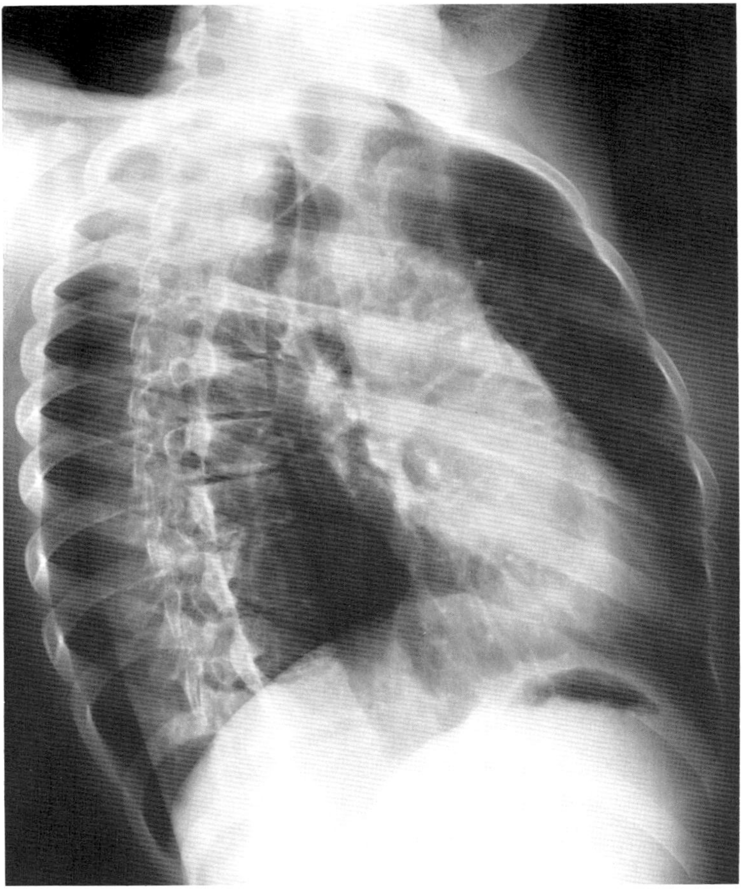

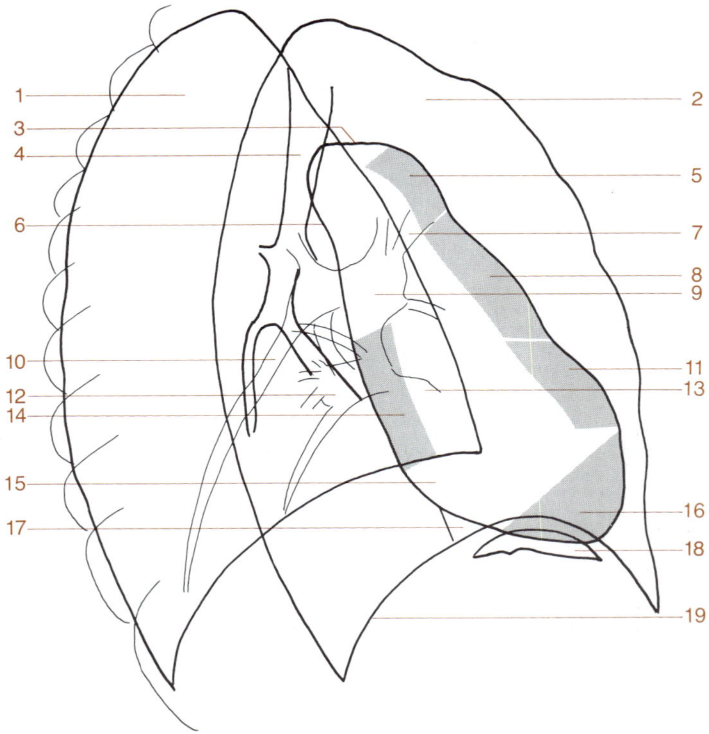

1 Right lung
2 Left lung
3 Aortic arch
4 Trachea
5 Ascending aorta
6 Descending aorta
7 Left upper lobe pulmonary vein, artery, and bronchus
8 Main pulmonary artery segment
9 Left pulmonary artery
10 Right lower lobe artery
11 Infundibulum (pulmonary outflow tract)
12 Inferior right pulmonary vein
13 Inferior left pulmonary vein
14 Left atrium
15 Right atrium
16 Left ventricle
17 Inferior vena cava
18 Stomach bubble
19 Diaphragm

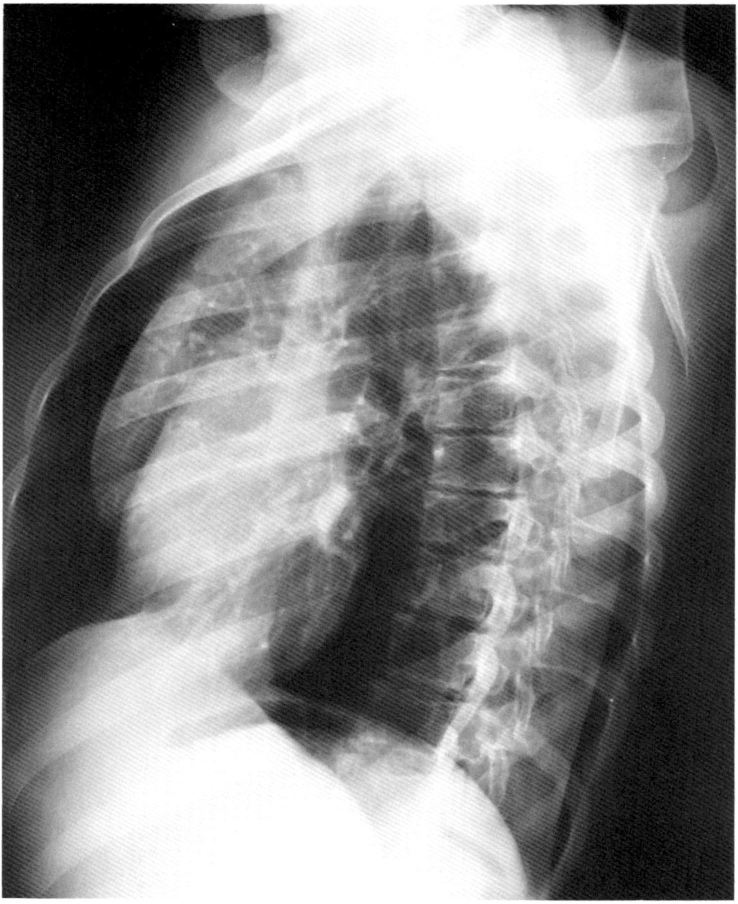

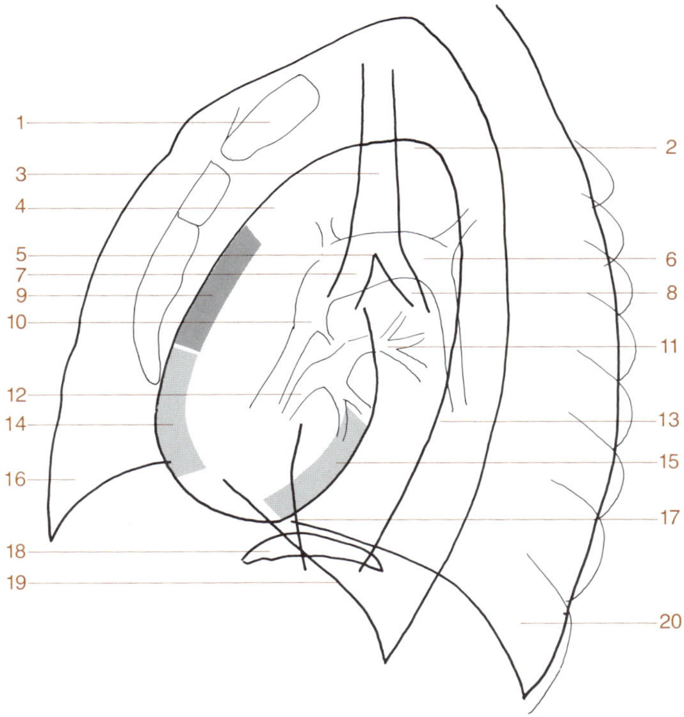

1 Sternum
2 Aortic arch
3 Trachea
4 Ascending aorta
5 Carina
6 Left pulmonary artery
7 Right main stem bronchus
8 Left main stem bronchus
9 Right atrium
10 Right pulmonary artery
11 Left pulmonary vein
12 Right pulmonary vein
13 Descending aorta
14 Right ventricle
15 Left ventricle
16 Right lung
17 Inferior vena cava
18 Stomach bubble (left hemidiaphragm)
19 Right hemidiaphragm
20 Left lung

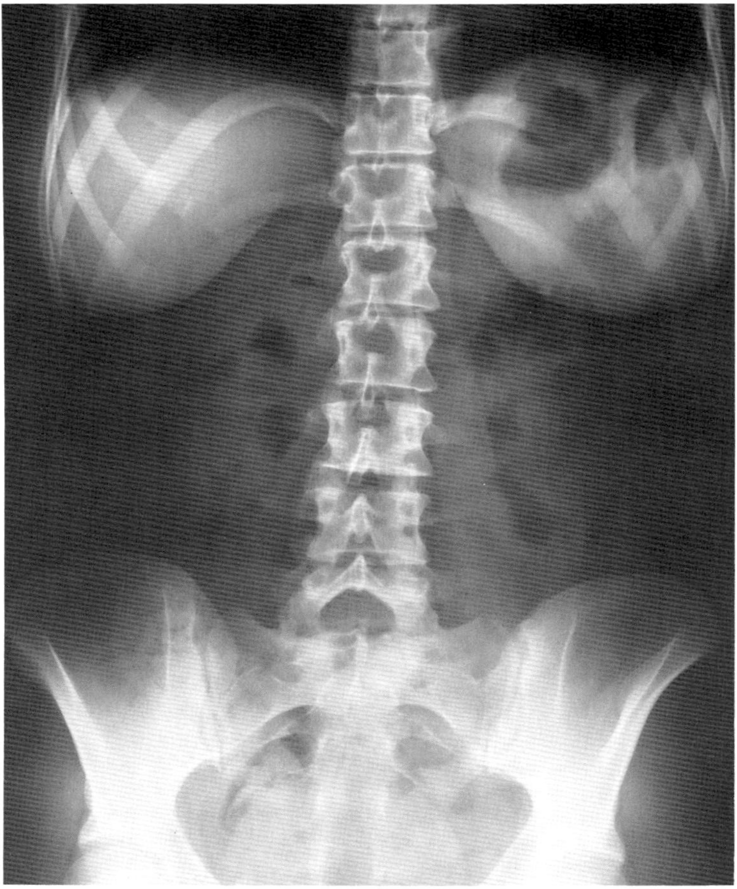

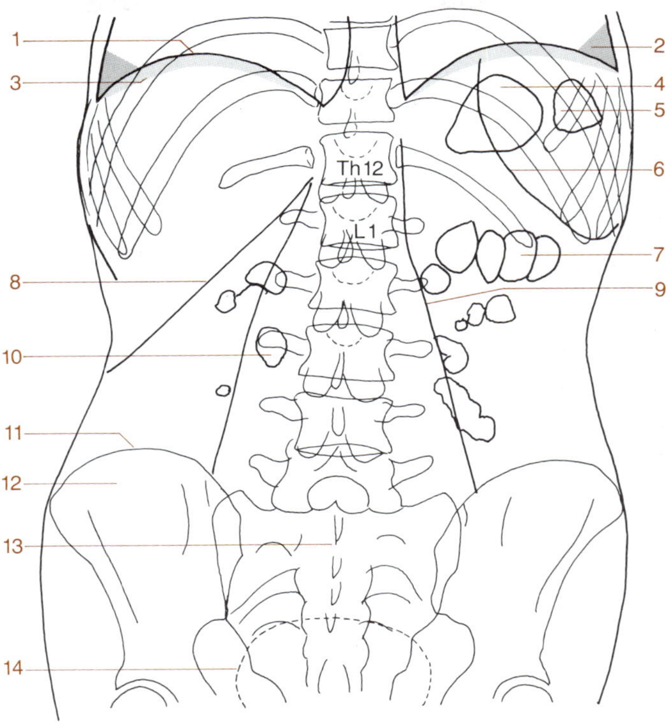

1 Dome of the abdomen
2 Costophrenic sulcus
3 Subphrenic space
4 Stomach bubble
5 Gas in the splenic flexure of the colon
6 Lower margin of the spleen
7 Gas in the transverse colon
8 Lower liver margin
9 Contour of the psoas muscle
10 Gas in the small intestine
11 Iliac crest
12 Iliac bone
13 Sacrum
14 Urinary bladder

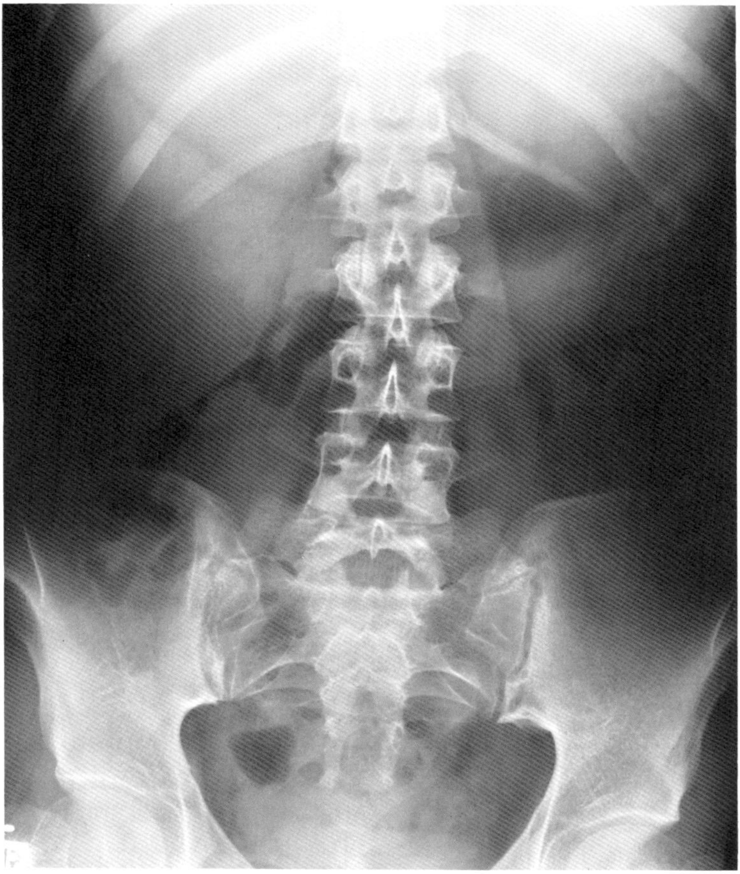

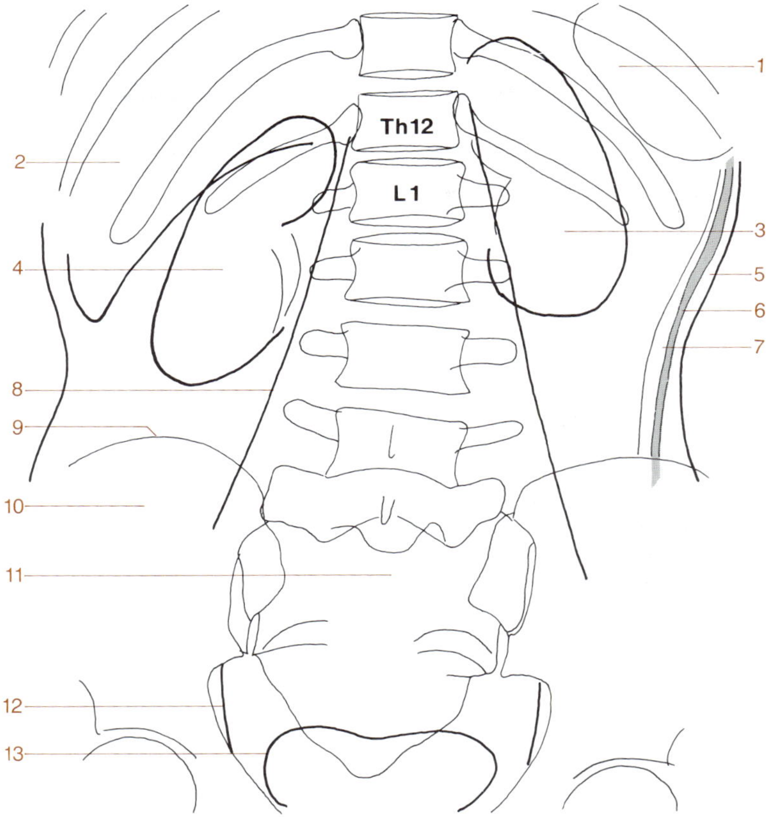

1 Spleen
2 Liver
3 Left kidney
4 Right kidney
5 Subcutaneous fat
6 Abdominal muscles
7 Properitoneal fat
8 Psoas muscle
9 Iliac crest
10 Iliac bone
11 Sacrum
12 Internal obturator muscle
13 Urinary bladder

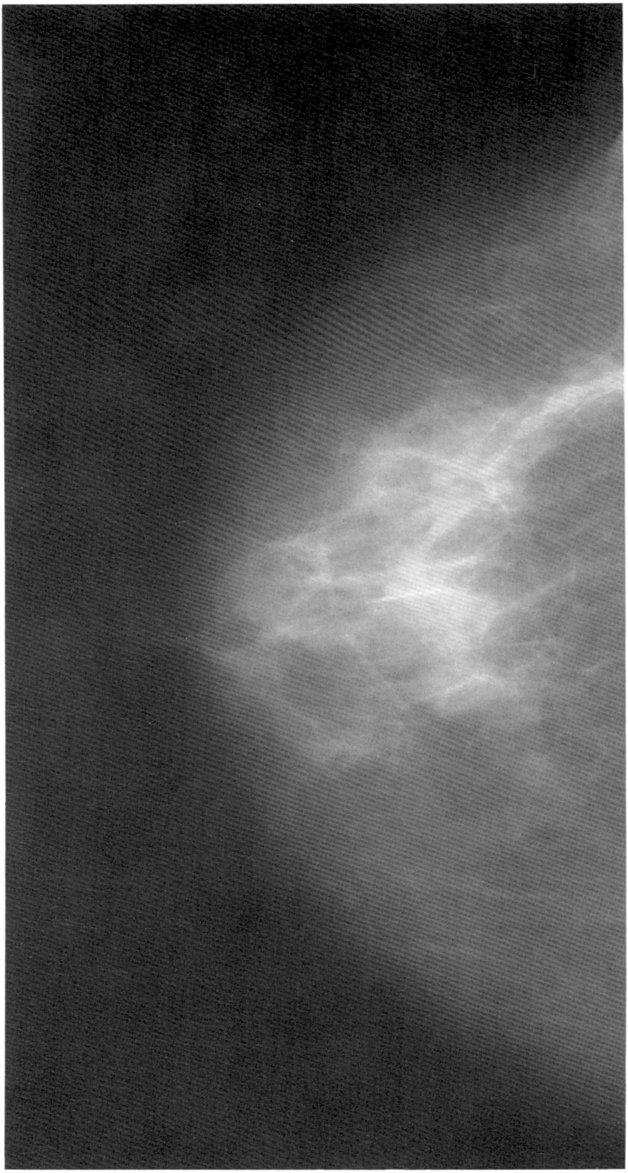

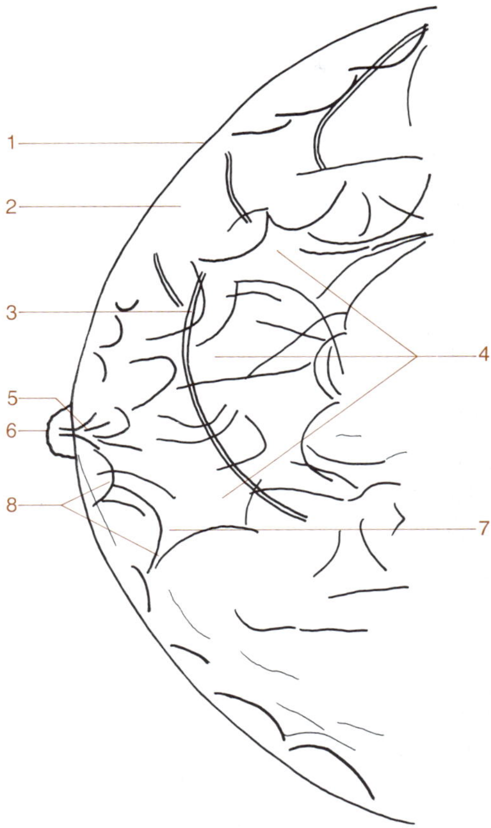

1 Skin
2 Subcutaneous fat
3 Veins
4 Glandular body
5 Mammary ducts and areolar ducts
6 Nipple
7 Contour of a glandular lobule
8 Cooper's ligaments

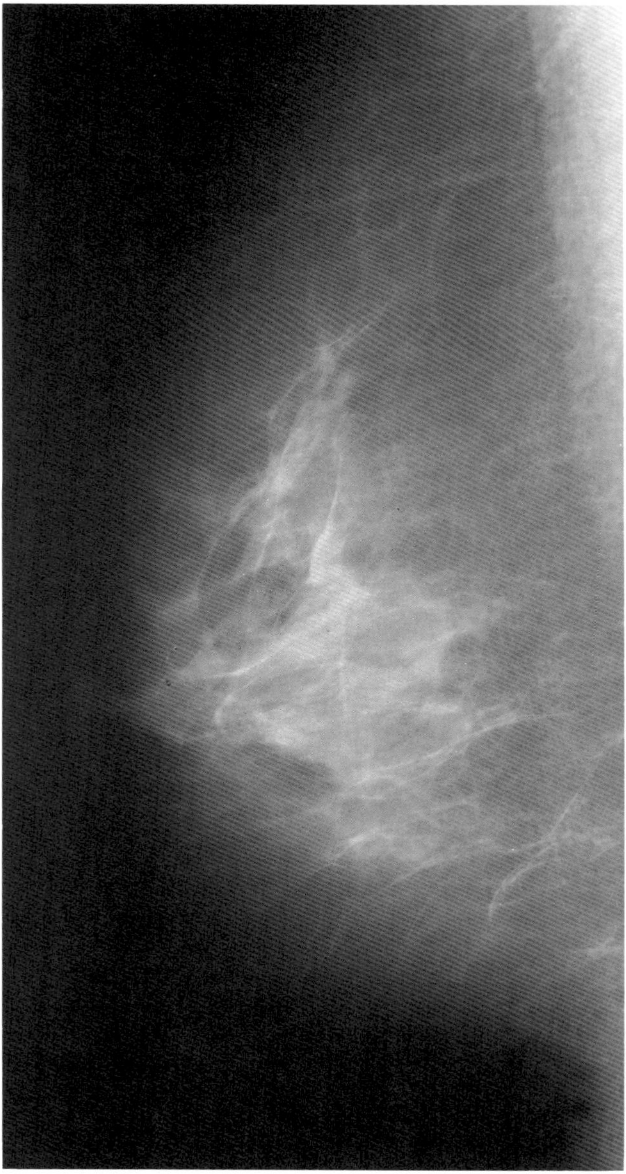

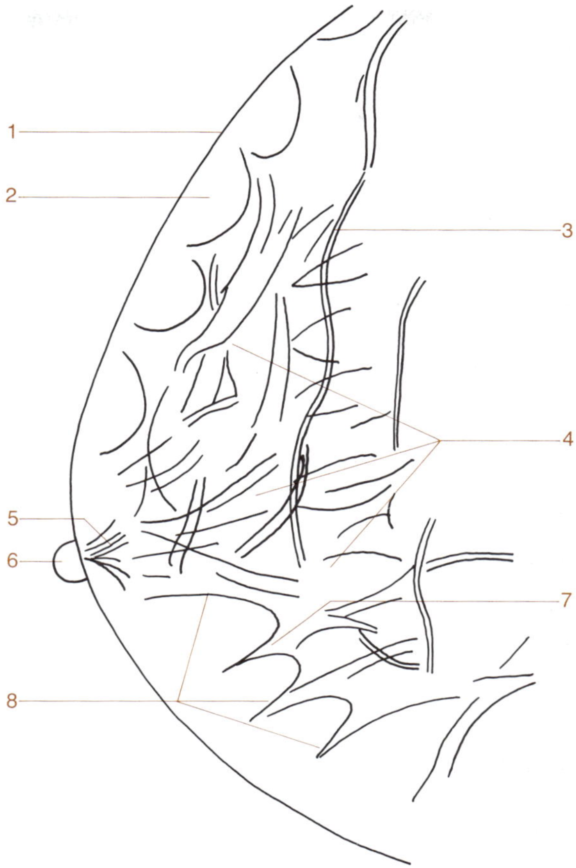

1 Skin
2 Subcutaneous fat
3 Veins
4 Glandular structures
5 Mammary ducts and areolar ducts
6 Nipple
7 Contour of a glandular lobule
8 Cooper's ligaments

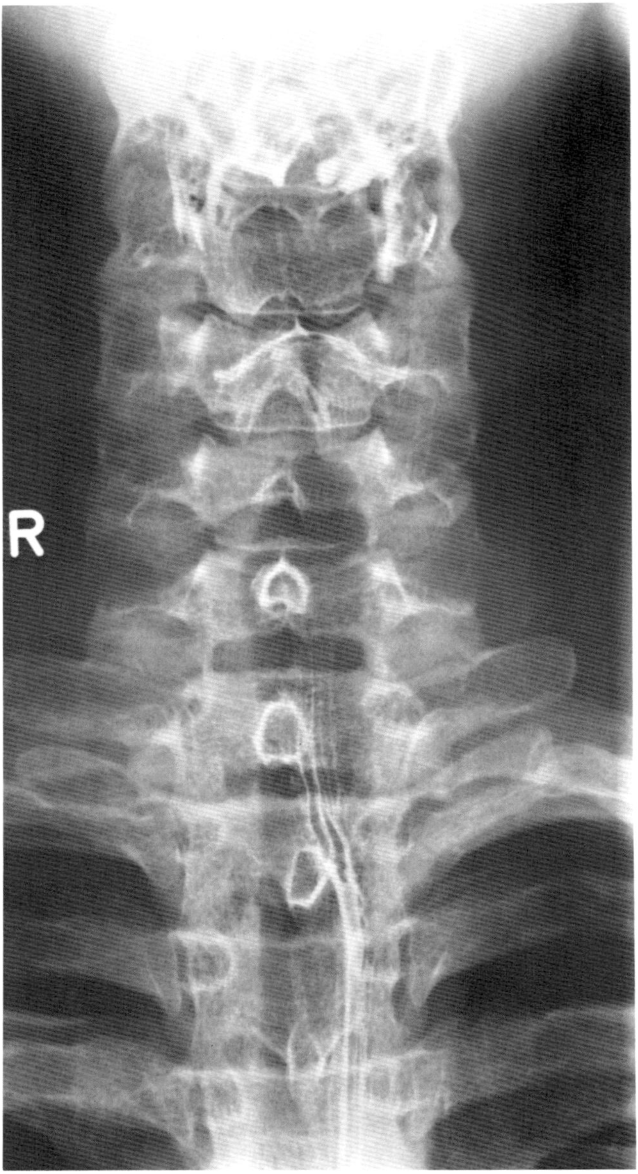
R

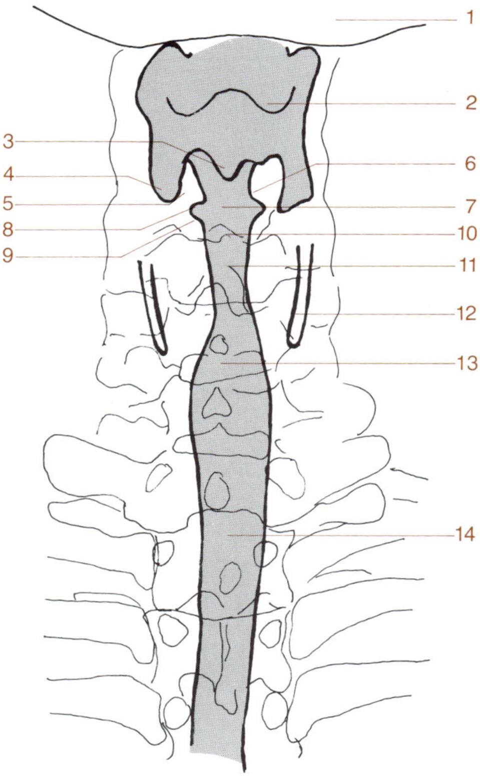

1 Mandible
2 Floor of the vallecula
3 Interarytenoid cleft
4 Piriform sinus
5 Arytenoid cartilage
6 False vocal cord
7 Laryngeal vestibule
8 Laryngeal ventricle
9 True vocal cord
10 Rima glottidis
11 Subglottic space
12 Thyroid cartilage
13 Proximal cervical trachea
14 Intrathoracic trachea

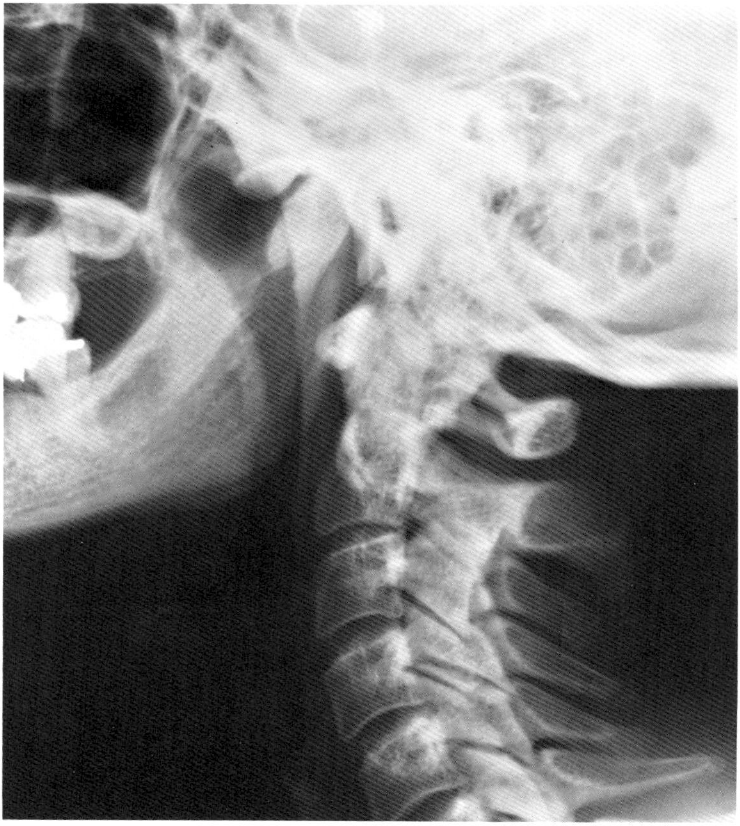

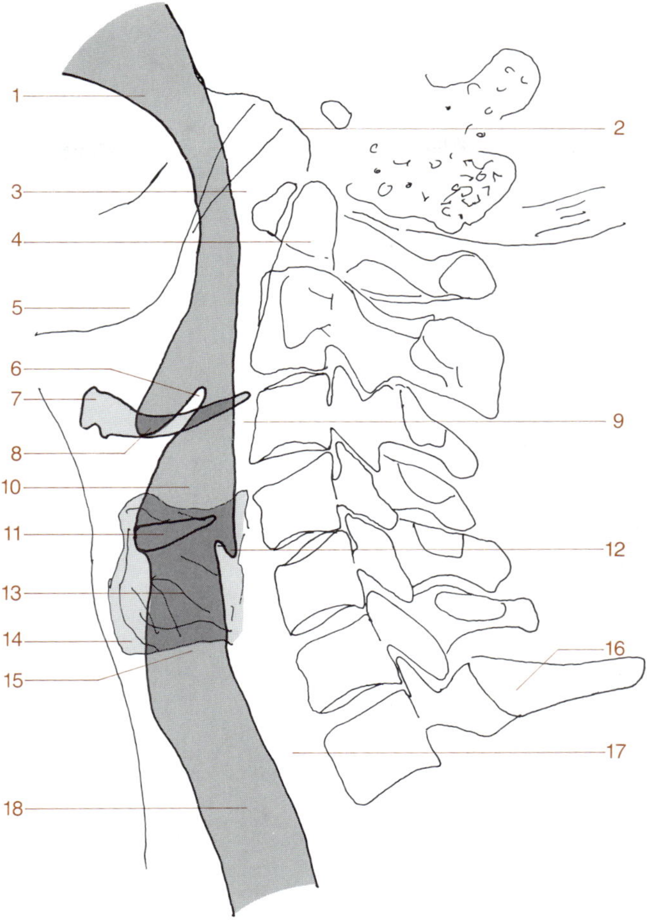

1 Oral cavity
2 Skull base
3 Posterior retropharyngeal space
4 Odontoid
5 Mandible
6 Epiglottis
7 Hyoid bone
8 Floor of the vallecula
9 Retropharyngeal space
10 Laryngeal vestibule
11 Laryngeal ventricle
12 Inferior posterior margin of the piriform sinus
13 Subglottic space
14 Thyroid cartilage
15 Cervical trachea
16 C7 vertebra
17 Retrotracheal space (esophagus)
18 Lower trachea

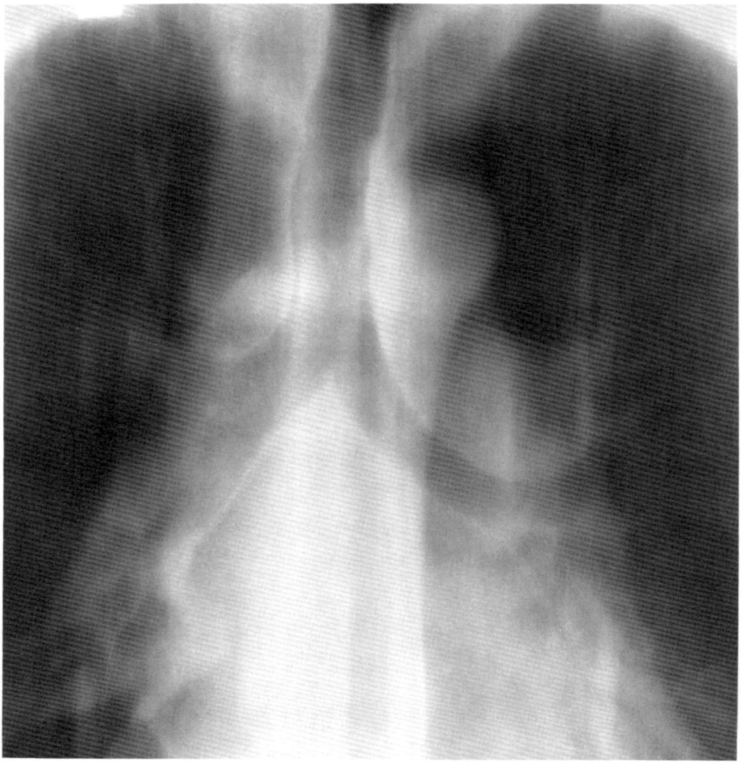

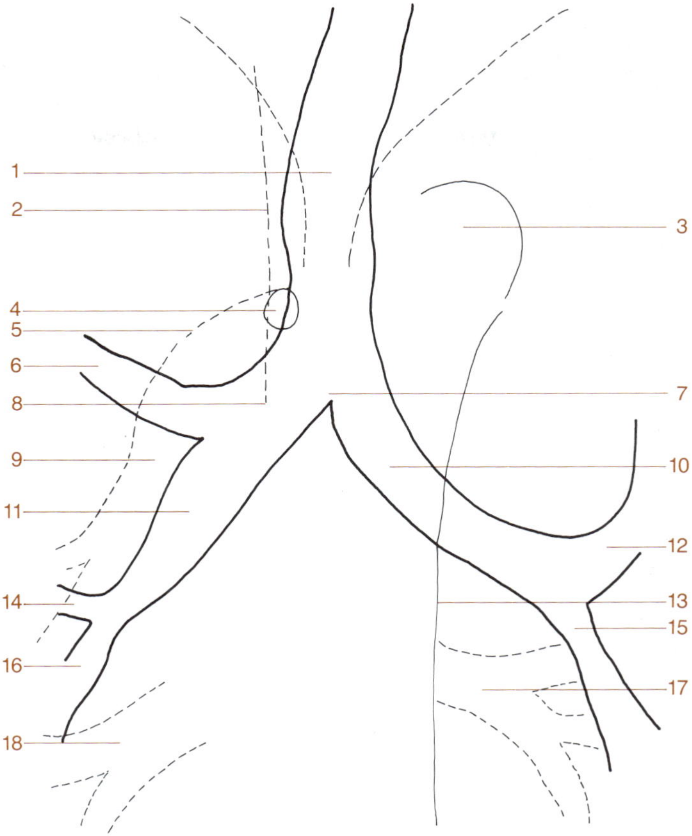

1 Trachea
2 Superior vena cava
3 Aortic arch
4 Azygos vein
5 Right superior pulmonary vein, apical-anterior branch
6 Right upper lobe bronchus
7 Bifurcation of the trachea
8 Right main stem bronchus
9 Lower lobe pulmonary artery
10 Left main stem bronchus
11 Bronchus intermedius
12 Left upper lobe bronchus
13 Descending aorta
14 Middle lobe bronchus
15 Left lower lobe bronchus
16 Right lower lobe bronchus
17 Left lower lobe pulmonary veins
18 Confluence of the right lower lobe pulmonary veins

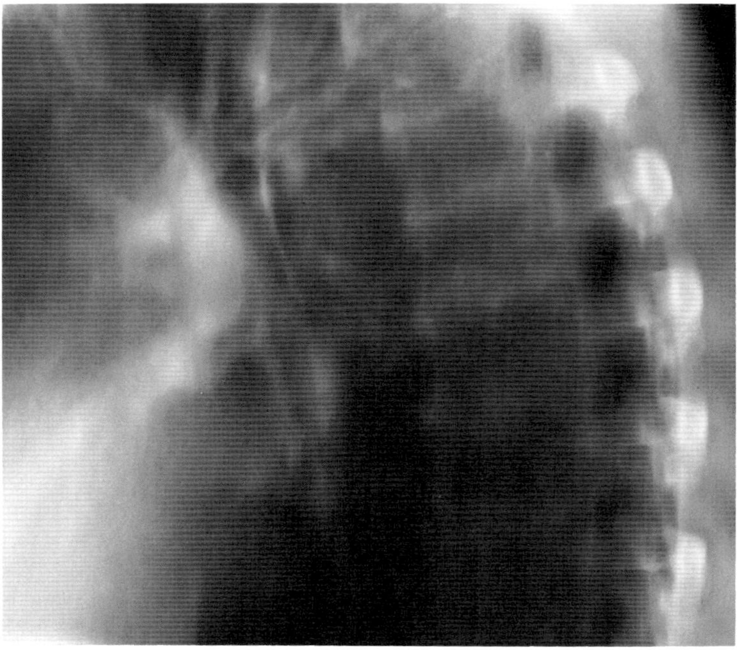

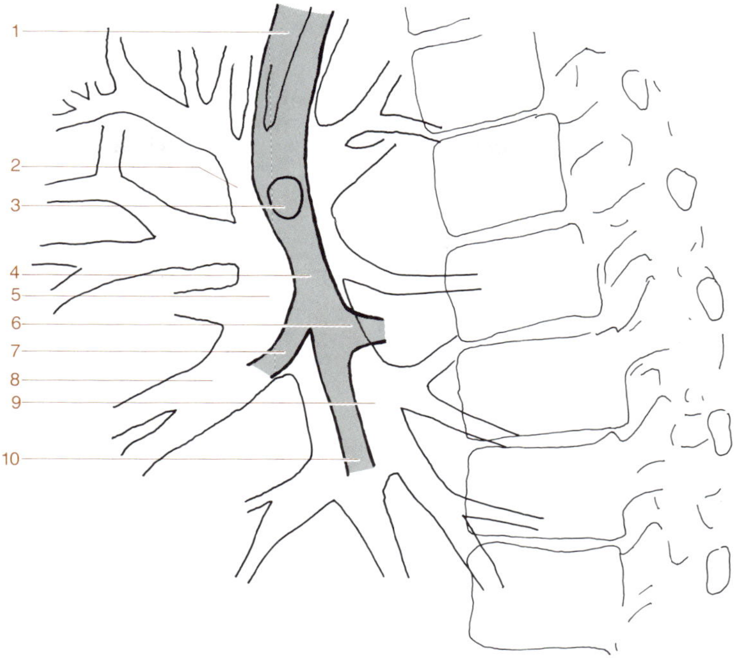

1 Trachea
2 Apical segmental branch of the right pulmonary artery
3 Origin of the right upper lobe bronchus
4 Bronchus intermedius
5 Right pulmonary artery
6 Superior segmental bronchus, right lower lobe
7 Middle lobe bronchus
8 Middle lobe branch of the right pulmonary artery
9 Right lower lobe pulmonary artery
10 Right lower lobe bronchus

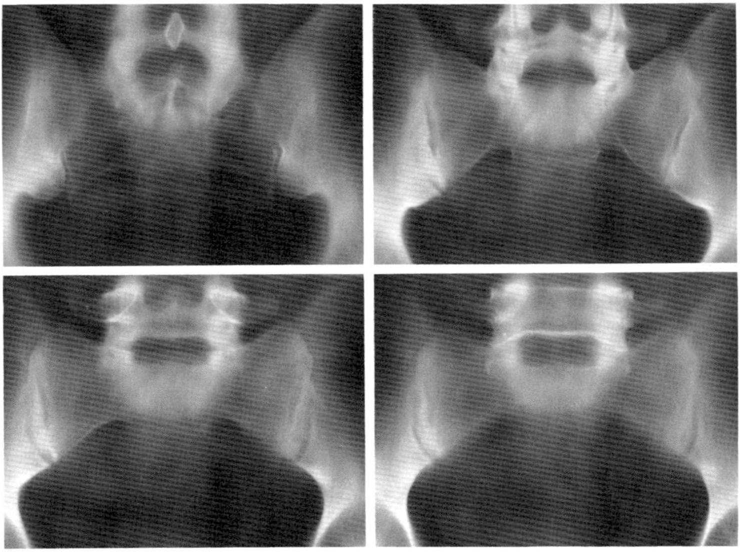

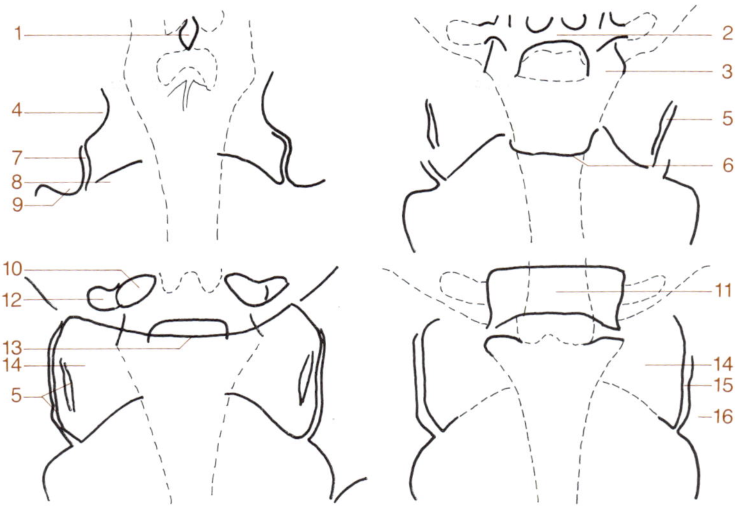

1 Spinous process
2 Lamina of the vertebral arch
3 Inferior articular process
4 Posterior superior iliac spine
5 Medial aspect of the sacroiliac joint
6 Sacrum (anterior surface)
7 Posterior inferior aspect of the sacroiliac joint
8 Sacral foramina
9 Posterior inferior iliac spine
10 Pedicle of the vertebral arch
11 L5
12 Transverse process
13 Promontory
14 Sacral ala
15 Anterior aspect of the sacroiliac joint
16 Iliac bone

Contrast Examinations

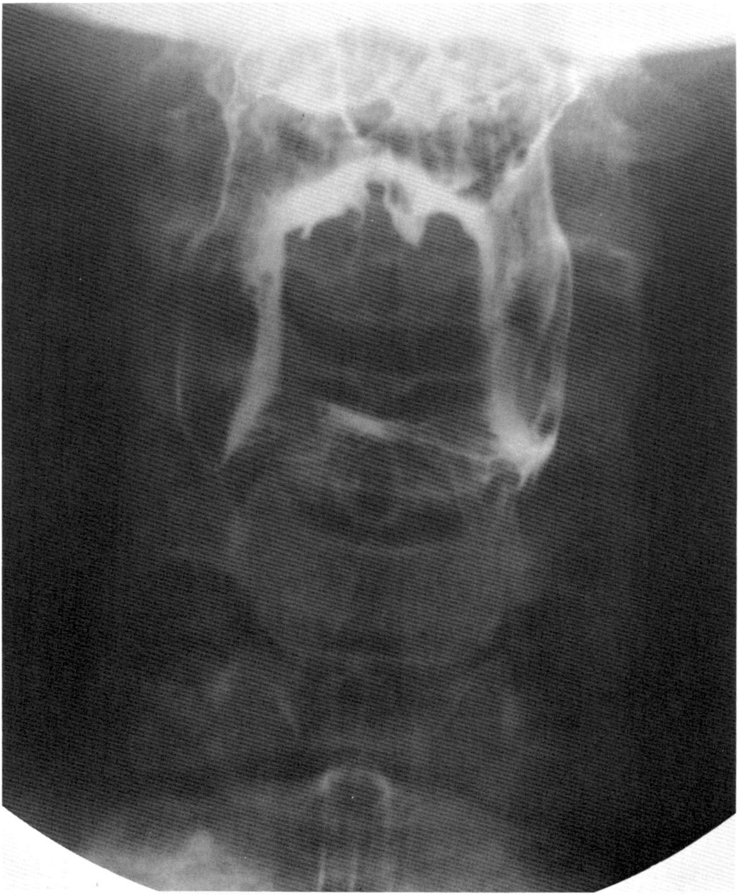

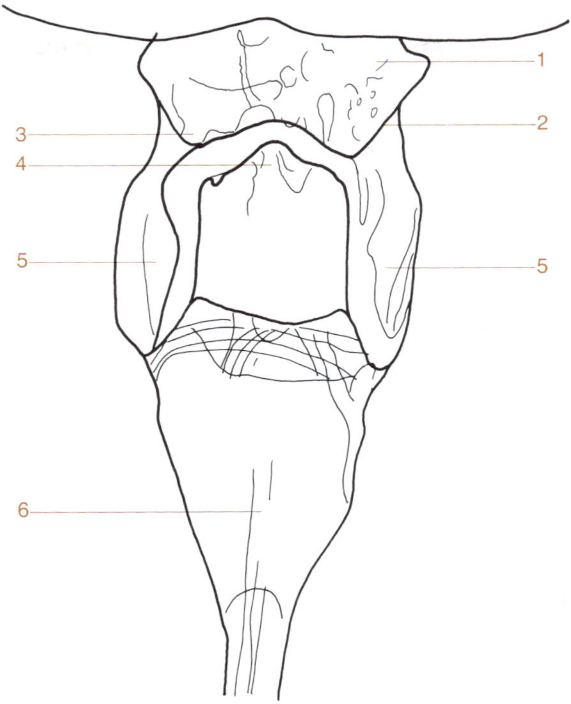

1 Pharynx
2 Lateral glossoepiglottic fold
3 Vallecula
4 Epiglottis
5 Piriform sinus
6 Esophagus

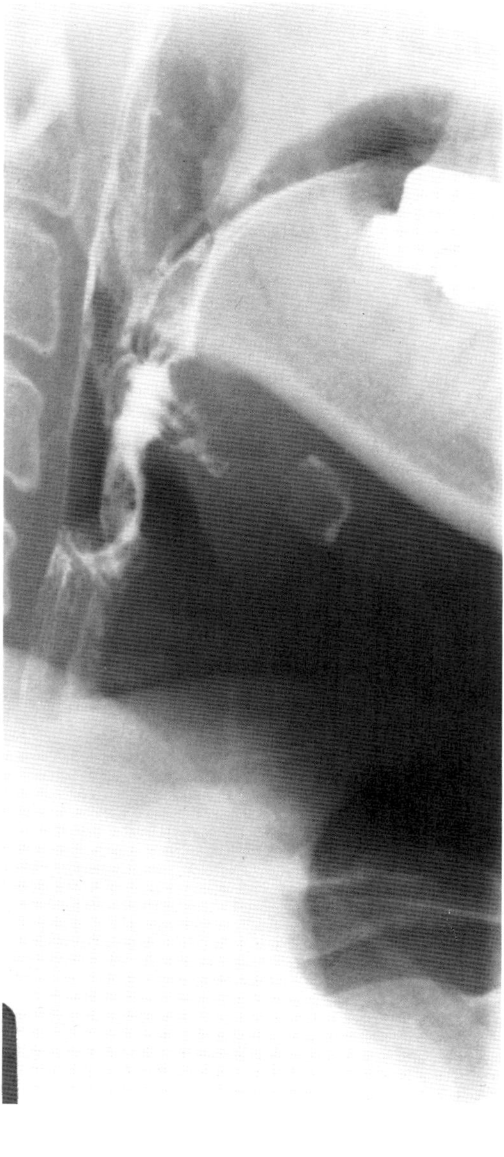

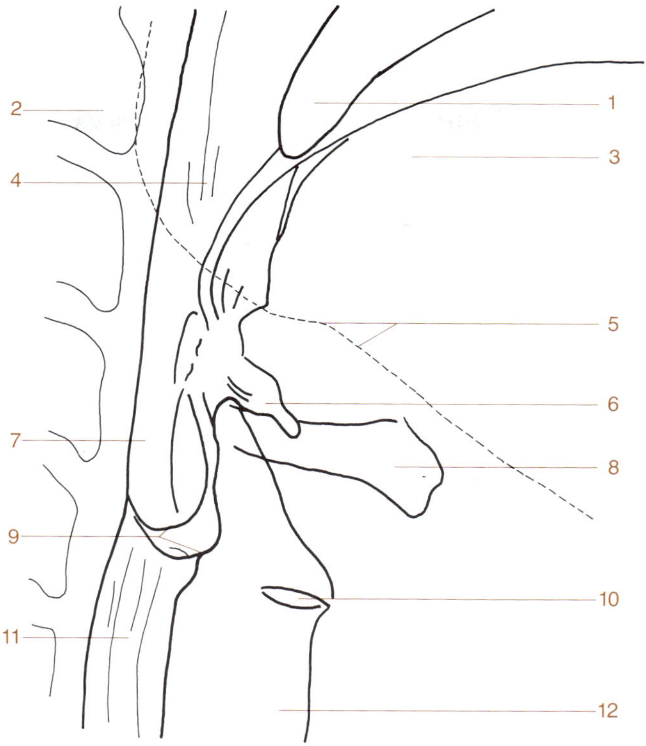

1 Uvula
2 Cervical spine (C2)
3 Base of tongue
4 Oropharynx
5 Mandible
6 Vallecula
7 Larynx
8 Hyoid bone
9 Piriform sinus
10 Laryngeal ventricle
11 Esophagus
12 Trachea

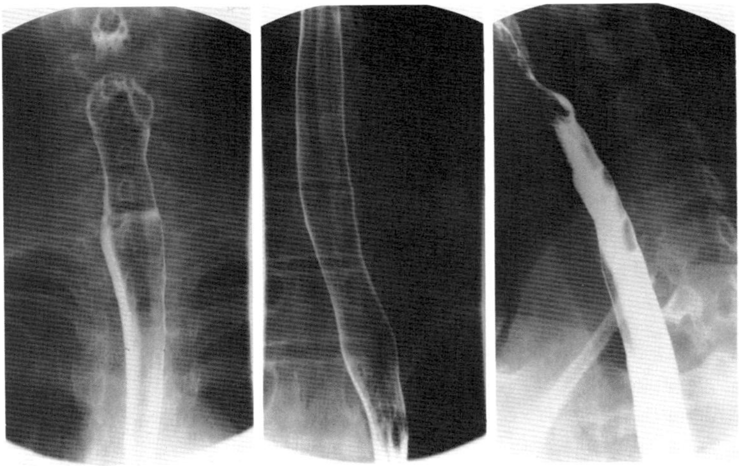

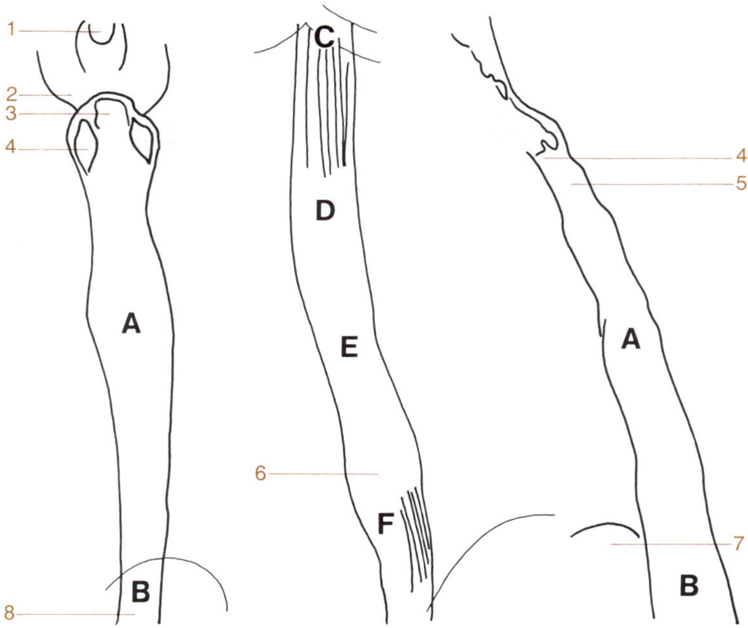

1 Uvula
2 Lateral glossoepiglottic fold
3 Epiglottis
4 Piriform sinus
5 Cardia
6 Esophageal ampulla
7 Aortic arch
8 Interaorticobronchial segment of the esophagus

A Paratracheal segment
B Aortic segment
C Bronchial segment
D Interbronchial segment
E Retrocardiac segment
F Epiphrenic segment

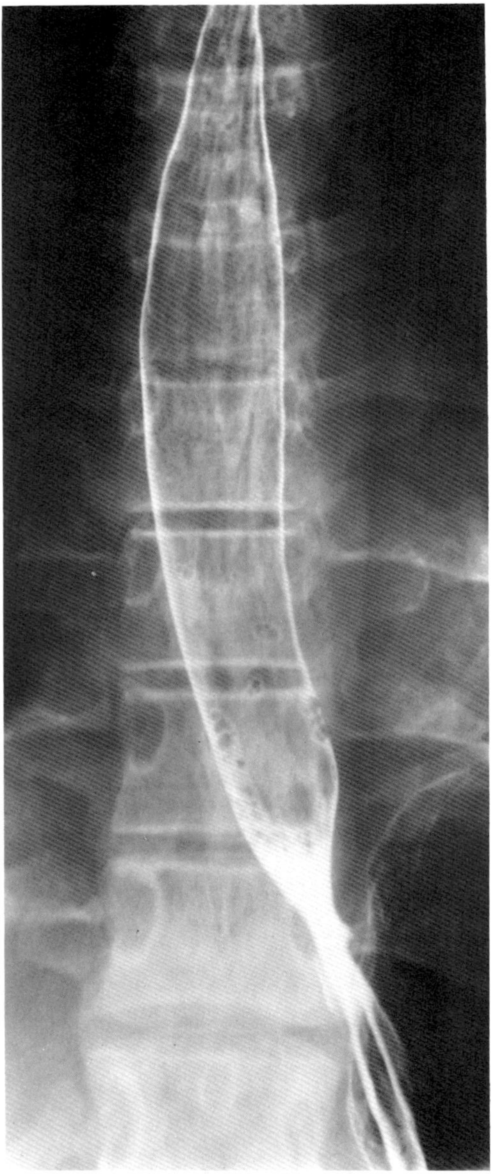

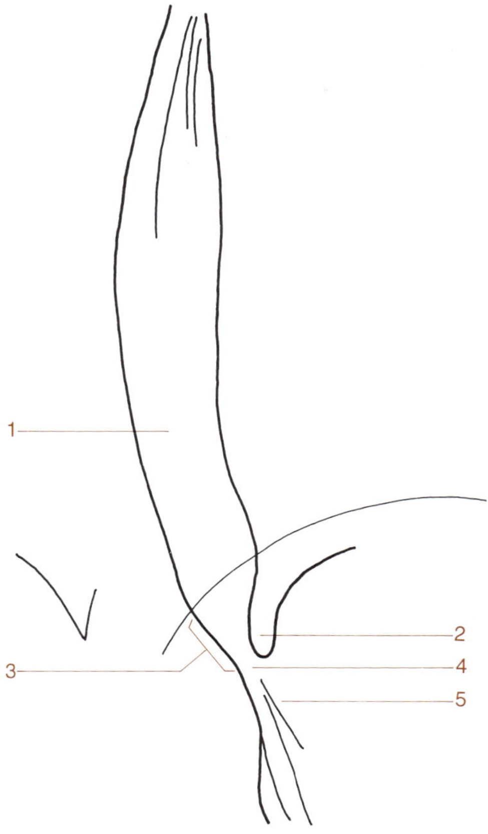

1 Distal (retrocardiac) esophagus
2 Gastroesophageal angle of His
3 Vestibule (abdominal esophagus)
4 Lower esophageal sphincter
5 Cardia (gastroesophageal junction)

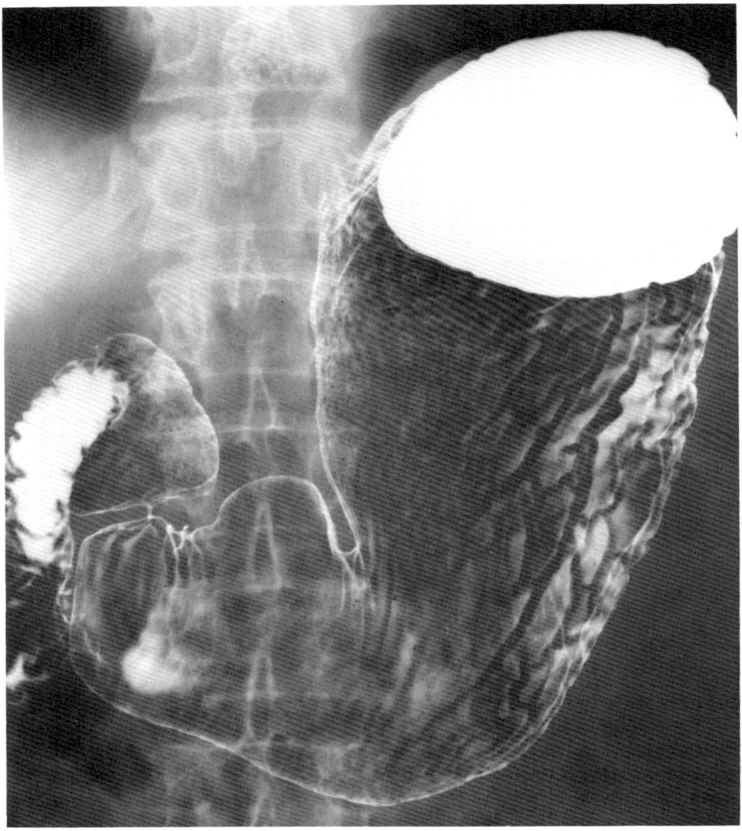

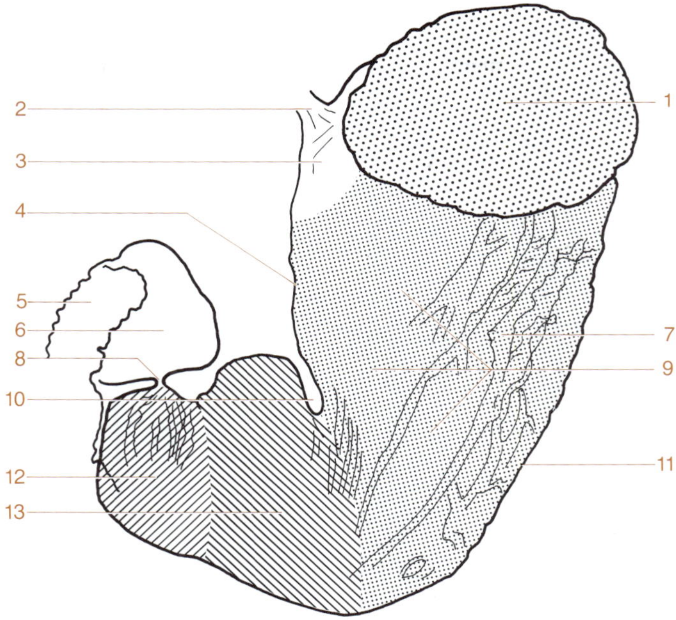

1 Gastric fundus	7 Gastric folds (posterior wall)
2 Esophagus, abdominal segment	8 Pylorus
3 Cardia (gastroesophageal segment)	9 Gastric body
4 Lesser curvature	10 Incisura angularis
5 Second part of the duodenum	11 Greater curvature
6 Duodenal bulb	12 Antrum
	13 Distal stomach

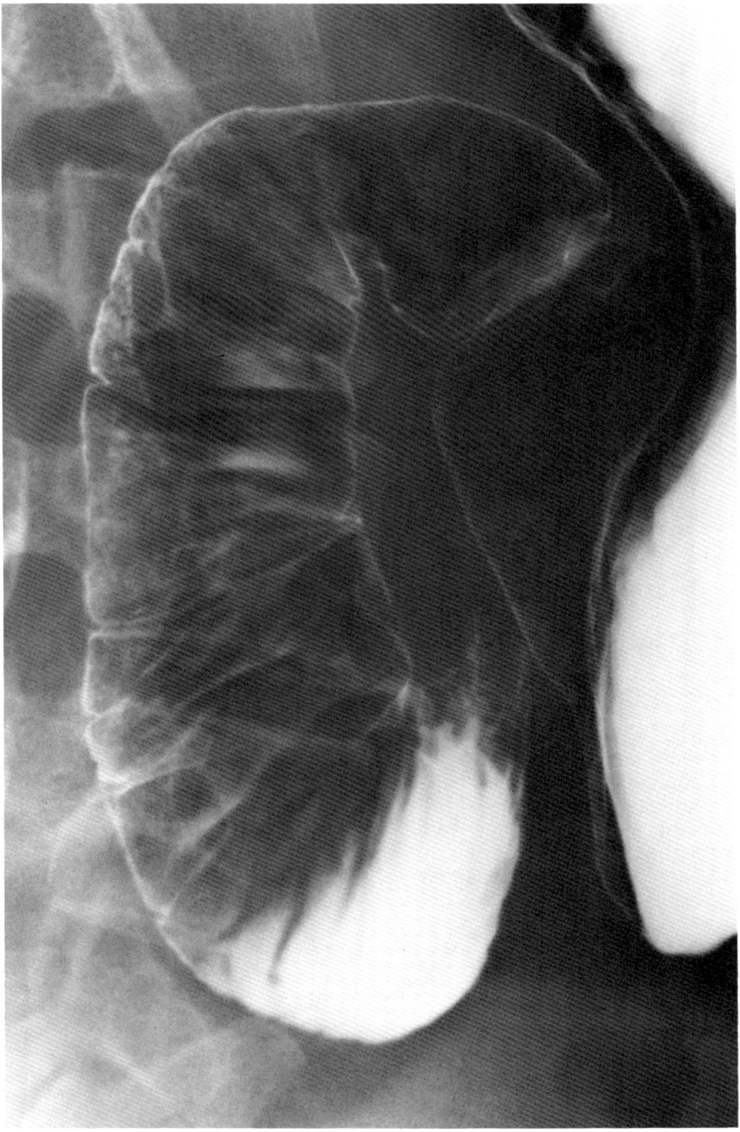

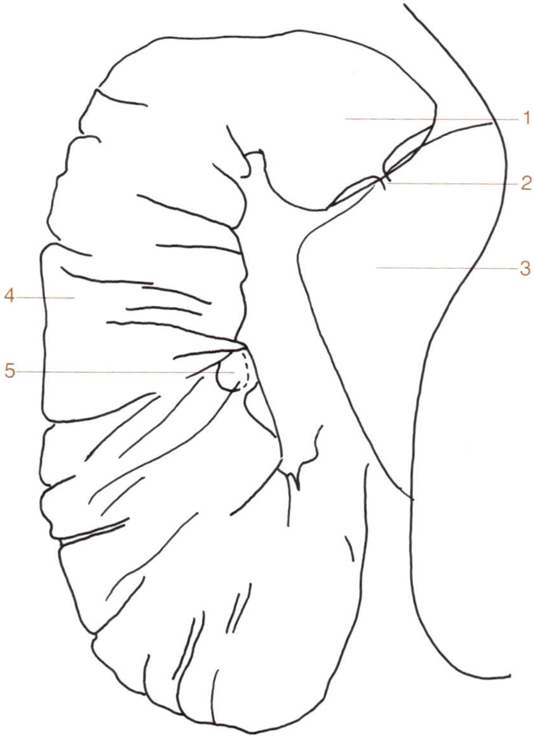

1 Duodenal bulb
2 Pylorus
3 Antrum
4 Second part of the duodenum
5 Duodenal papilla (Vater)

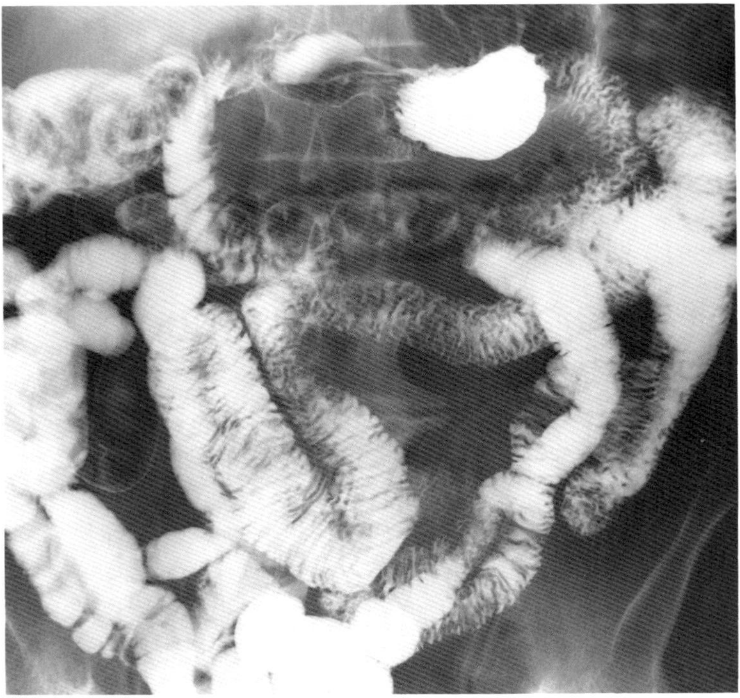

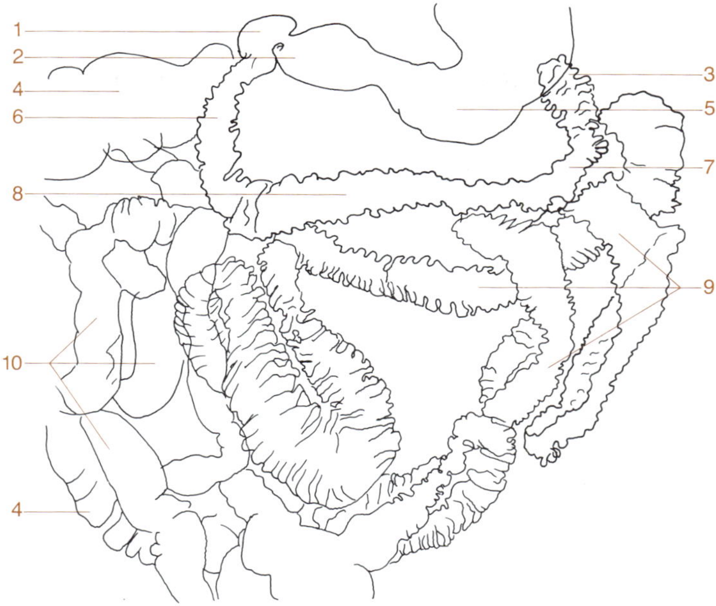

1 Duodenal bulb
2 Antrum
3 Ligament of Treitz (duodeno-jejunal junction)
4 Ascending colon
5 Stomach
6 Second part of the duodenum
7 Fourth part of the duodenum
8 Third part of the duodenum
9 Jejunum
10 Ileum

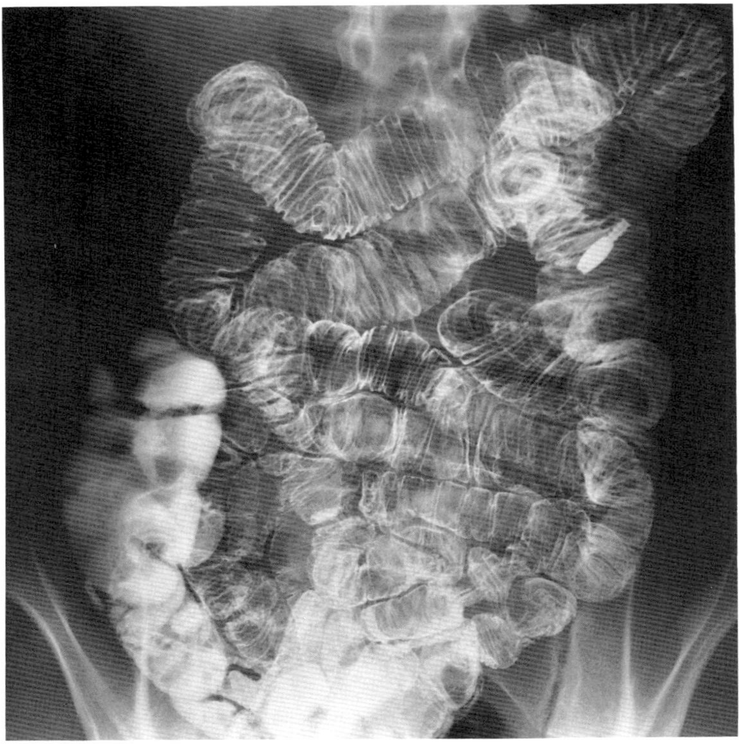

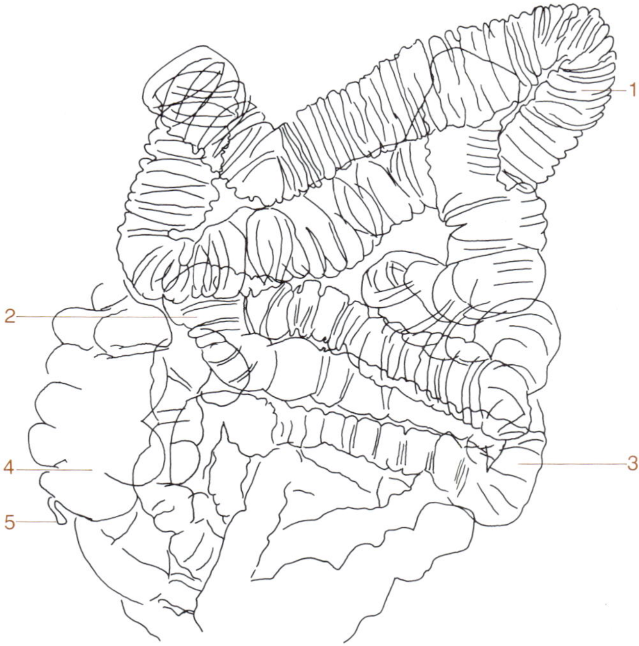

1 Jejunum
2 Jejunoileal junction
3 Ileum
4 Cecum
5 Appendix

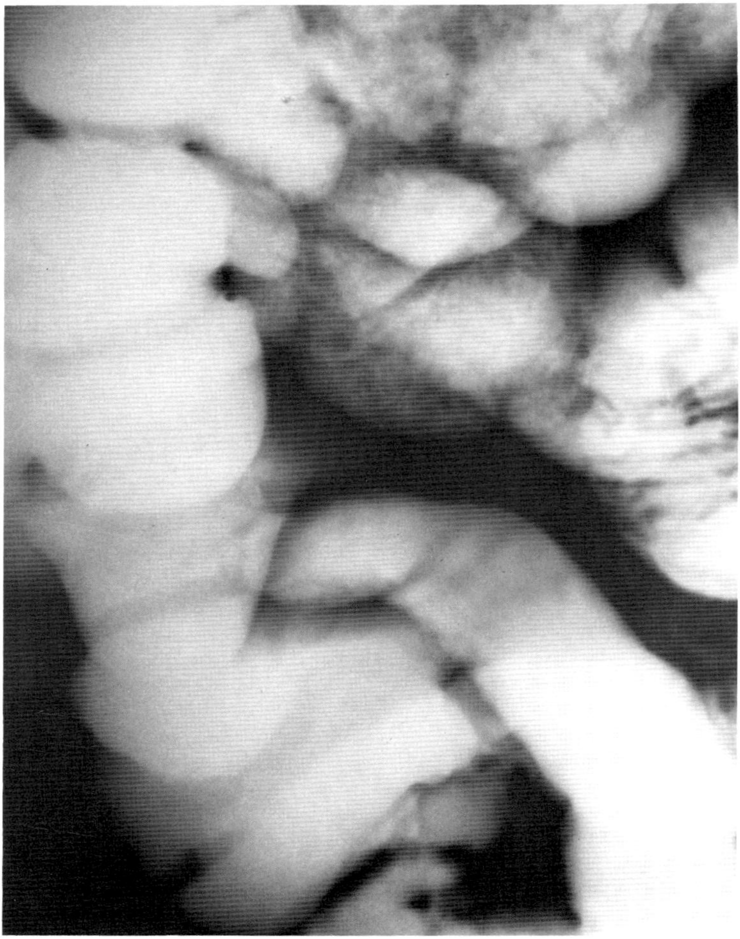

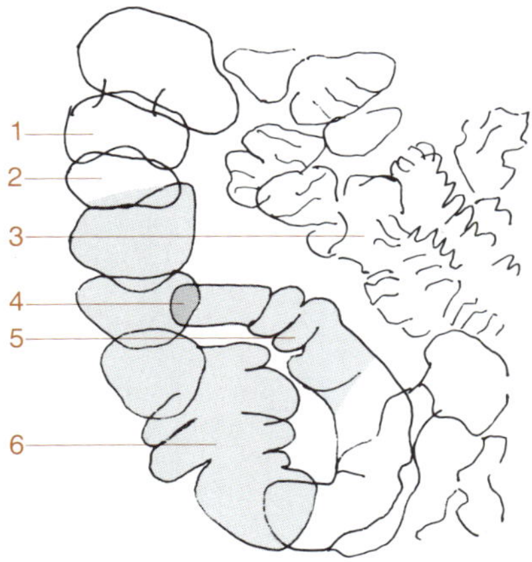

1 Haustra of the colon
2 Ascending colon
3 Ileum
4 Ileocecal valve
5 Terminal ileum
6 Cecum

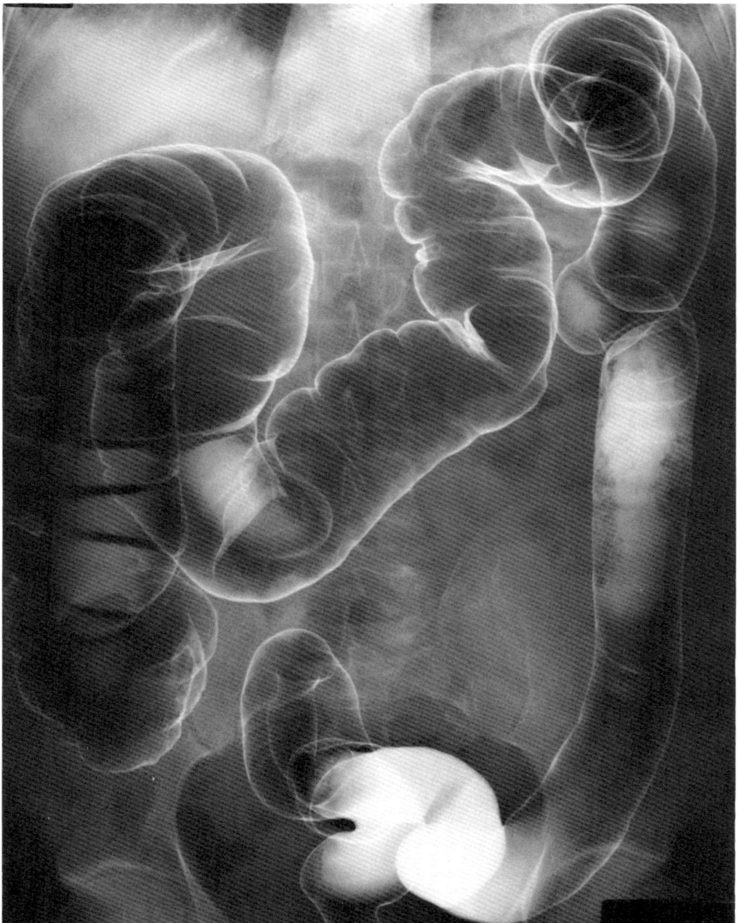

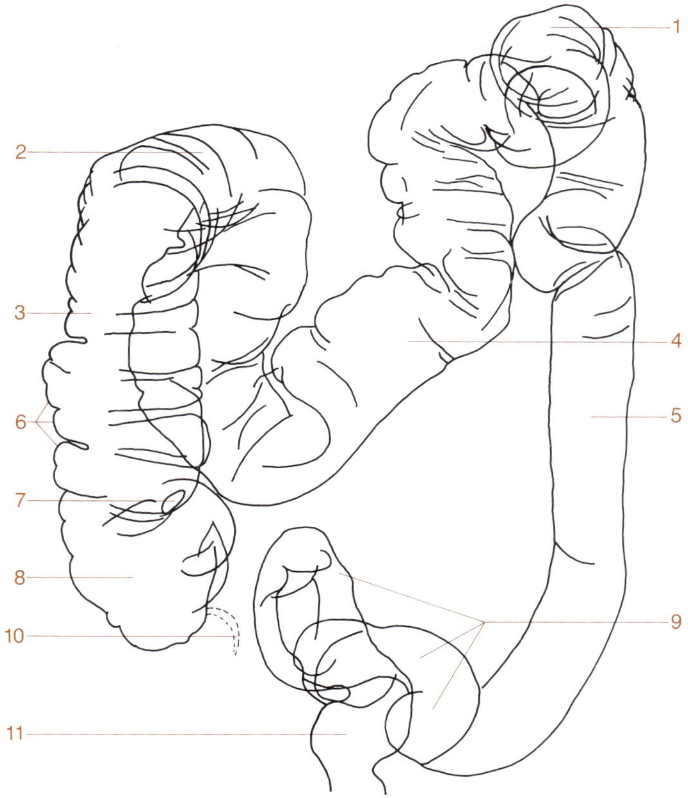

1 Splenic flexure of the colon
2 Hepatic flexure of the colon
3 Ascending colon
4 Transverse colon
5 Descending colon
6 Haustra
7 Ileocecal valve
8 Cecum
9 Sigmoid colon
10 Appendix
11 Rectum

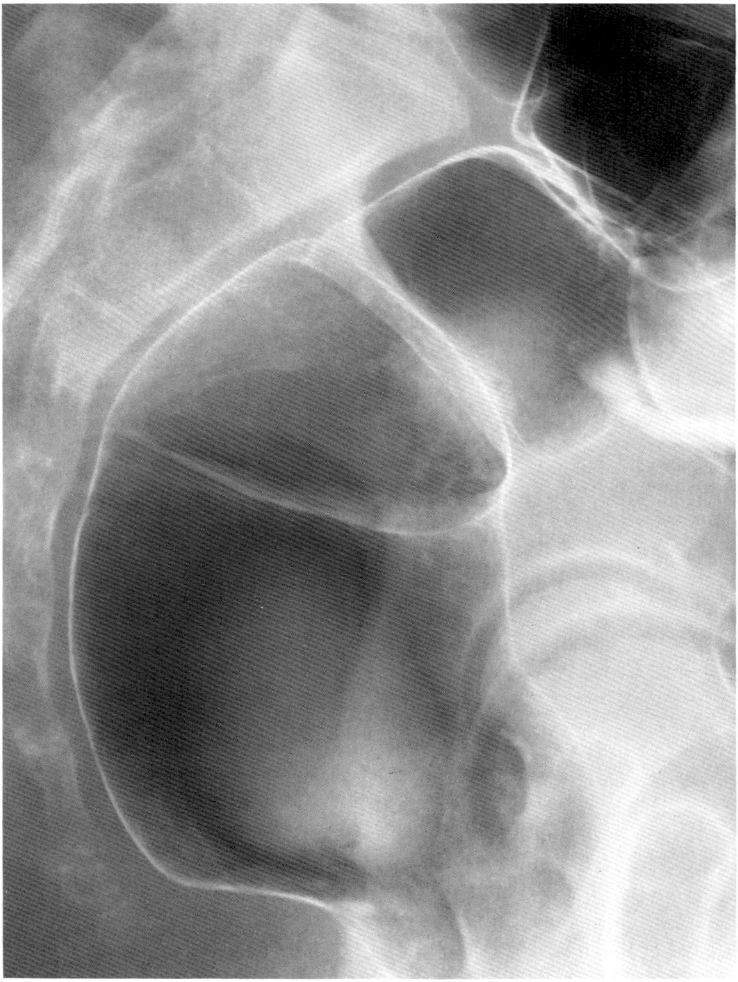

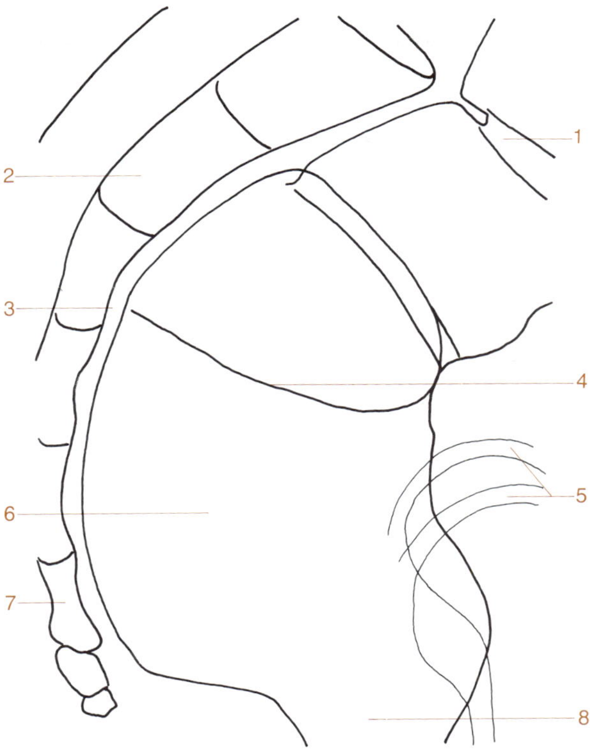

1 Rectosigmoid junction
2 Sacrum
3 Retrorectal space
4 Transverse fold of the rectum (valve of Houston)
5 Femoral head
6 Rectal ampulla
7 Coccygeal bone
8 Anorectal junction

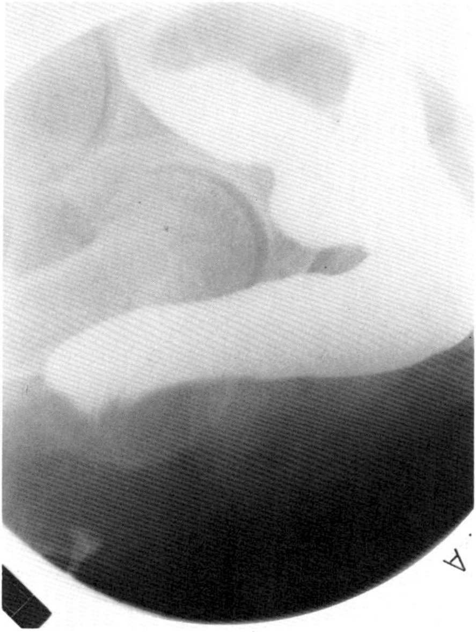

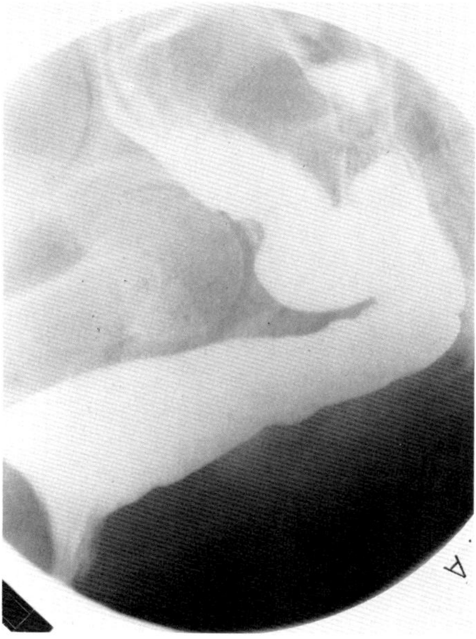

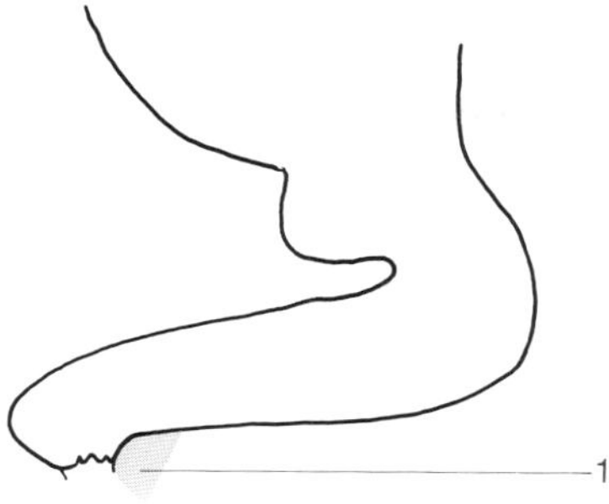

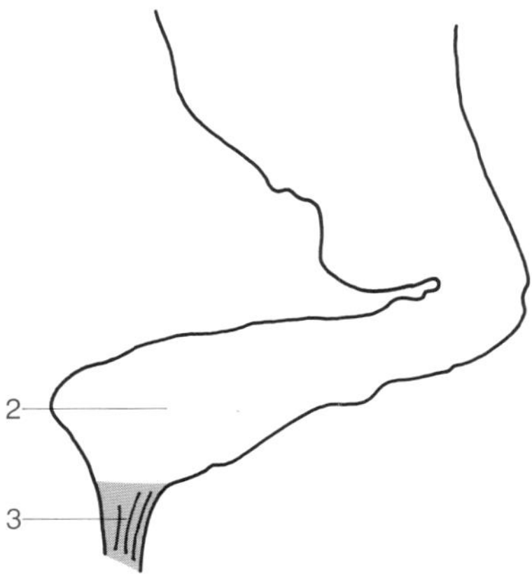

1 Imprint of the puborectal muscle

2 Rectal ampulla
3 Anal canal

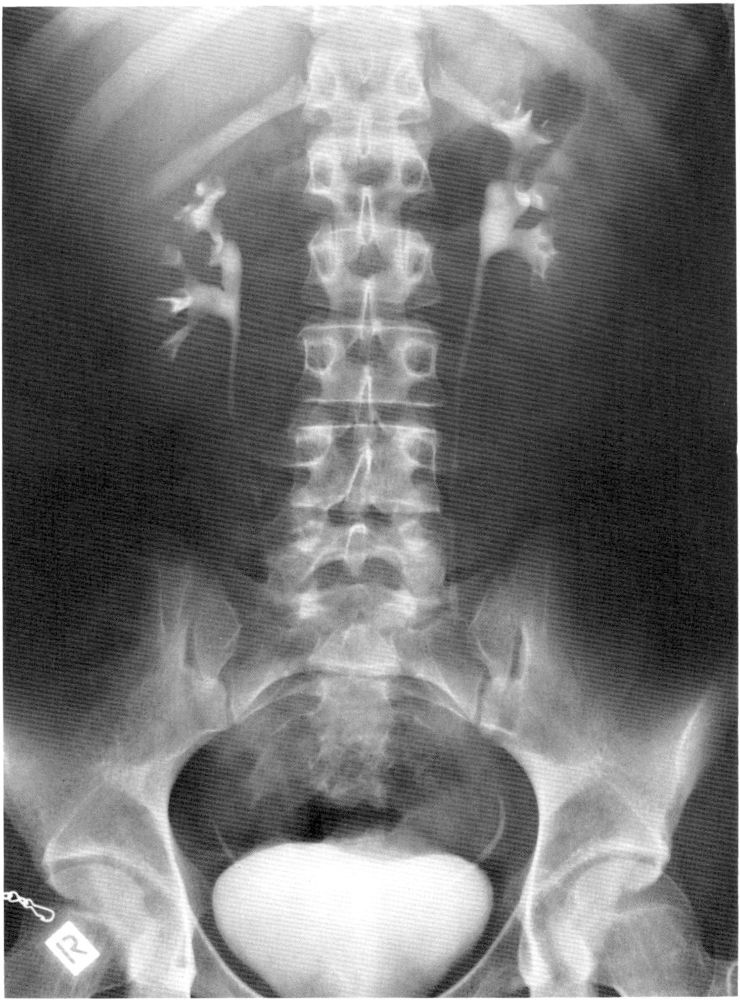
R

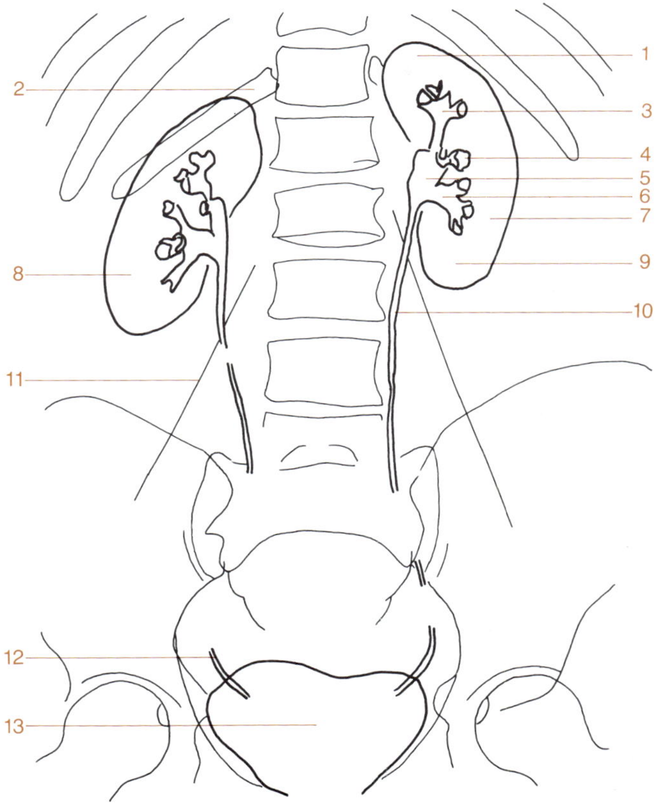

1 Upper pole of the kidney
2 Twelfth rib
3 Superior calyces
4 Middle calyces
5 Renal pelvis
6 Inferior calyces
7 Left nephrogram
8 Right nephrogram
9 Lower pole of the kidney
10 Ureter
11 Psoas muscle
12 Distal ureter
13 Urinary bladder

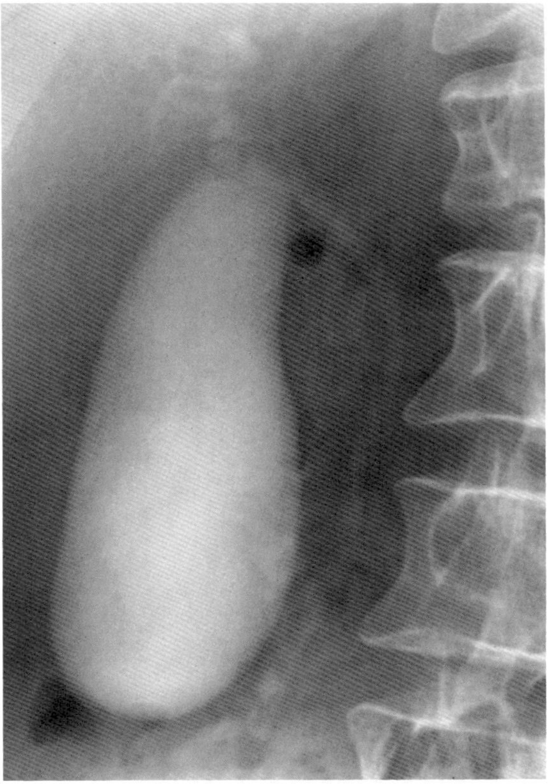

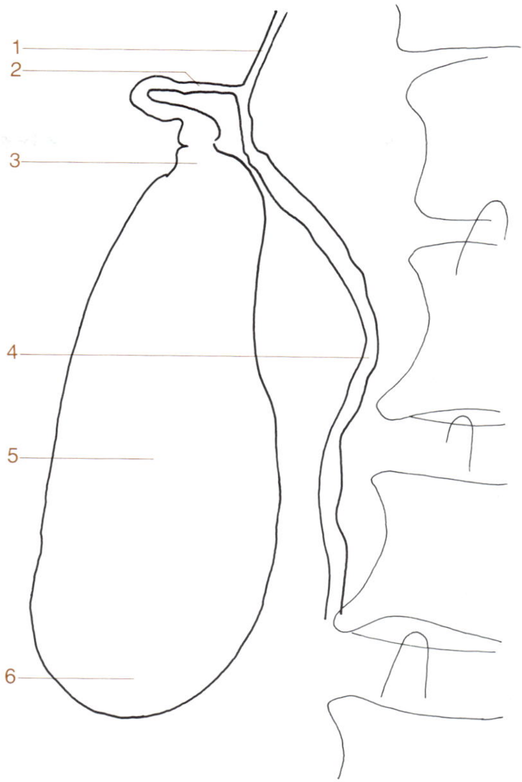

1 Common hepatic duct
2 Cystic duct
3 Neck of the gallbladder
4 Common bile duct
5 Body of the gallbladder
6 Fundus of the gallbladder

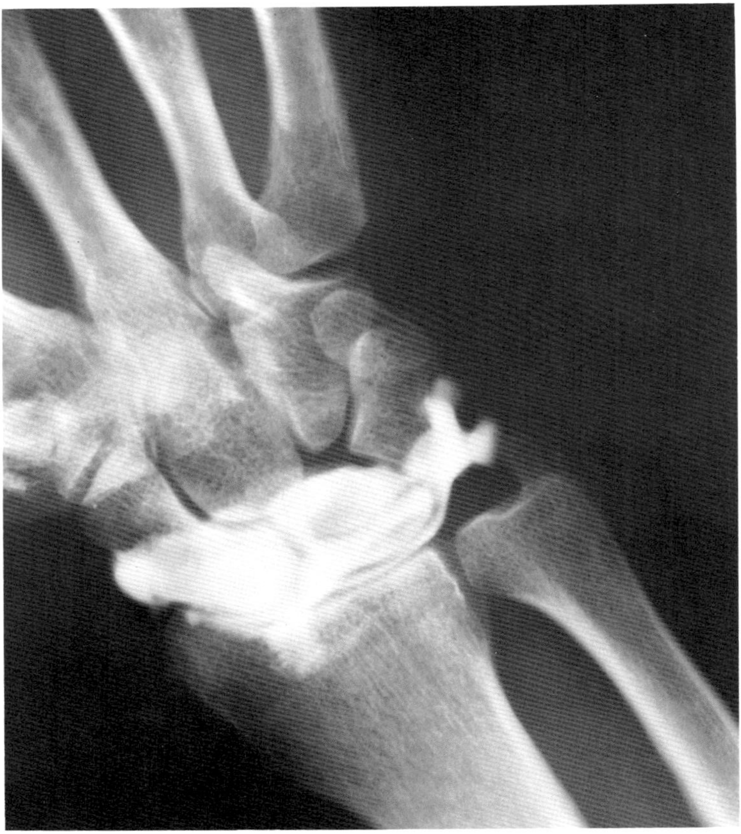

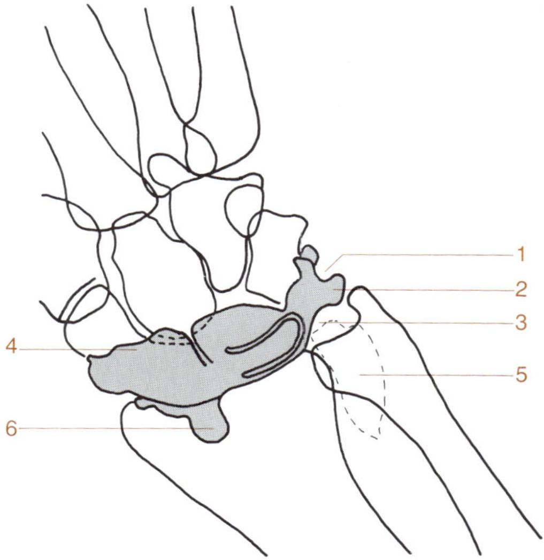

1 Meniscal imprint
2 Prestyloid recess
3 Triangular cartilage
4 Dorsal recess
5 Saccular recess
6 Volar recess

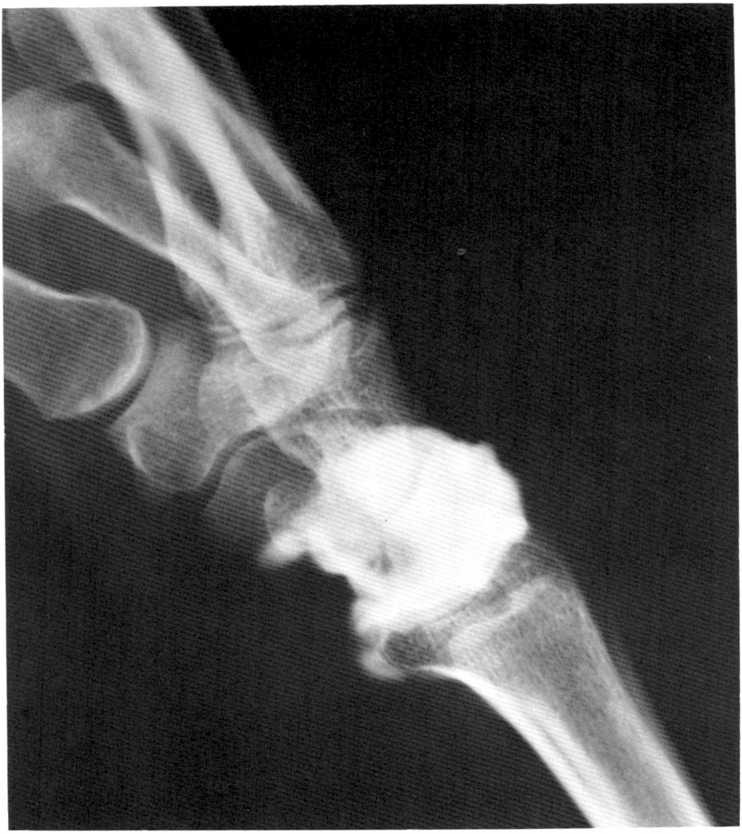

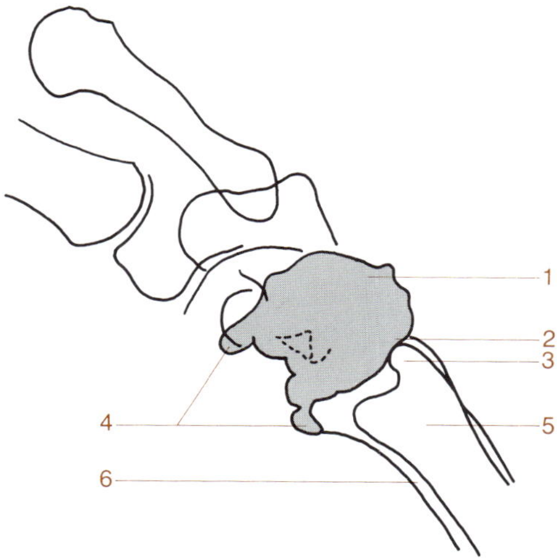

1 Dorsal recess
2 Prestyloid recess
3 Styloid process of the ulna
4 Volar recesses
5 Ulna
6 Radius

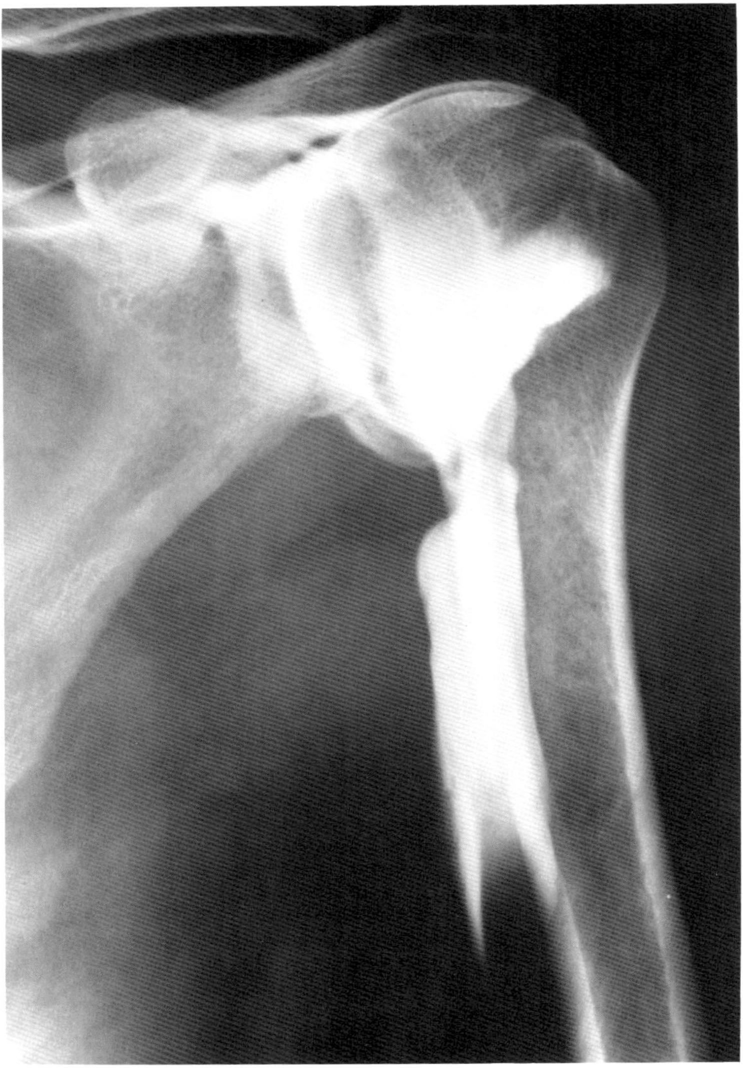

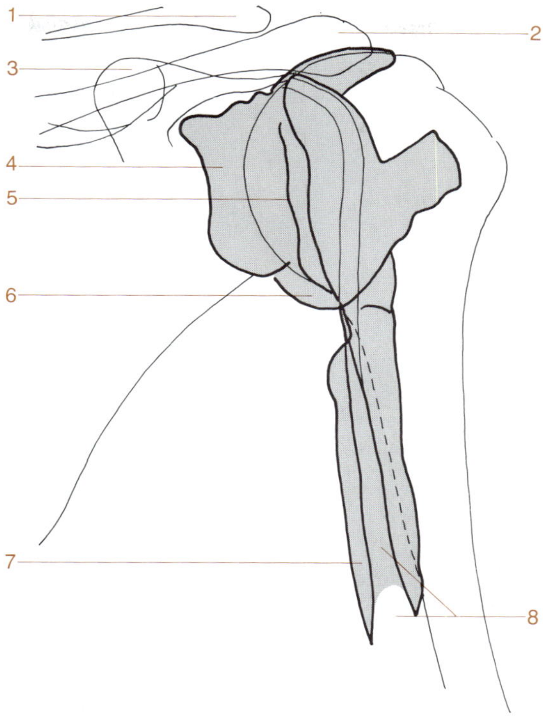

1 Clavicle
2 Acromion
3 Coracoid process
4 Subtendinous bursa of the subscapularis muscle (subcoracoid bursa)
5 Labium glenoidale
6 Axillary recess
7 Intertubercular tendon sheath
8 Tendon sheath of the long head of the biceps muscle

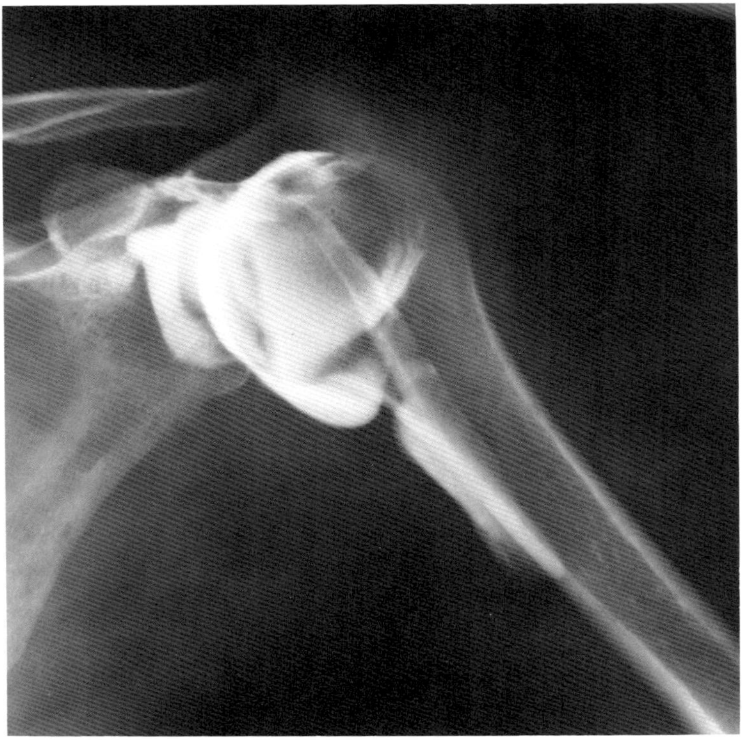

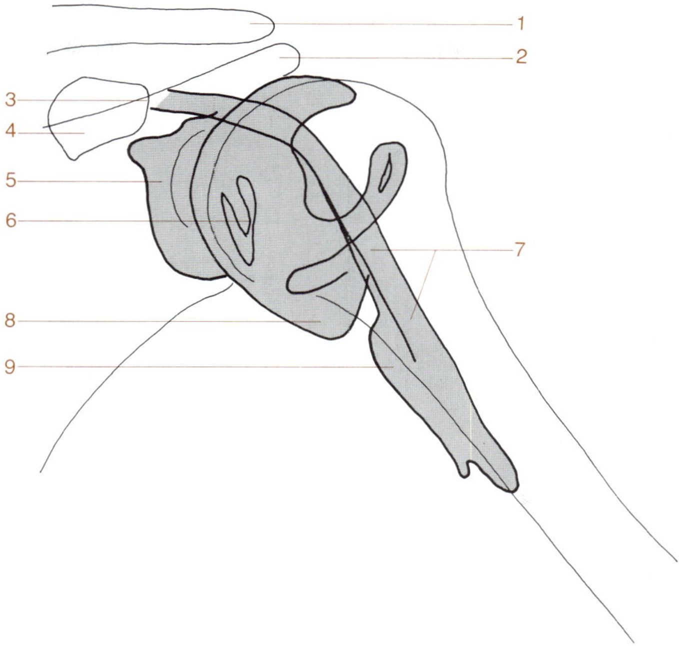

1 Clavicle
2 Acromion
3 Insertion of the biceps tendon
4 Coracoid process
5 Subscapular bursa
6 Labium glenoidale
7 Tendon sheath of the long head of the biceps muscle
8 Axillary recess
9 Intertubercular tendon sheath

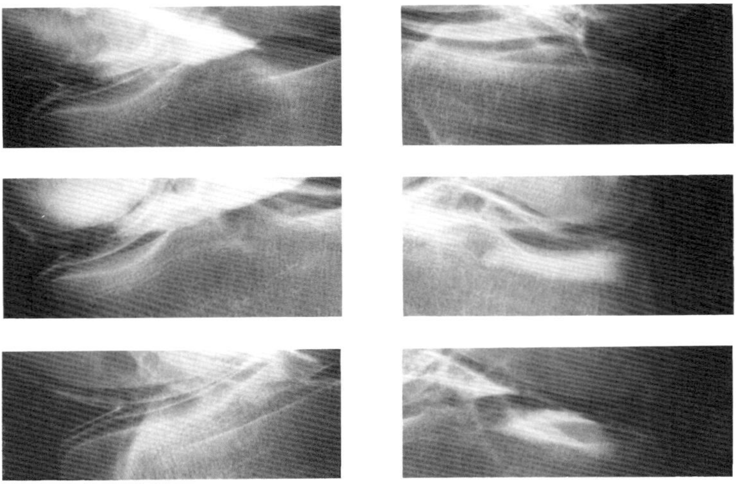

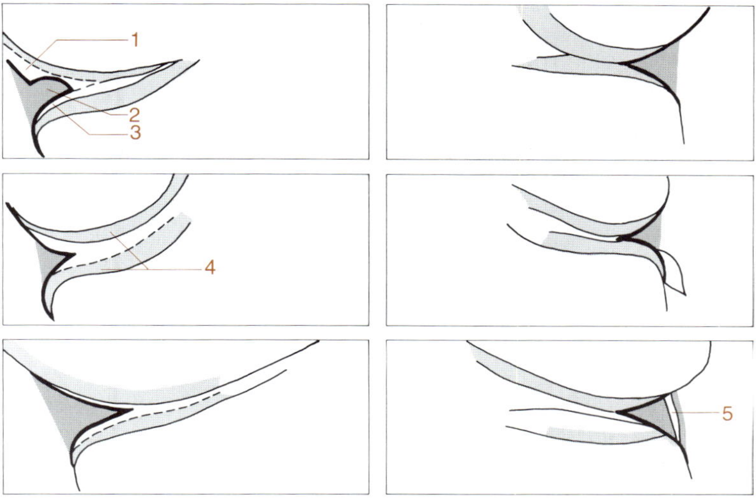

1 Superior capsular recess
2 Meniscus
3 Inferior capsular recess
4 Cartilage
5 Popliteal bursa

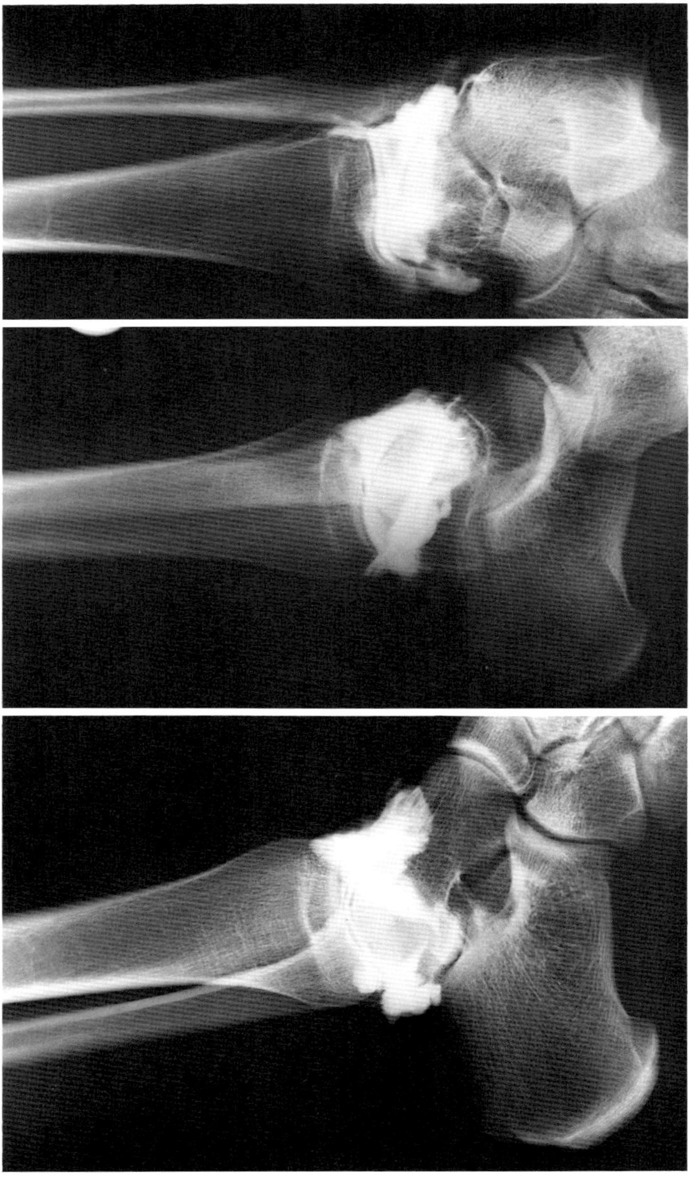

1 Tibia
2 Fibula
3 Tibiofibular joint
4 Joint space
5 Dorsal recess
6 Ventral recess
7 Scalloping due to tendons (normal variant)
8 Talus
9 Supracalcaneal recess
10 Calcaneus
11 Medial malleolus
12 Lateral malleolus

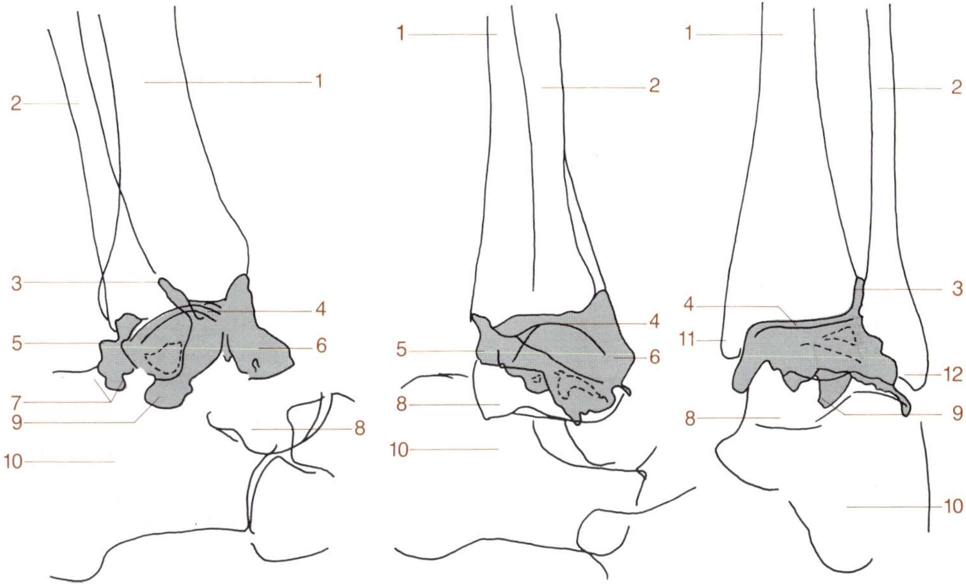

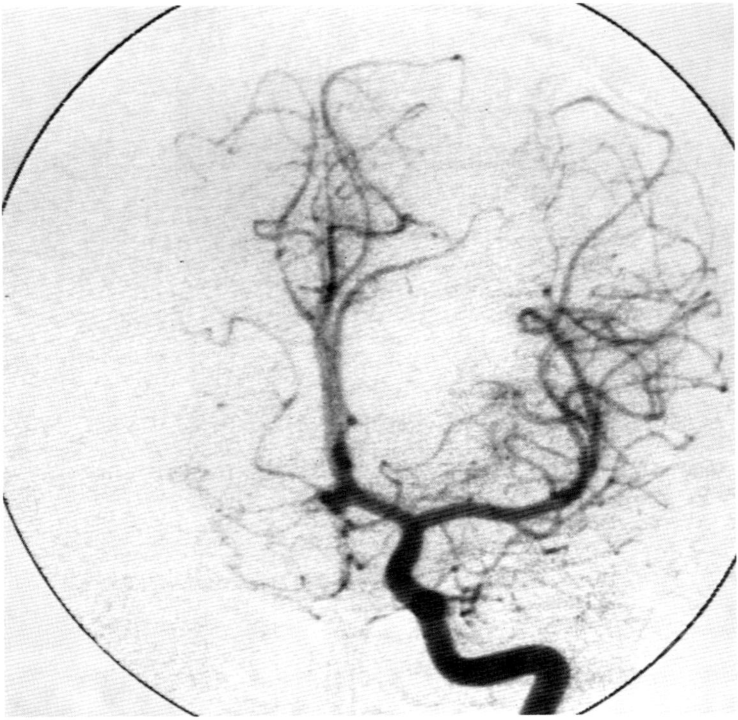

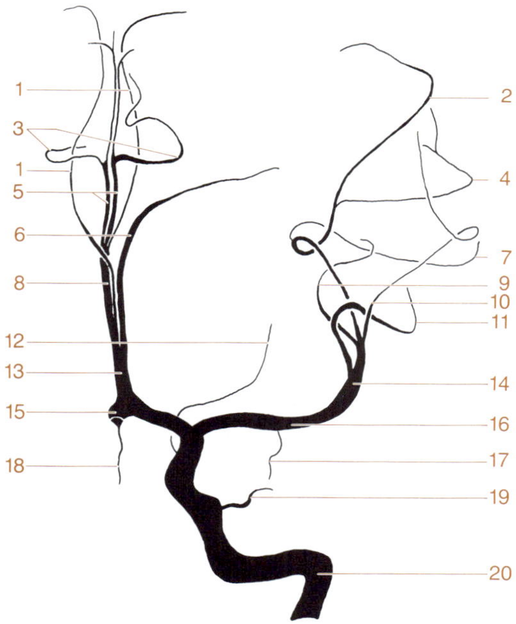

1 Callosomarginal artery
2 Anterior parietal artery
3 Moustache-shaped pericallosal artery
4 Posterior parietal artery
5 Pericallosal artery (fourth segment of the anterior cerebral artery, superior to the corpus callosum)
6 Frontopolar artery
7 Prerolandic artery
8 Third segment of the anterior cerebral artery or pericallosal artery
9 Angular gyrus artery
10 Posterior temporal artery
11 Prefrontal arteries
12 Anterior choroidal artery
13 Second segment of the anterior cerebral artery (from here on termed the pericallosal artery)
14 Second segment of the middle cerebral artery (pars insularis)
15 Anterior communicating artery of the cerebrum (hidden by a vascular loop)
16 First segment of the middle cerebral artery (pars sphenoidalis)
17 Temporopolar artery
18 Fronto-orbital artery
19 Ophthalmic artery
20 Internal carotid artery

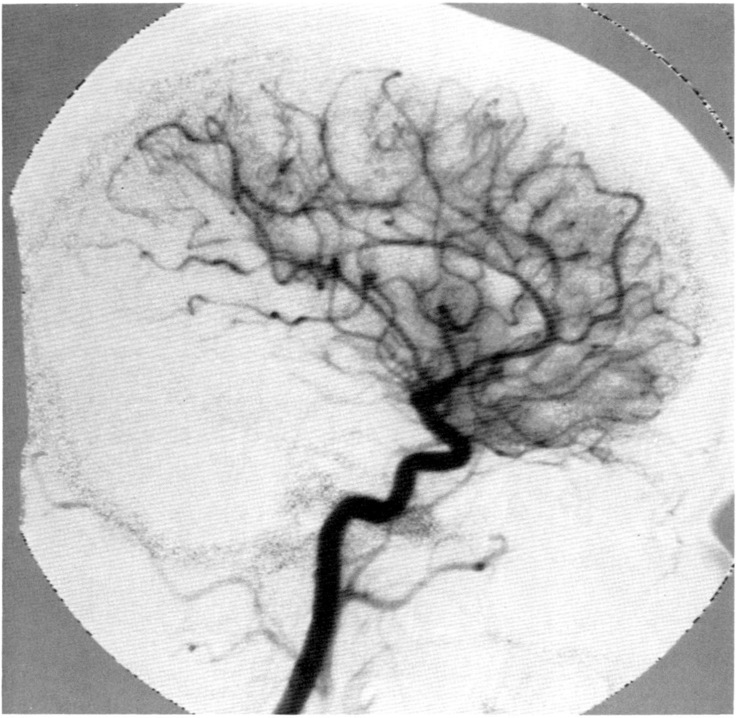

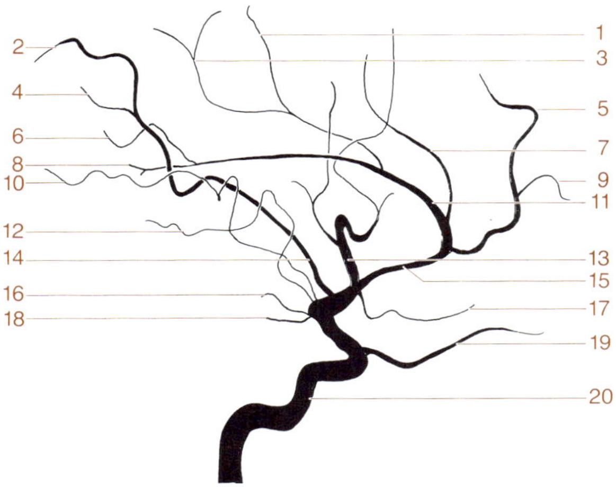

Variant (40%)

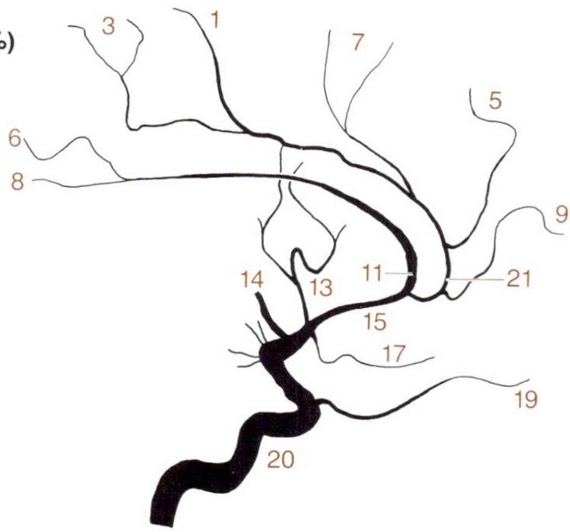

1 Internal posterior frontal artery
2 Anterior parietal artery
3 Paracentral artery
4 Posterior parietal artery
5 Internal anterior frontal artery
6 Internal superior parietal artery
7 Internal medial frontal artery
8 Internal inferior parietal artery
9 Frontopolar artery
10 Angular gyrus artery
11 Pericallosal artery
12 Posterior temporal artery
13 Prefrontal arteries
14 Second segment of the middle cerebral artery
15 Second segment of the anterior cerebral artery
16 Anterior choroidal artery
17 Fronto-orbital artery
18 Posterior communicating artery
19 Ophthalmic artery
20 Internal carotid artery
21 Callosomarginal artery

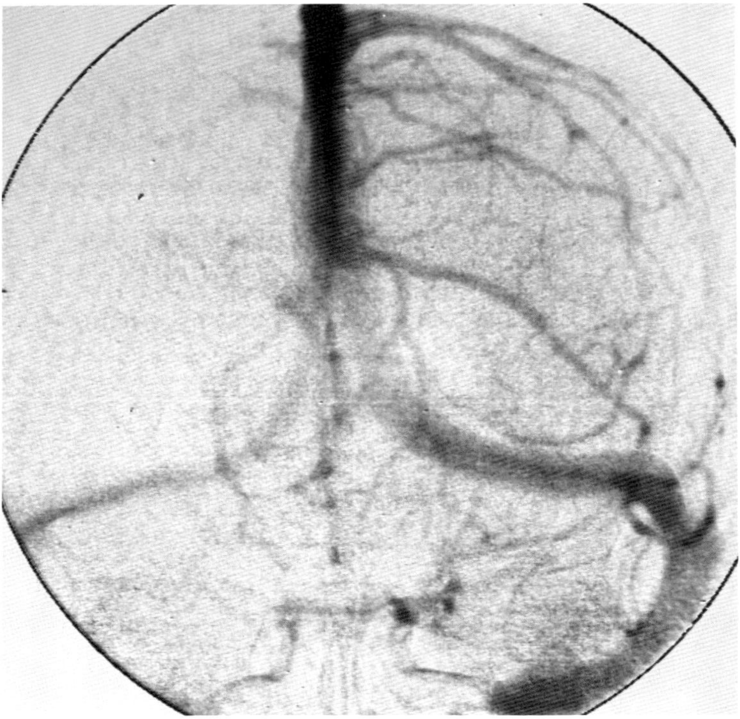

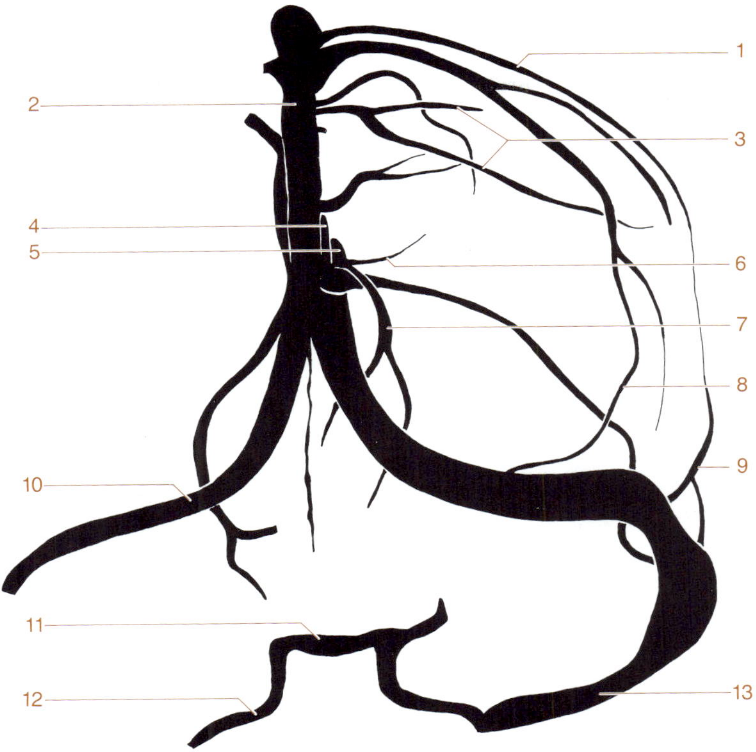

1 Parietal vein (vein of Roland)
2 Superior sagittal sinus
3 Superior anastomotic vein (vein of Trolard)
4 Vein of Galen
5 Internal cerebral vein
6 Superior thalamostriate vein
7 Basal vein of Rosenthal
8 Sylvian veins
9 Sphenoparietal sinus
10 Transverse sinus
11 Intercavernous sinus
12 Inferior petrosal sinus
13 Sigmoid sinus

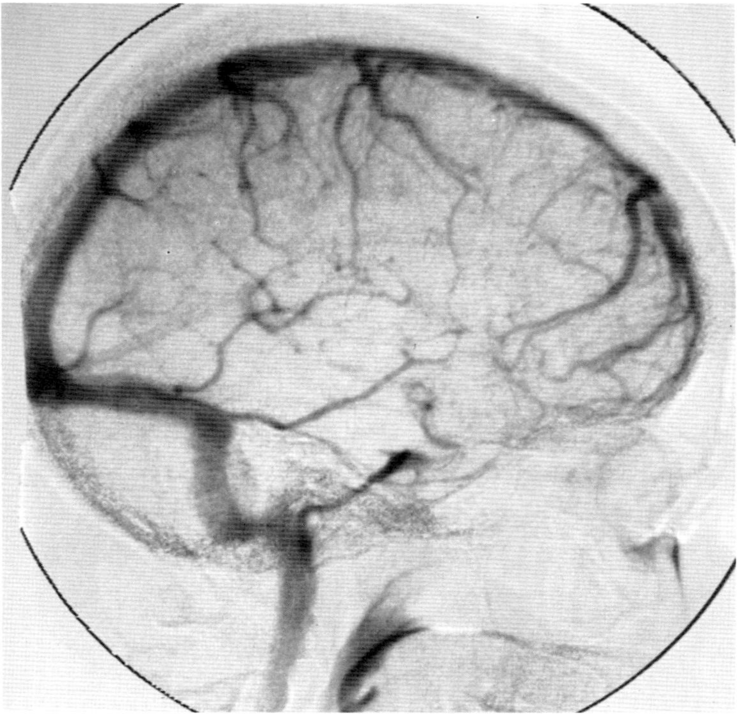

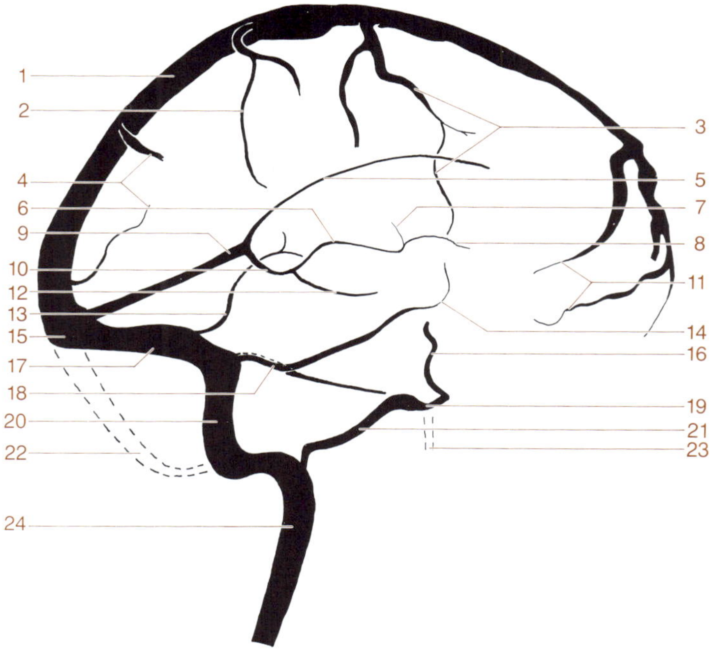

1 Superior sagittal sinus
2 Parietal vein
3 Superior anastomotic vein (vein of Trolard)
4 Occipital veins
5 Inferior sagittal sinus
6 Internal cerebral vein
7 Superior thalamostriate veins
8 Vein of the septum pellucidum
9 Straight sinus (sinus rectus)
10 Vein of Galen
11 Ascending frontal veins
12 Basal vein of Rosenthal
13 Inferior anastomotic vein (Labbé vein)
14 Sylvian veins
15 Torcular Herophili
16 Cavernous sinus (anterior drainage)
17 Transverse sinus
18 Superior petrosal sinus
19 Cavernous sinus (posterior drainage)
20 Sigmoid sinus
21 Inferior petrosal sinus
22 Occipital sinus
23 Pterygoid plexus
24 Internal jugular vein

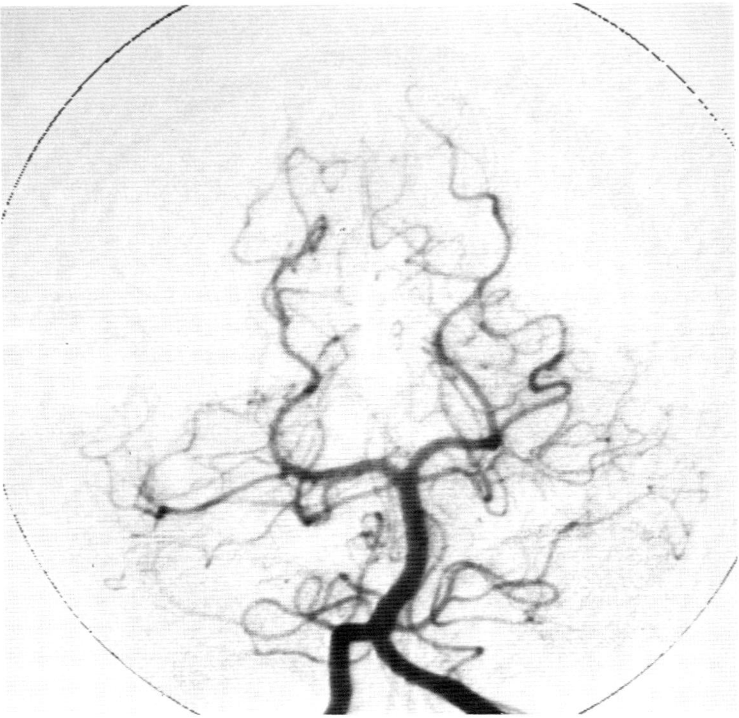

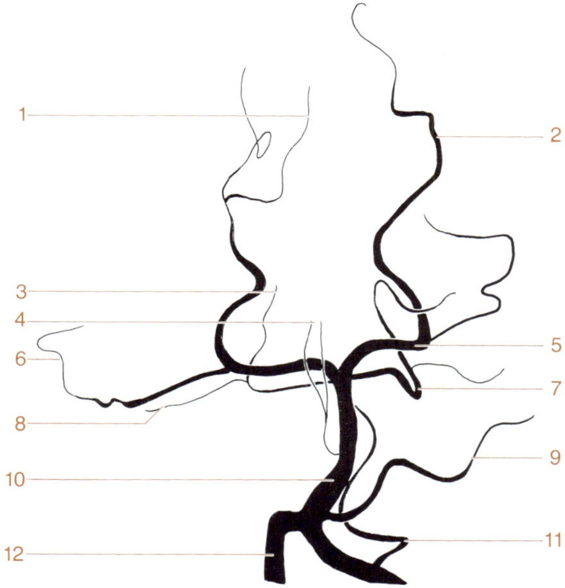

1 Calcarine artery
2 Parieto-occipital artery
3 Anterior vermian branch
4 Thalamoperforate arteries
5 Posterior cerebral artery
6 Temporo-occipital artery
7 Superior cerebellar artery
8 Marginal artery
9 Anterior inferior cerebellar artery
10 Basilar artery
11 Posterior inferior cerebellar artery
12 Vertebral artery

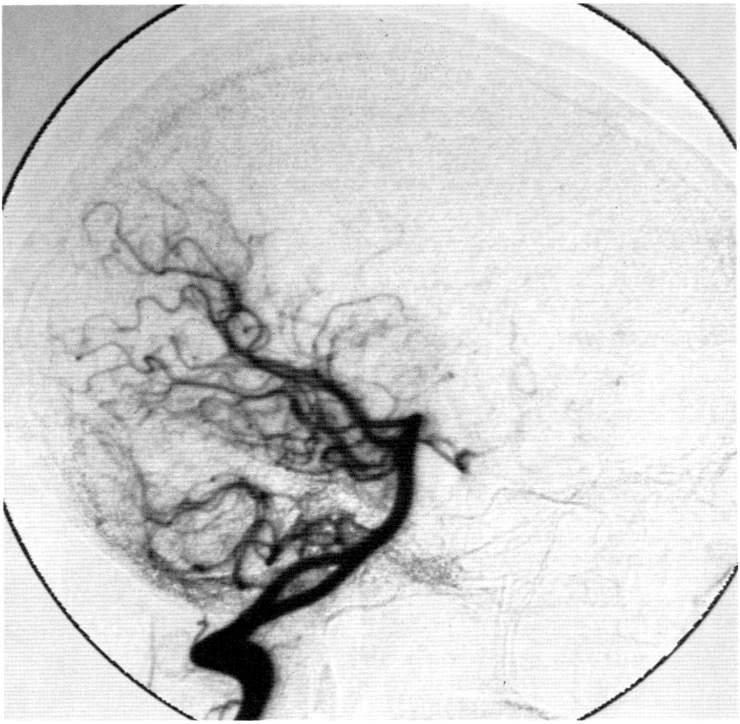

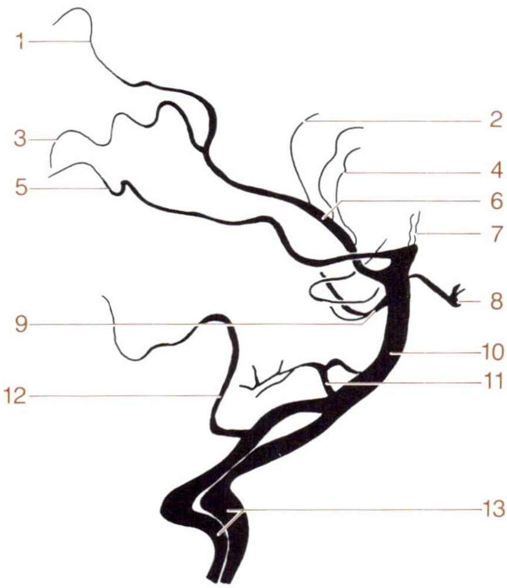

1 Parieto-occipital artery
2 Posterior callosal branch
3 Calcarine artery
4 Choroidal arteries (posterior, medial, and lateral)
5 Temporo-occipital artery
6 Posterior cerebral artery
7 Thalamic branches
8 Posterior communicating artery
9 Superior cerebellar artery
10 Basilar artery
11 Anterior inferior cerebellar artery
12 Posterior inferior cerebellar artery
13 Vertebral arteries

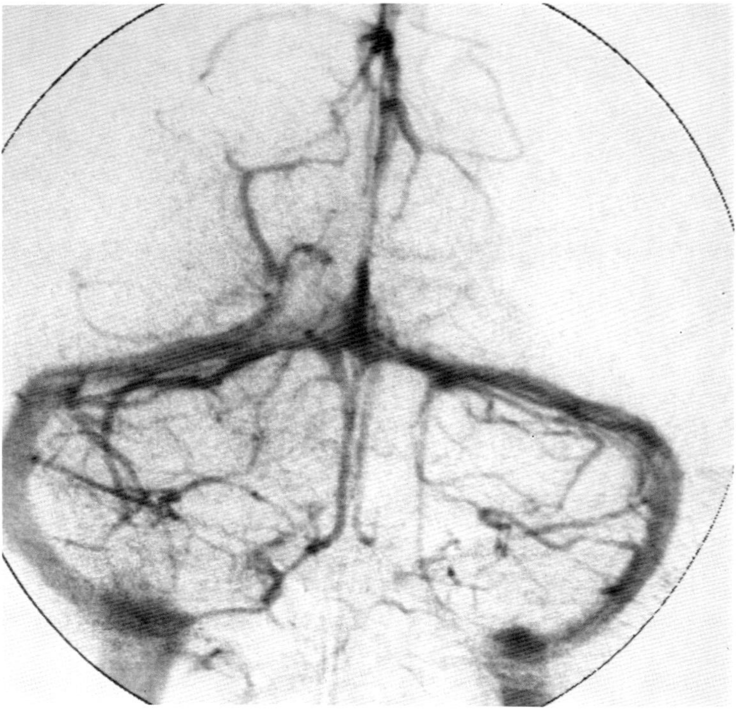

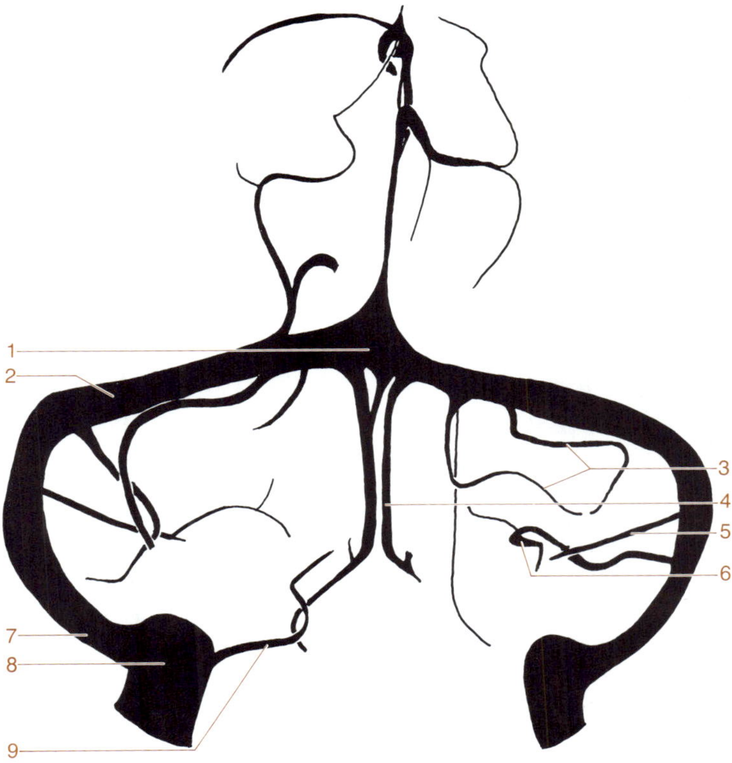

1 Torcular Herophili
2 Transverse sinus
3 Hemispheric cerebellar veins
4 Inferior vein of the vermis
5 Inferior hemispheric cerebellar vein
6 Petrosal vein (joining the superior petrosal sinus)
7 Sigmoid sinus
8 Jugular vein bulb
9 Inferior petrosal sinus

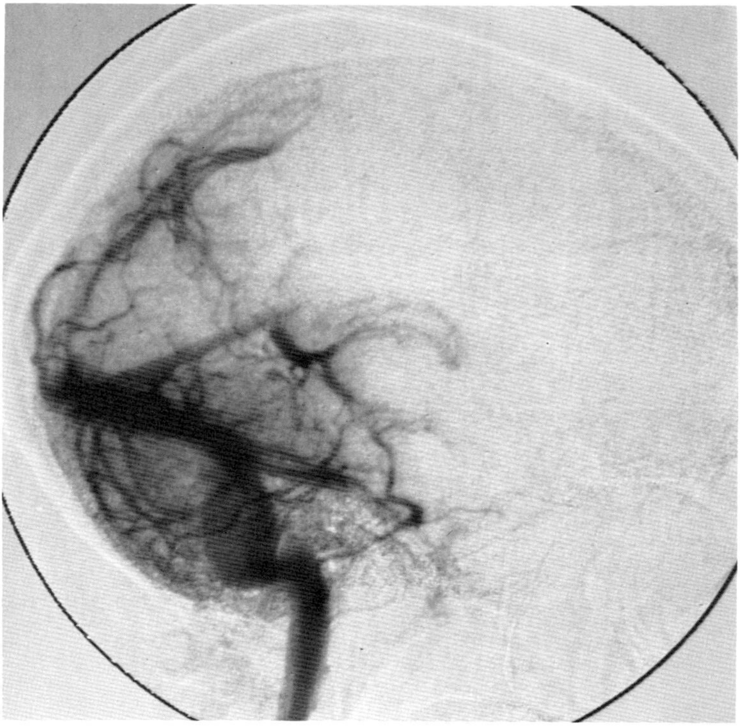

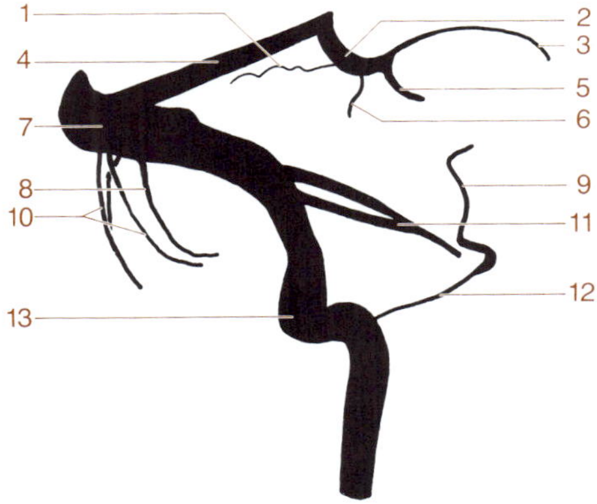

1 Superior cerebellar veins
2 Vein of Galen
3 Internal cerebral vein
4 Straight sinus (sinus rectus)
5 Basal vein of Rosenthal
6 Precentral cerebellar vein
7 Torcular Herophili
8 Inferior veins of the cerebellar hemisphere
9 Cavernous sinus
10 Inferior cerebellar veins
11 Superior petrosal sinus
12 Inferior petrosal sinus
13 Sigmoid sinus

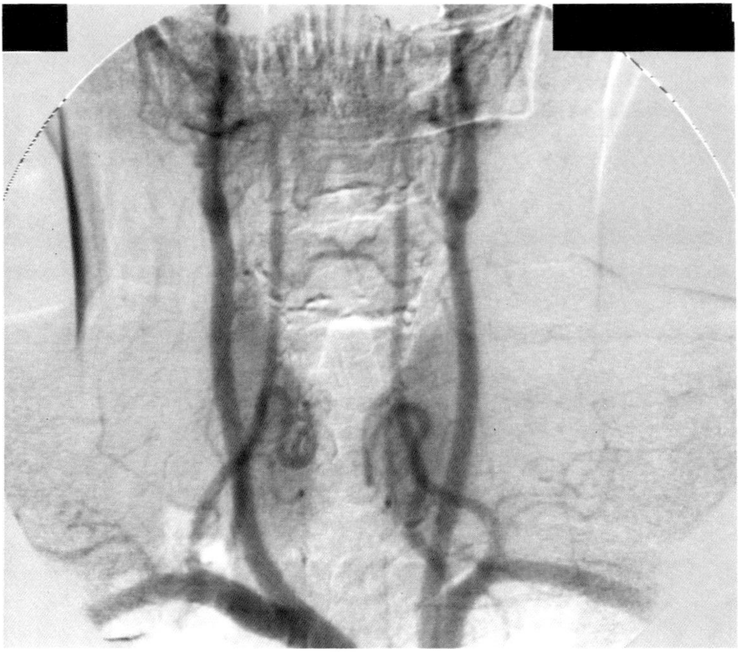

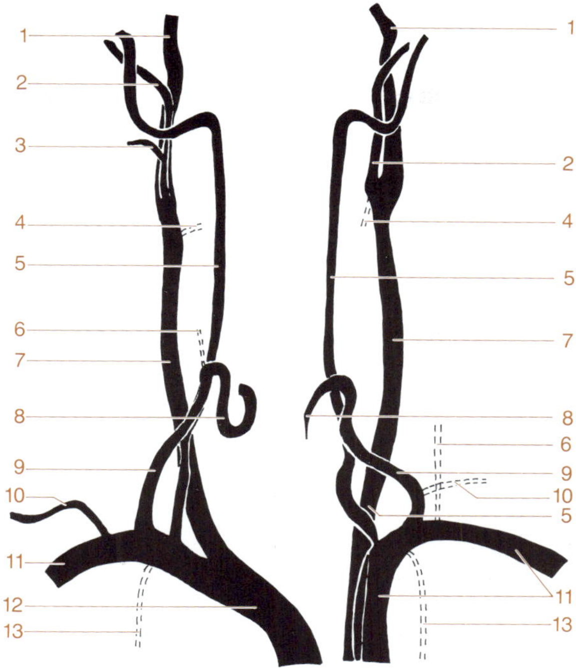

1 Internal carotid artery
2 External carotid artery
3 Facial artery
4 Superior thyroid artery
5 Vertebral artery
6 Ascending cervical artery
7 Common carotid artery
8 Inferior thyroid artery
9 Thyrocervical trunk
10 Suprascapular artery
11 Subclavian artery
12 Brachiocephalic trunk
13 Internal mammary artery

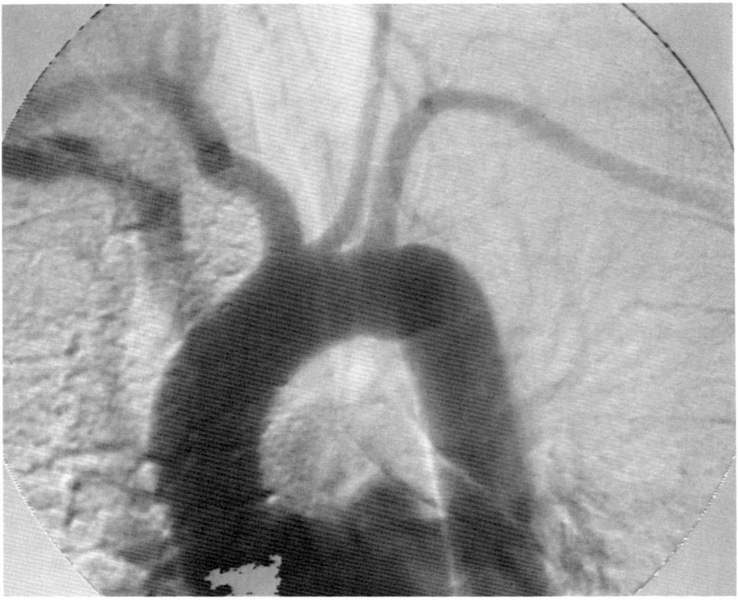

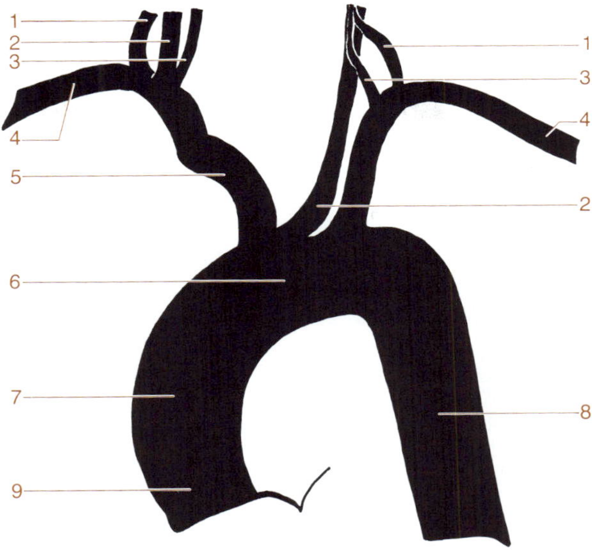

1 Thyrocervical trunk
2 Common carotid artery
3 Vertebral artery
4 Subclavian artery
5 Brachiocephalic trunk
6 Arch of the aorta
7 Ascending aorta
8 Descending aorta
9 Aortic root

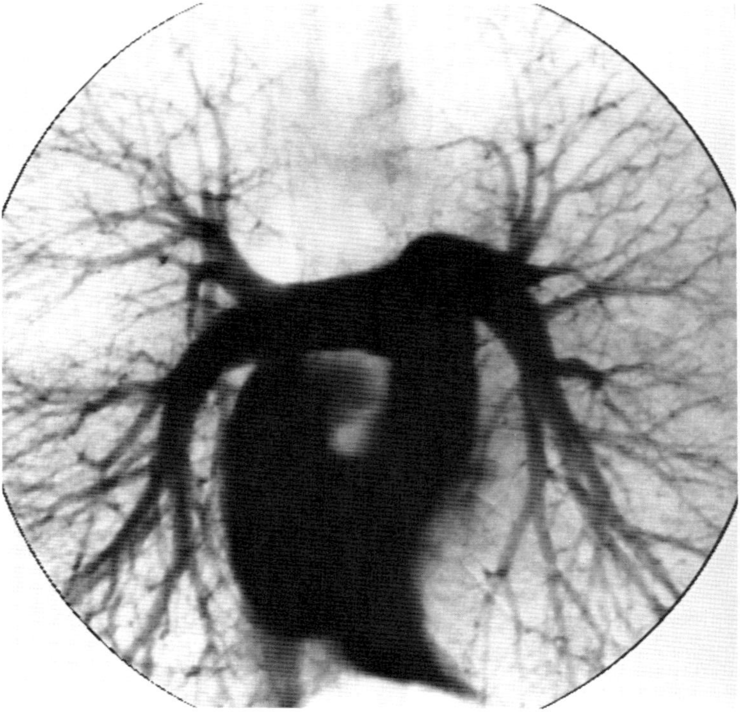

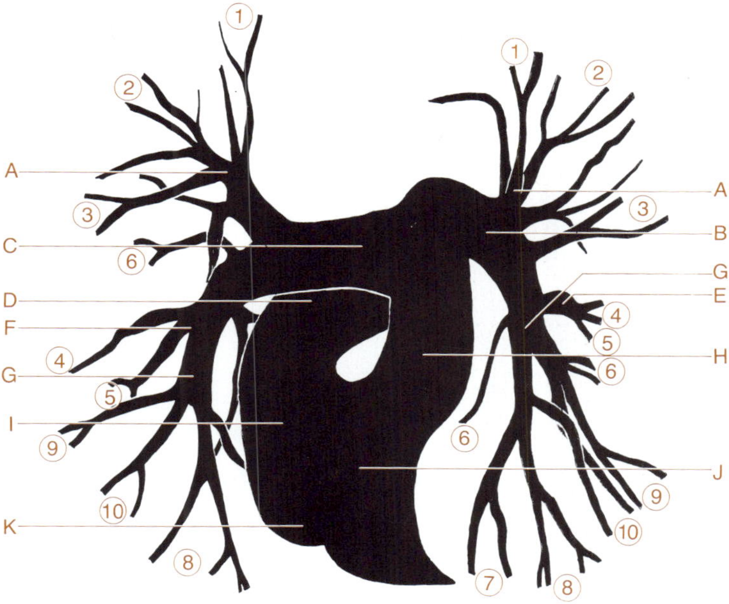

○ = Segmental artery 1–10

A Truncus anterior
B Left pulmonary artery
C Intrapericardiac segment of the right pulmonary artery
D Superior vena cava
E Lingular artery
F Middle lobe artery
G Right lower lobe artery
H Main pulmonary artery segment
I Right atrium
J Right ventricle
K Inferior vena cava

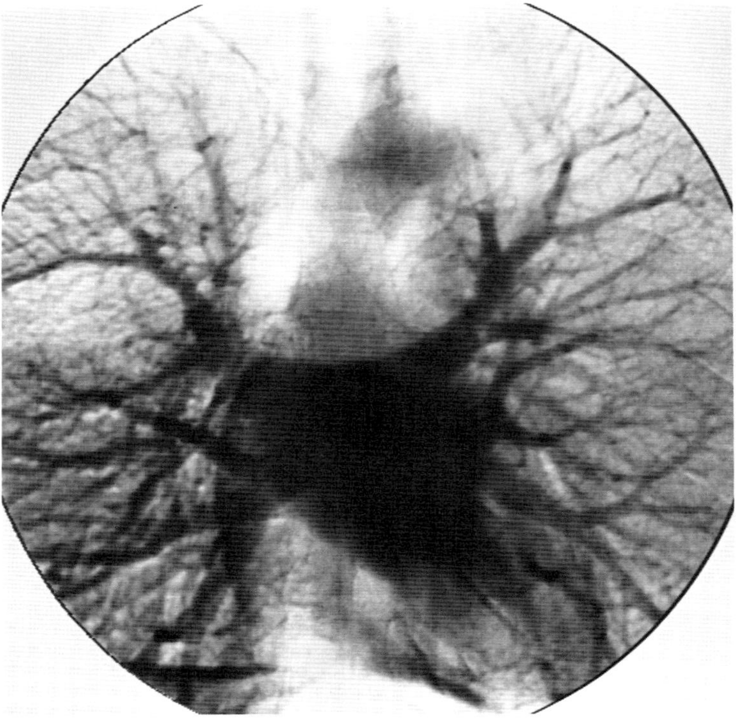

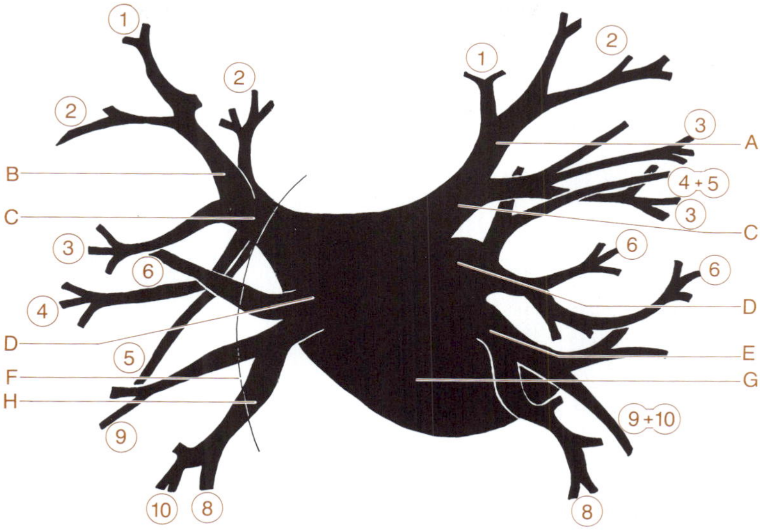

○ = Segmental artery 1–10

A Apicoposterior branch of left superior pulmonary vein
B Apical branch of right superior pulmonary vein
C Superior pulmonary veins
D Inferior pulmonary veins
E Left lower lobe vein
F Contour of the right atrium
G Left atrium
H Right lower lobe vein

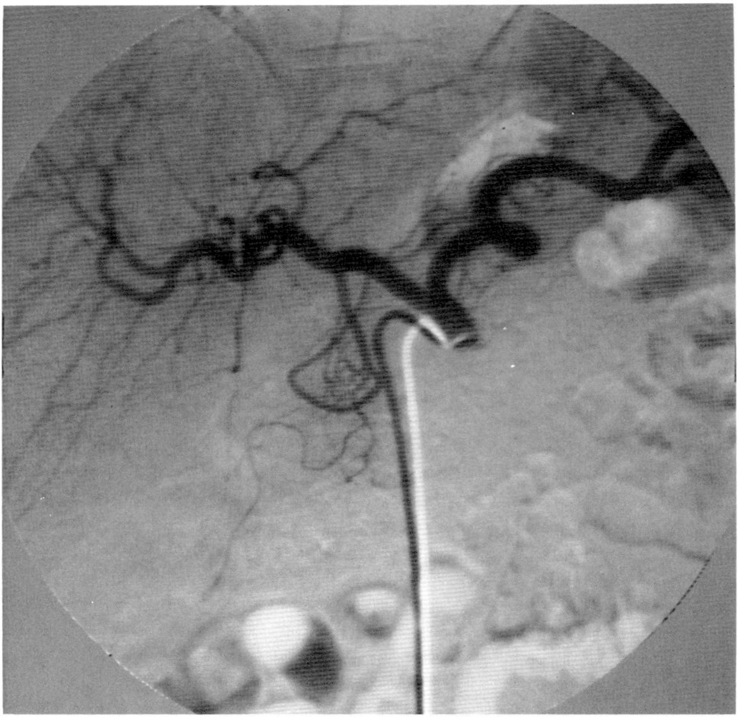

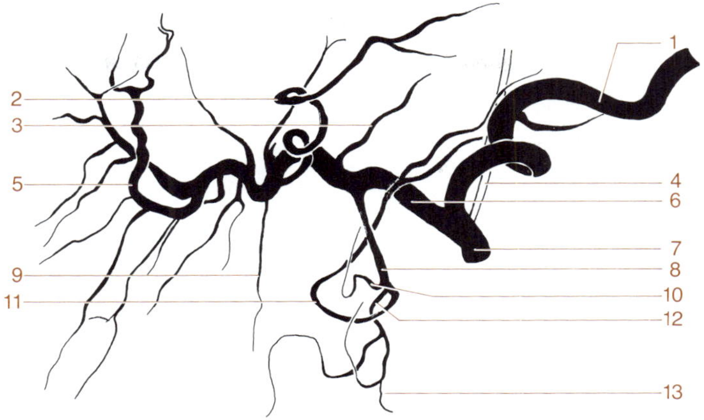

1 Splenic artery
2 Left hepatic artery
3 Right gastric artery
4 Left gastric artery
5 Right hepatic artery
6 Common hepatic artery
7 Celiac trunk
8 Gastroduodenal artery
9 Cystic artery
10 Superior supraduodenal artery
11 Right gastroepiploic artery
12 Superior pancreaticoduodenal artery
13 Inferior pancreaticoduodenal artery (anastomosis with the superior mesenteric artery)

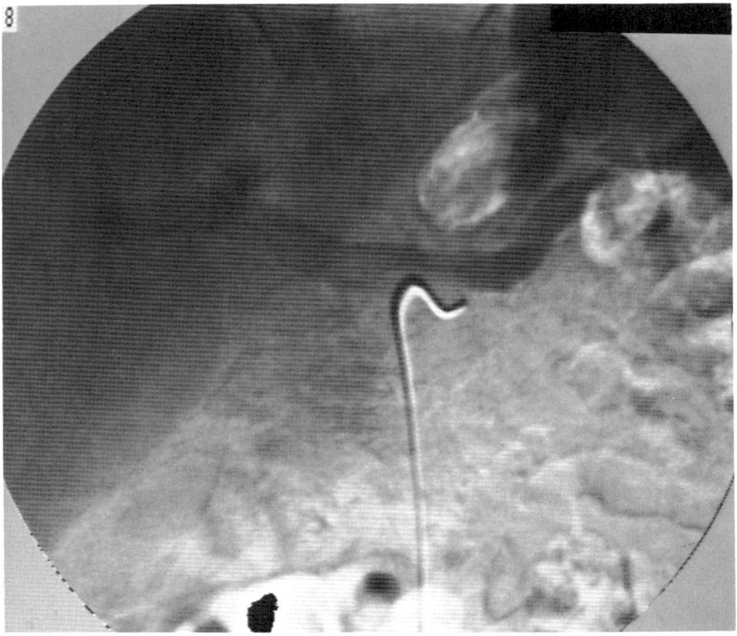
8

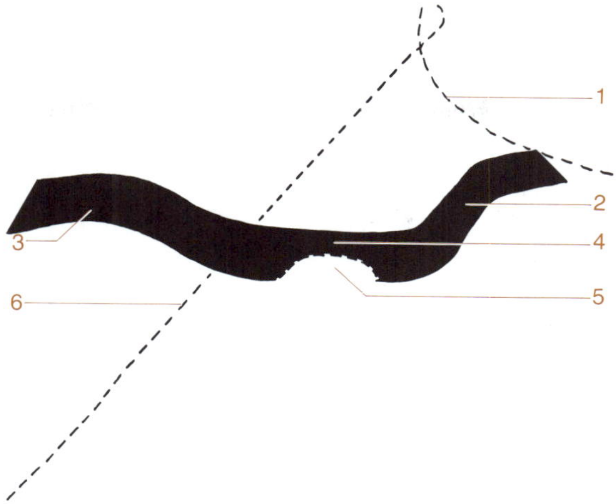

1 Spleen
2 Splenic vein
3 Portal vein
4 Confluence
5 Wash-out at the junction with the mesenteric vein
6 Liver

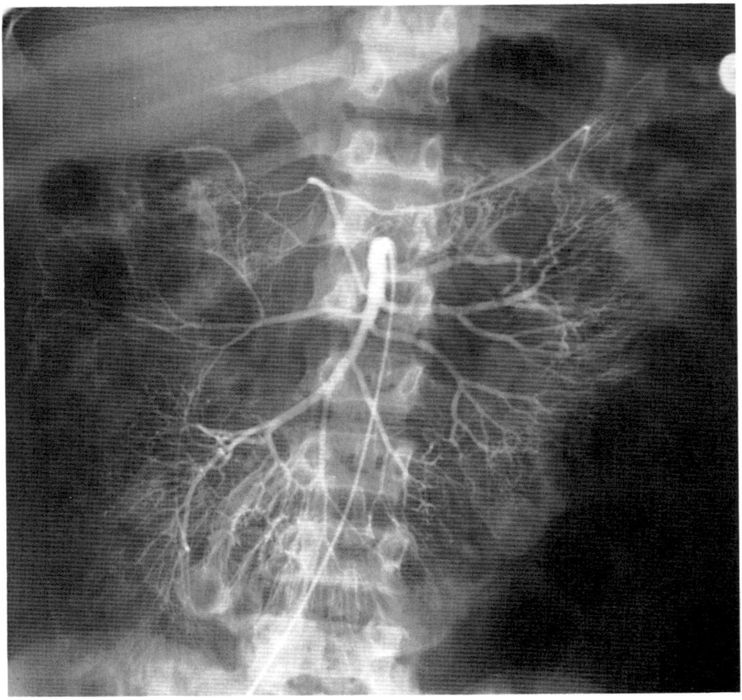

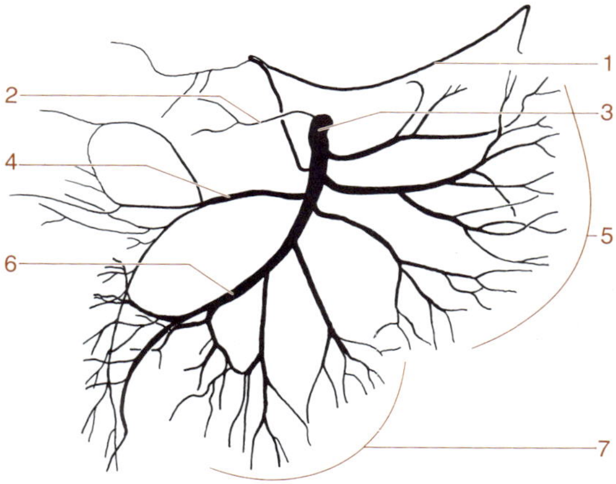

1 Middle colic artery
2 Inferior pancreaticoduodenal artery
3 Superior mesenteric artery
4 Right colic artery
5 Jejunal arteries
6 Ileocolic artery
7 Ileal arteries

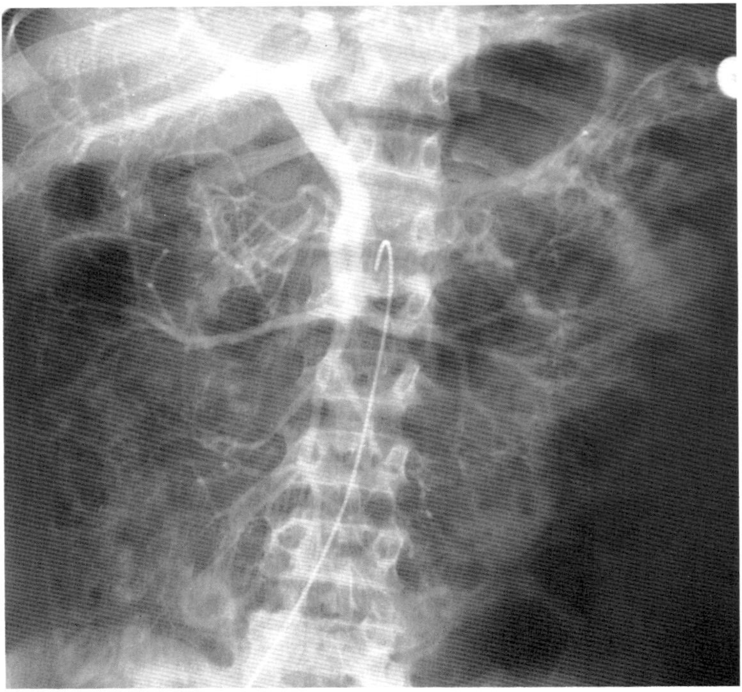

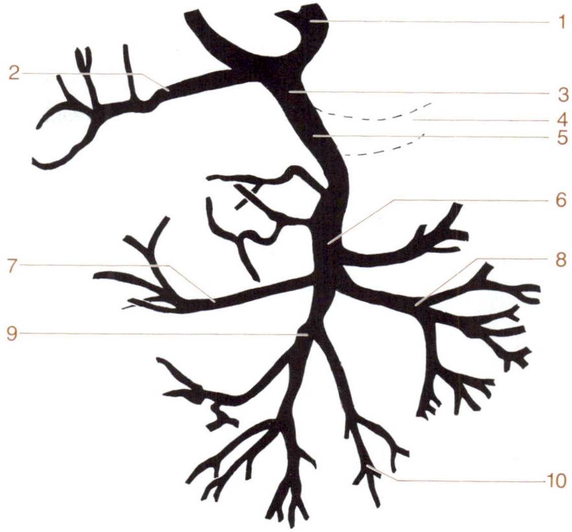

1 Left branch of the portal vein
2 Right branch of the portal vein
3 Portal vein
4 Splenic vein
5 Confluence
6 Superior mesenteric vein
7 Right colic vein
8 Jejunal veins
9 Ileocolic vein
10 Ileal veins

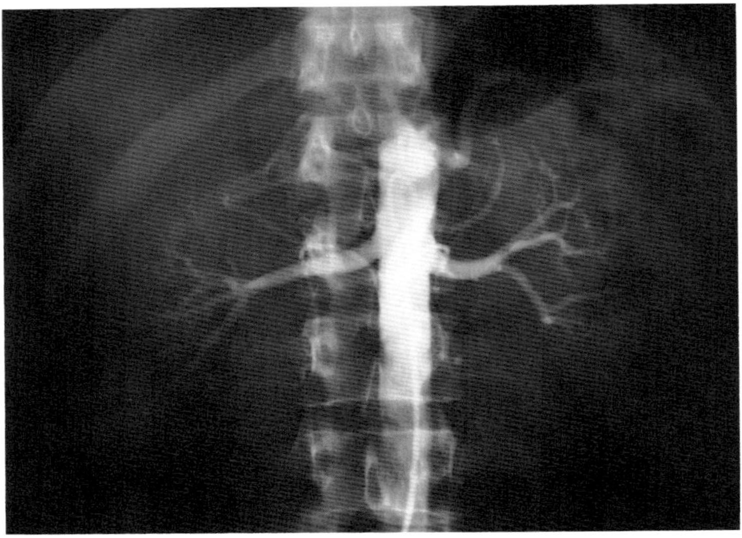

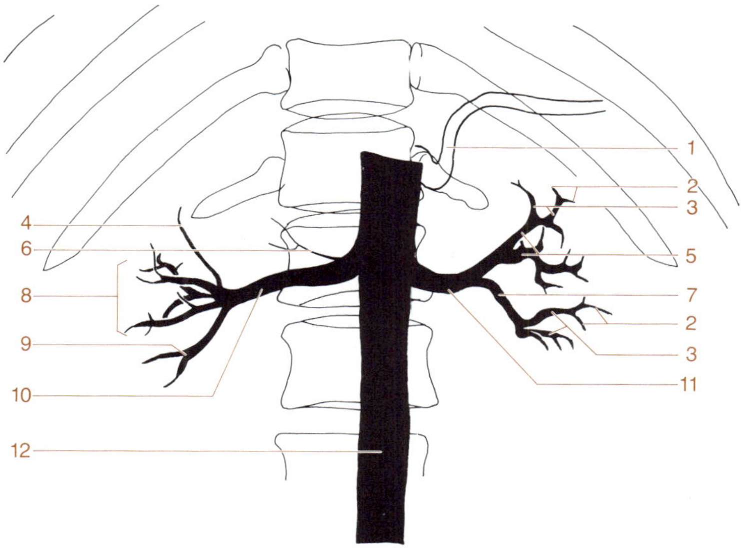

1 Splenic artery
2 Arcuate arteries
3 Interlobular arteries
4 Superior segmental artery
5 Segmental arteries (anterior branch)
6 Inferior adrenal artery
7 Segmental arteries (posterior branch)
8 Middle segmental artery
9 Inferior segmental artery
10 Right renal artery
11 Left renal artery
12 Abdominal aorta

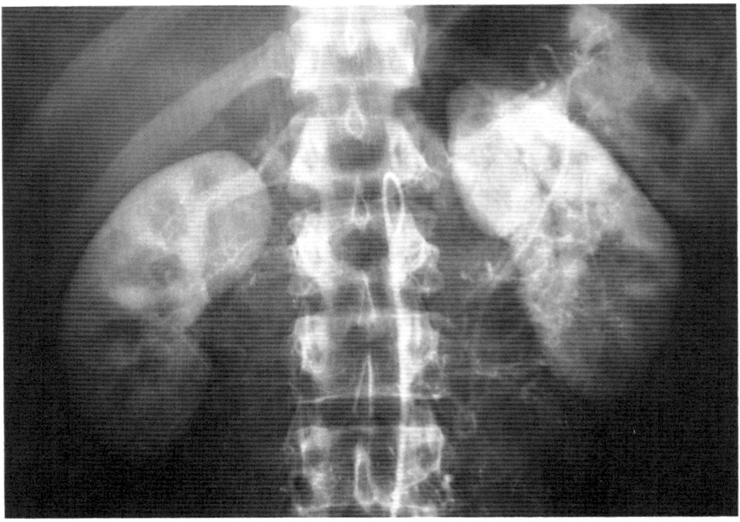

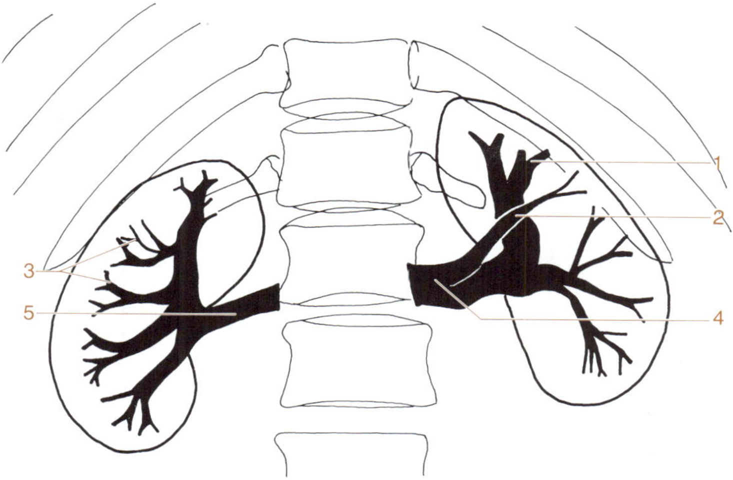

1 Interlobular vein
2 Superior branch of the renal vein
3 Arcuate vein
4 Left renal vein
5 Right renal vein

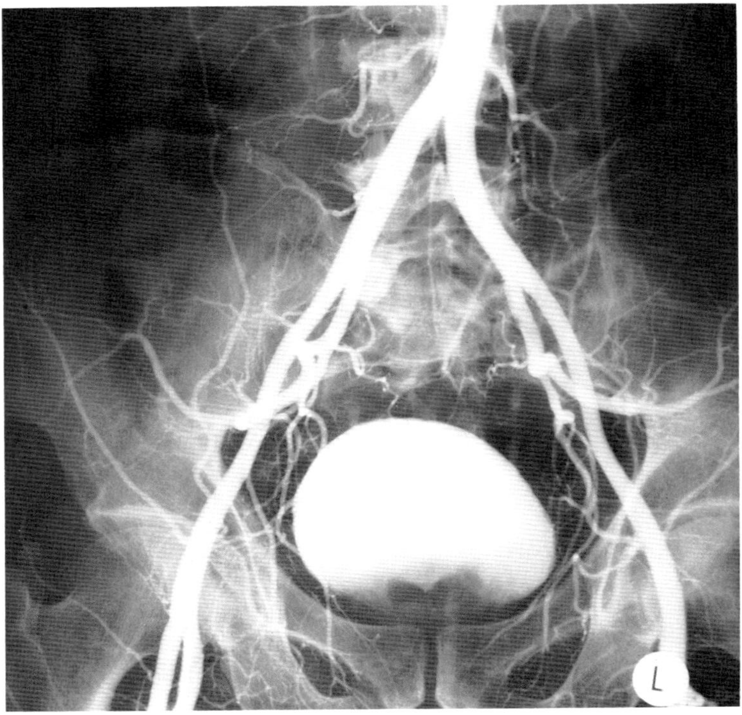
L

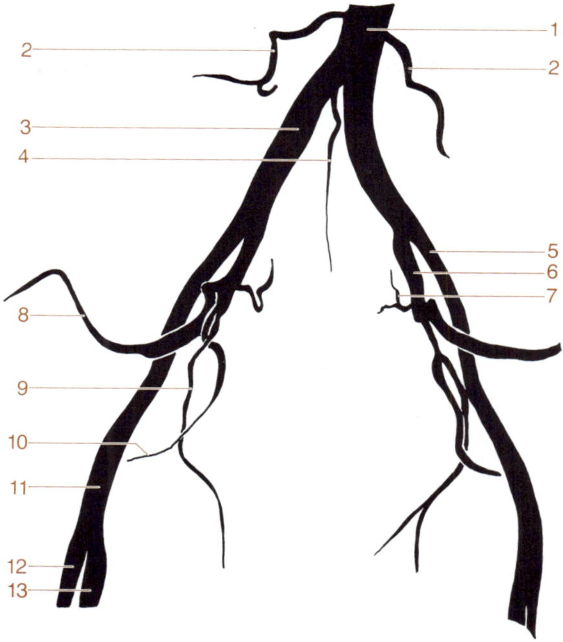

1 Abdominal aorta
2 Lumbar artery
3 Common iliac artery
4 Median sacral artery
5 External iliac artery
6 Internal iliac artery
7 Lateral sacral artery
8 Superior gluteal artery
9 Obturator artery
10 Inferior gluteal artery
11 Common femoral artery
12 Deep femoral artery
13 Superficial femoral artery

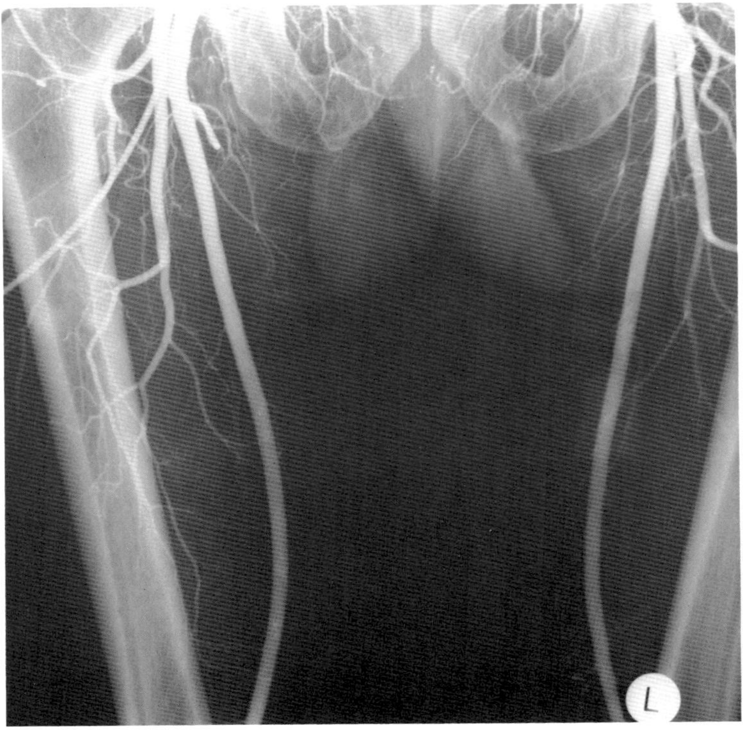
L

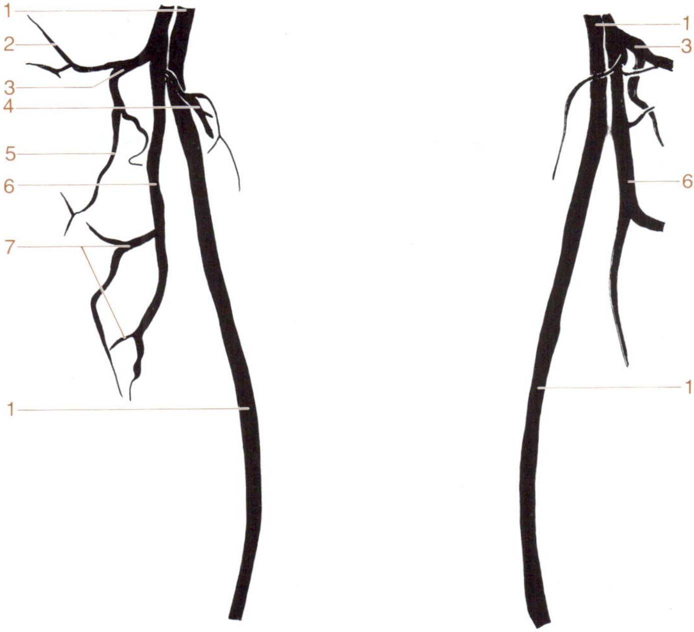

1 Superficial femoral artery
2 Ascending branch of the lateral circumflex femoral artery
3 Lateral circumflex femoral artery
4 Medial circumflex femoral artery
5 Descending branch of the lateral circumflex femoral artery
6 Deep femoral artery
7 Perforating artery

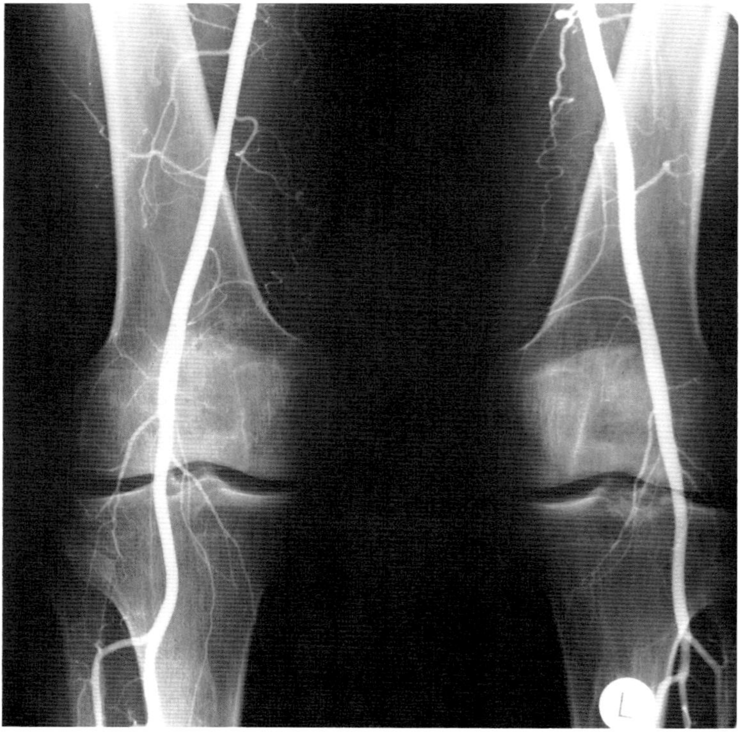

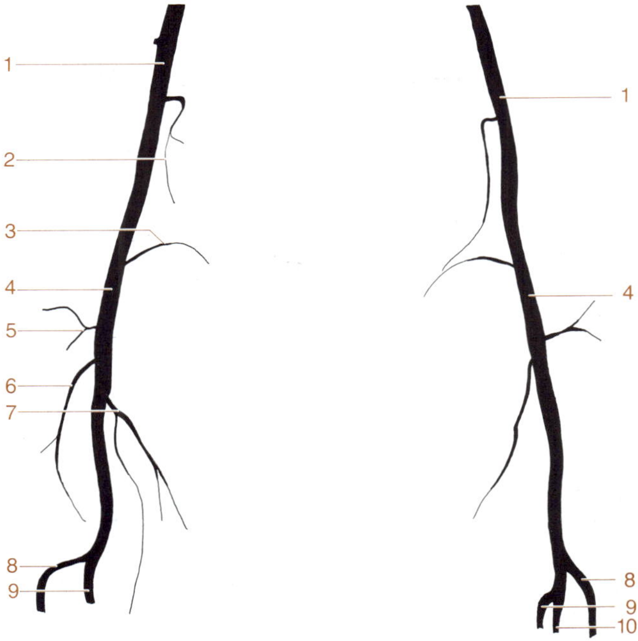

1 Superficial femoral artery
2 Descending genicular artery
3 Medial superior genicular artery
4 Popliteal artery
5 Lateral superior genicular artery
6 Middle genicular artery
7 Medial inferior genicular artery
8 Anterior tibial artery
9 Posterior tibial artery
10 Fibular artery

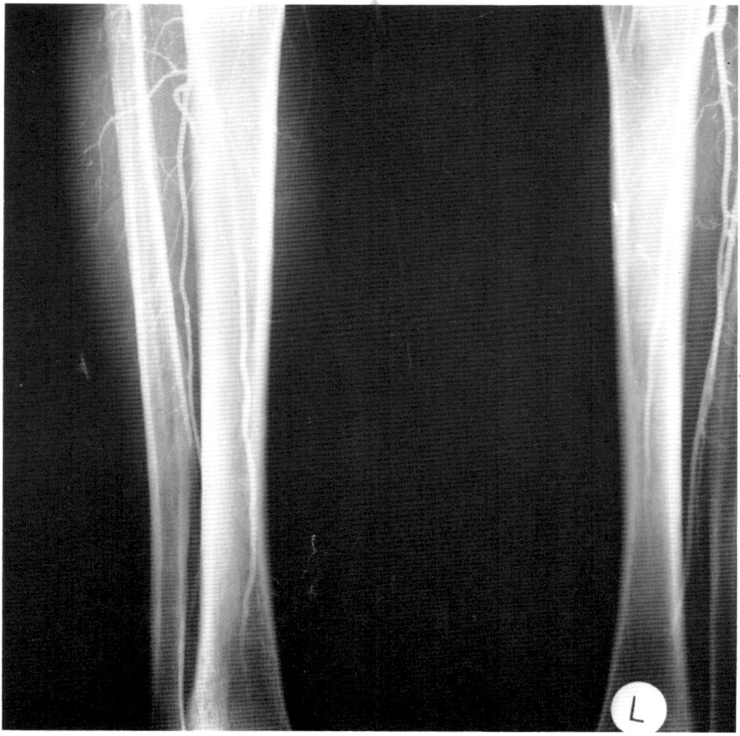
L

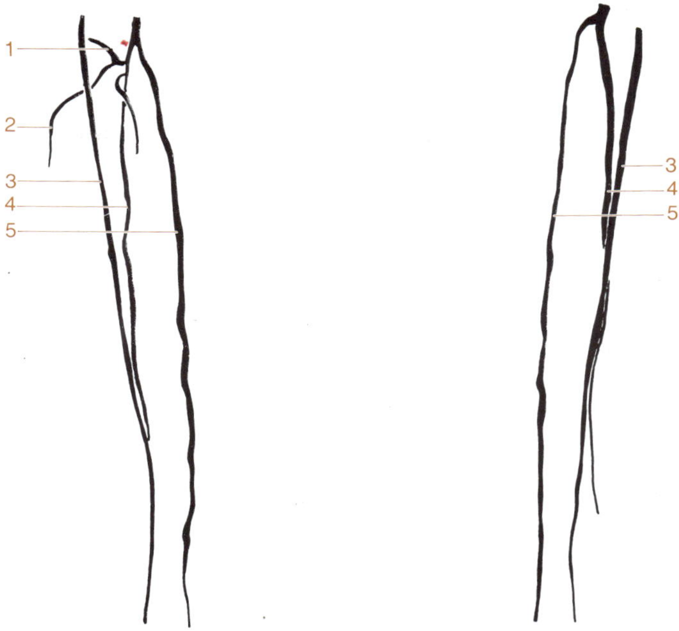

1 Peroneal circumflex branch
2 Muscular branch
3 Anterior tibial artery
4 Peroneal artery
5 Posterior tibial artery

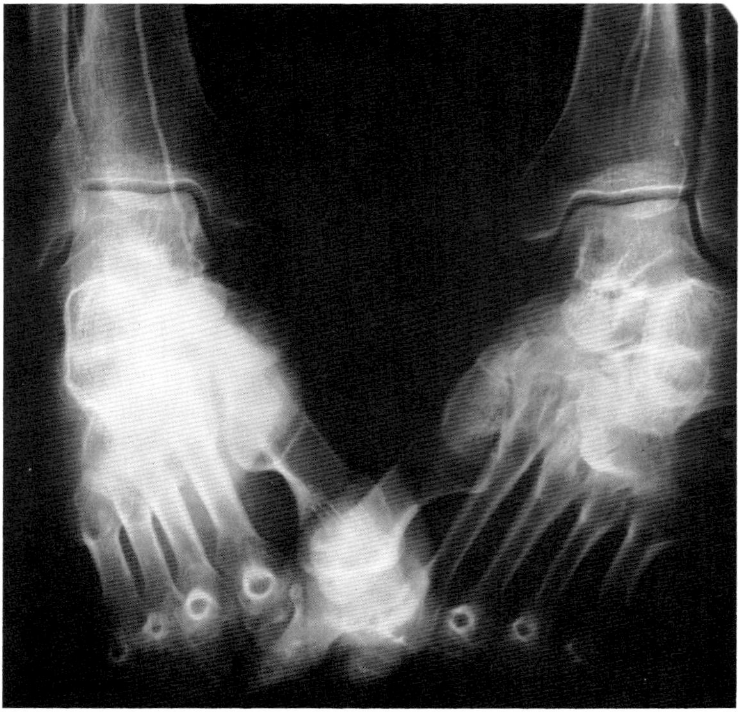

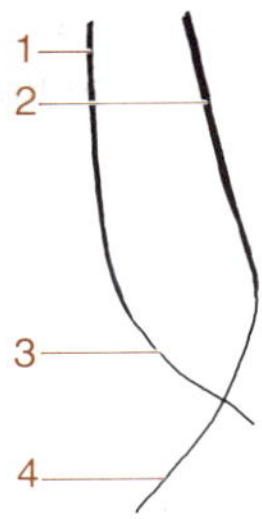

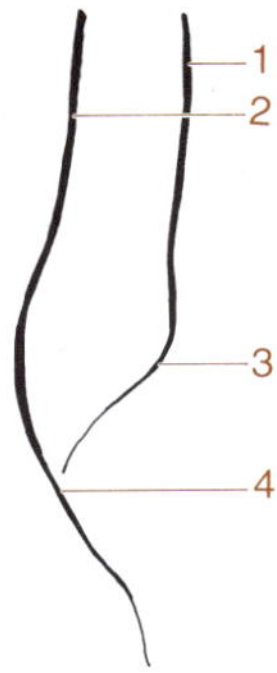

1 Anterior tibial artery
2 Posterior tibial artery
3 Dorsalis pedis artery
4 Plantar artery

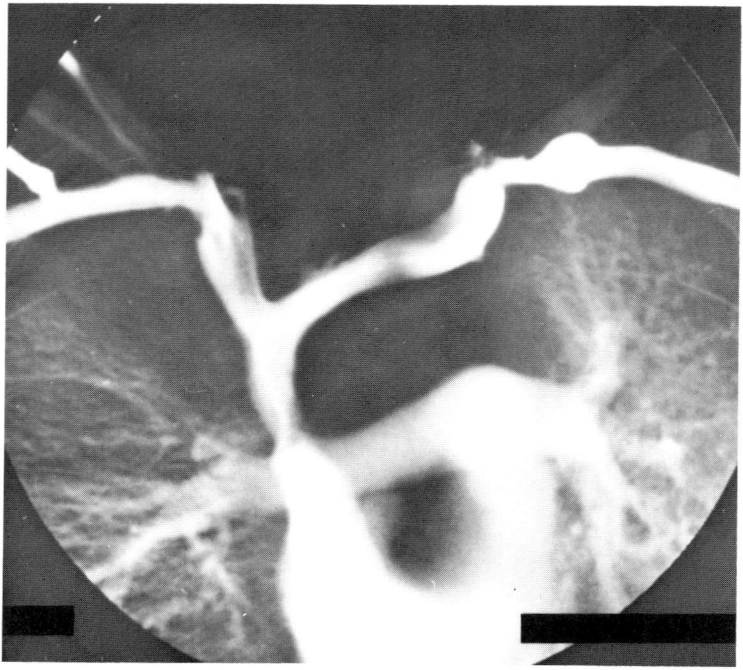

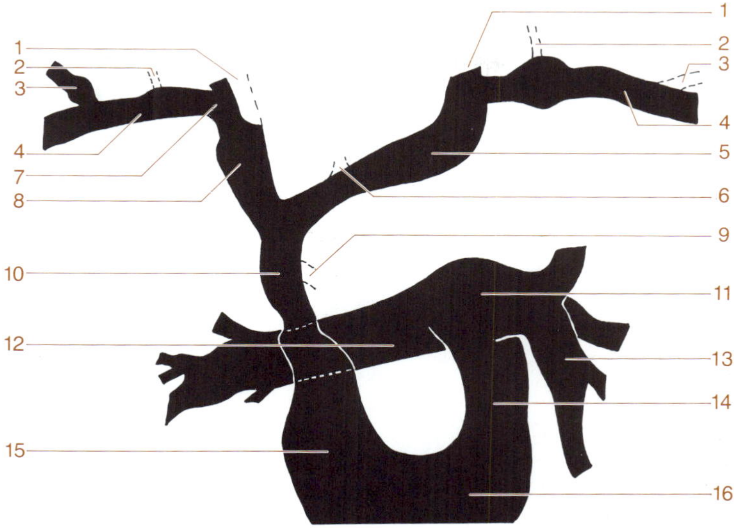

1 Internal jugular vein
2 External jugular vein
3 Cephalic vein
4 Subclavian vein
5 Left brachiocephalic vein
6 Vena thyroidea ima
7 Venous angle
8 Right brachiocephalic vein
9 Azygos vein
10 Superior vena cava
11 Main pulmonary artery segment
12 Right pulmonary artery
13 Left pulmonary artery
14 Conus pulmonalis
15 Right atrium
16 Right ventricle

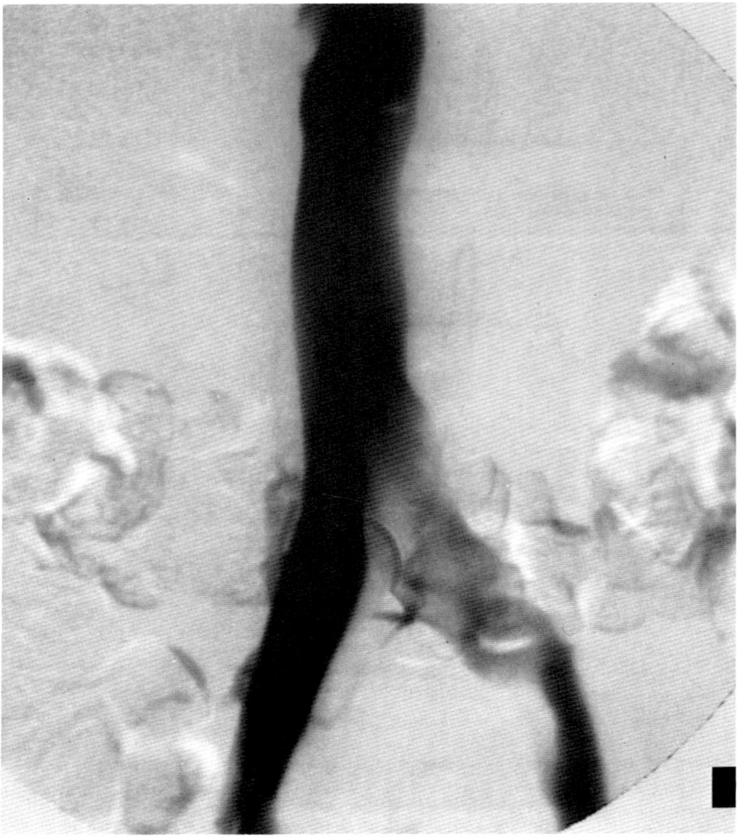

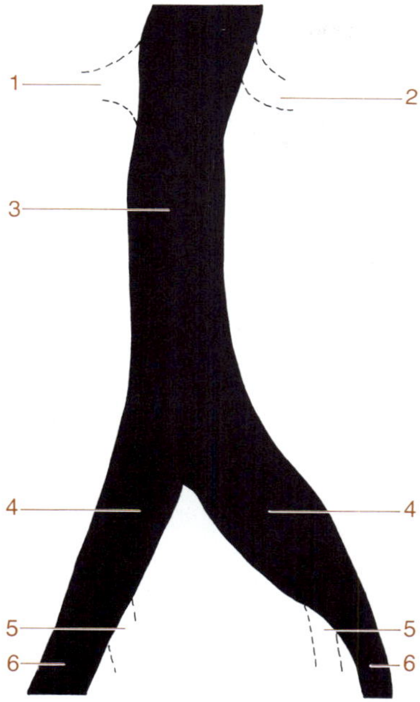

1 Right renal vein
2 Left renal vein
3 Inferior vena cava
4 Common iliac vein
5 Internal iliac vein
6 External iliac vein

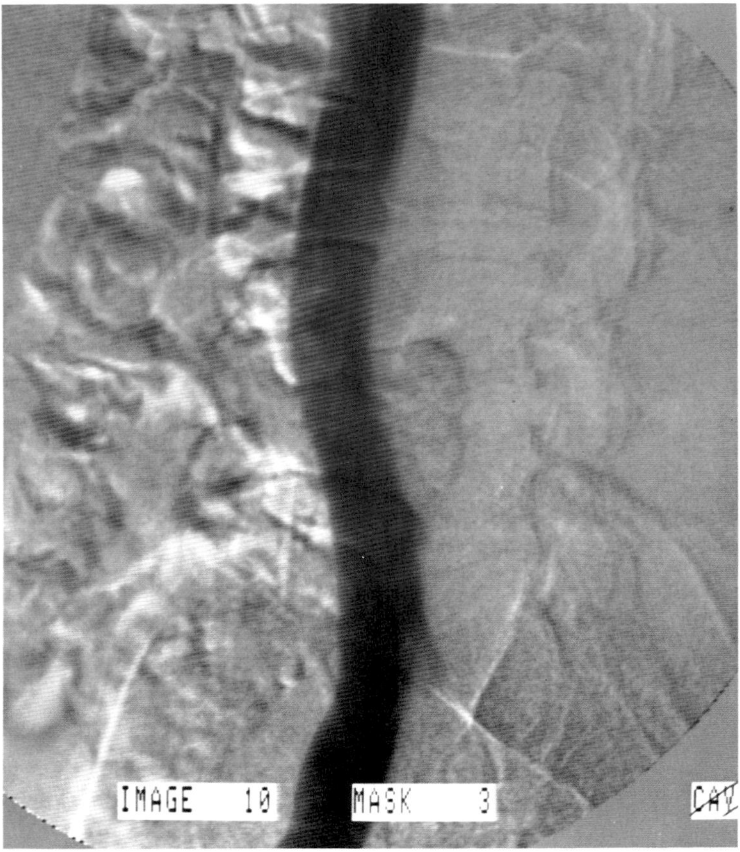
IMAGE 10
MASK 3

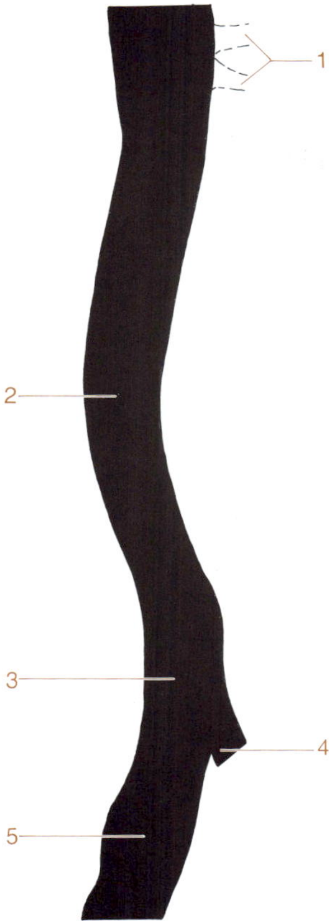

1 Renal veins
2 Inferior vena cava
3 Common iliac vein
4 Internal iliac vein
5 External iliac vein

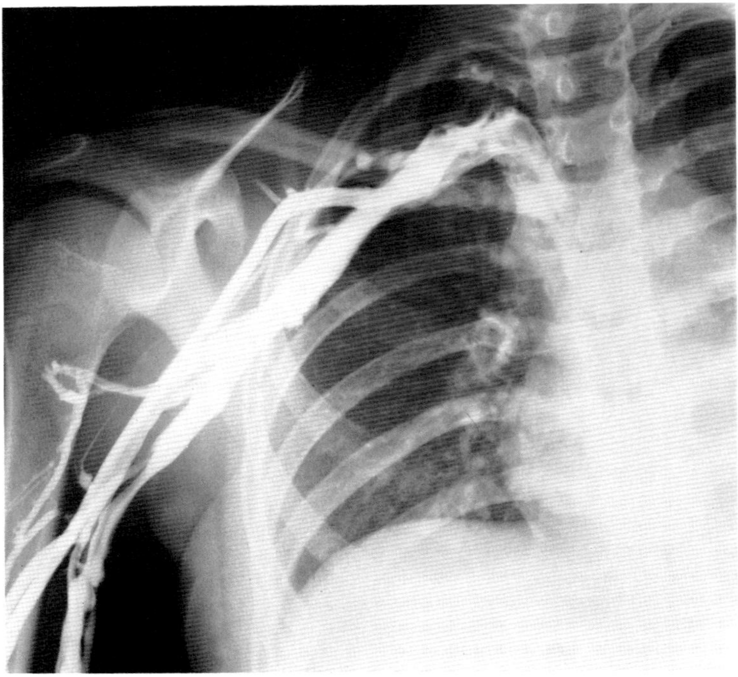

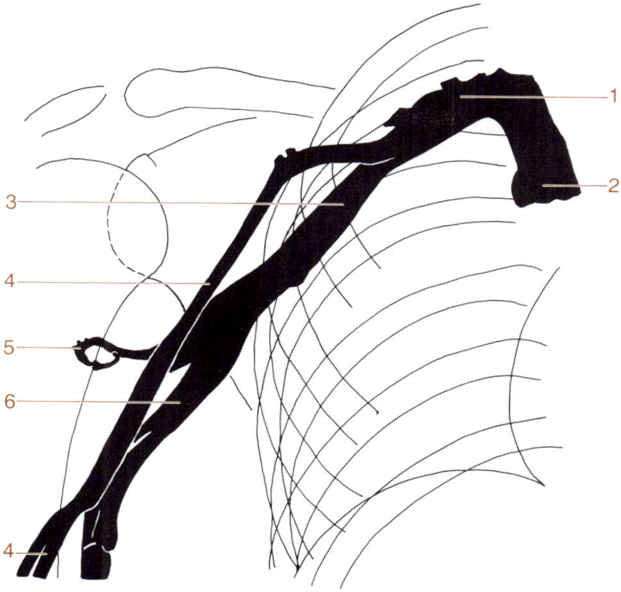

1 Subclavian vein
2 Superior vena cava
3 Axillary vein
4 Cephalic vein
5 Deep veins of the arm
6 Brachial veins

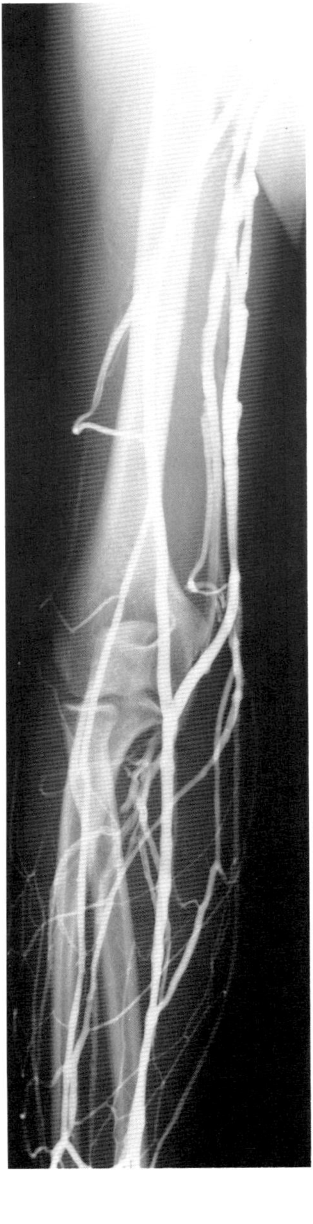

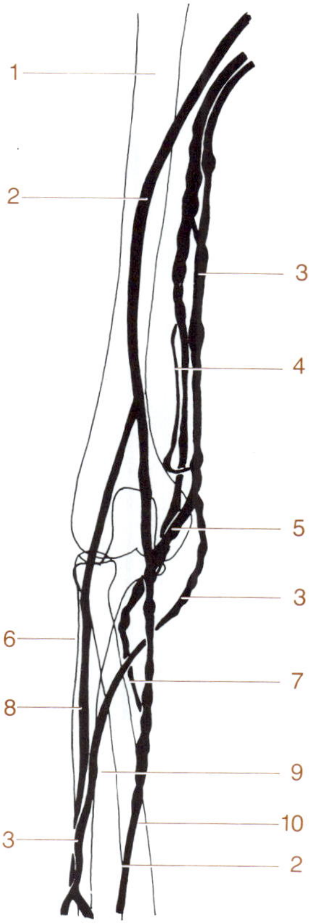

Pronation

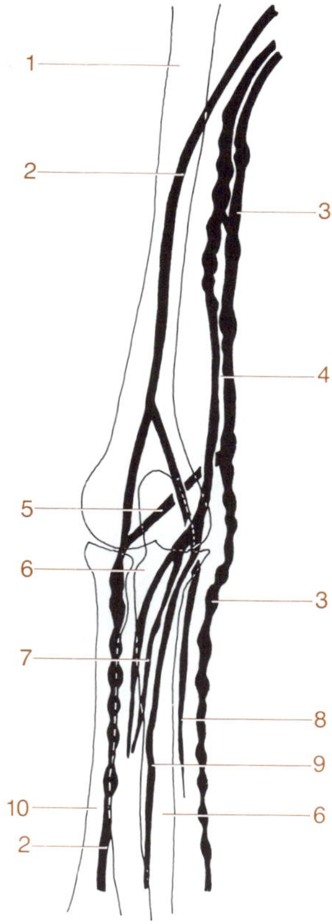

Supination

1 Humerus
2 Cephalic vein
3 Basilar vein
4 Brachial vein
5 Median cubital vein
6 Ulna
7 Radial veins
8 Ulnar veins
9 Median forearm vein
10 Radius

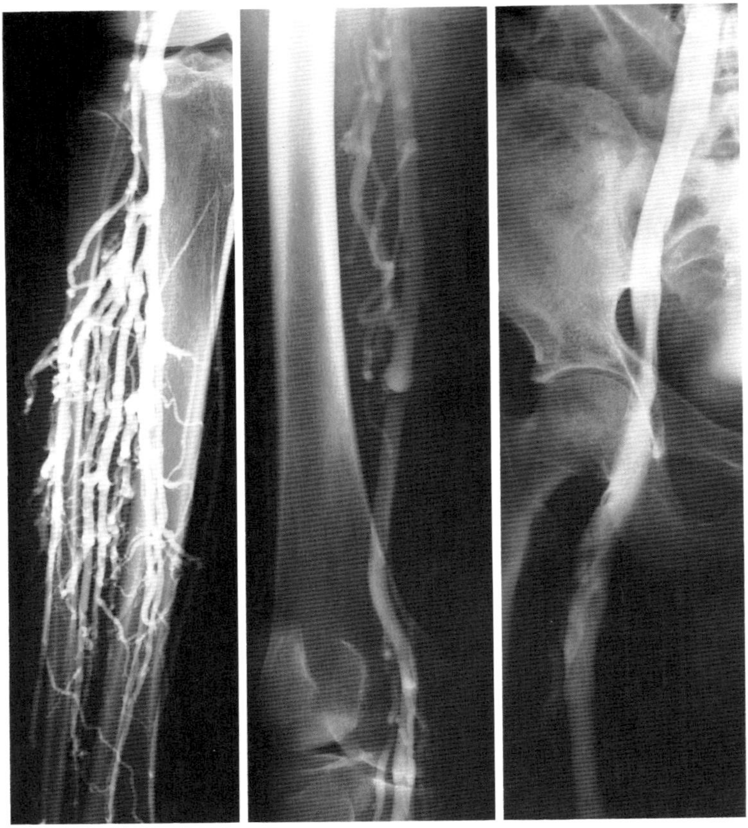

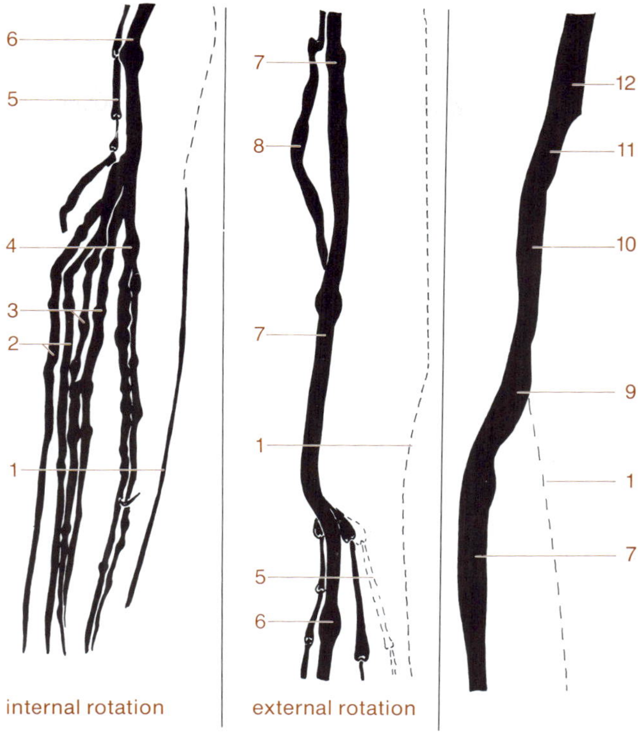

1 Greater saphenous vein
2 Anterior tibial veins
3 Peroneal veins
4 Posterior tibial veins
5 Lesser saphenous vein
6 Popliteal vein
7 Superficial femoral vein
8 Deep femoral vein
9 Common femoral vein
10 External iliac vein
11 Common iliac vein
12 Inferior vena cava

Special Examinations

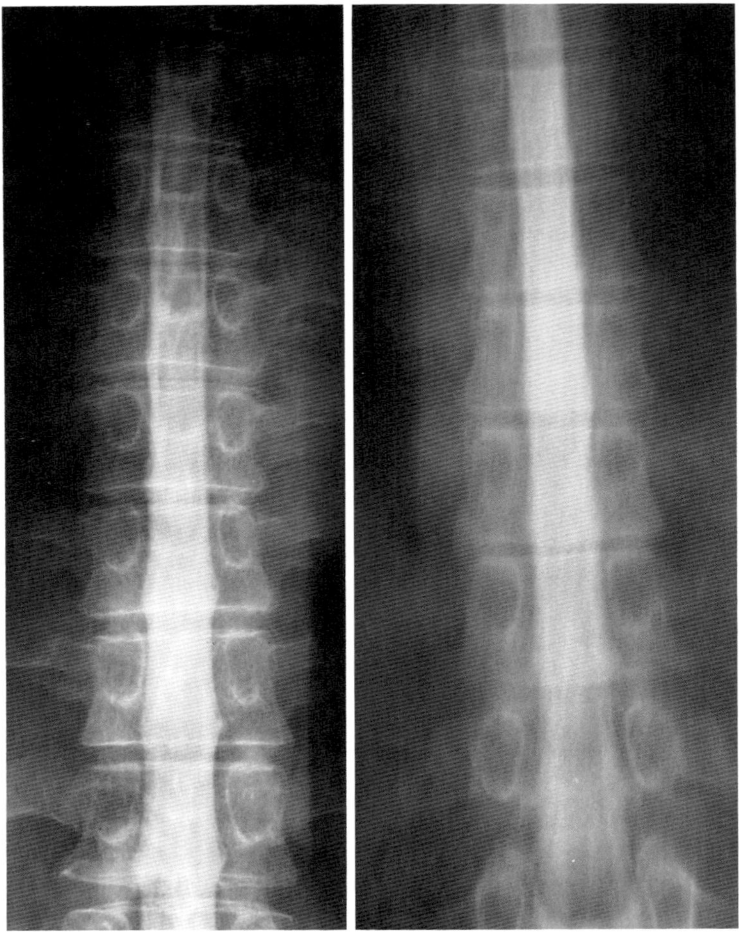

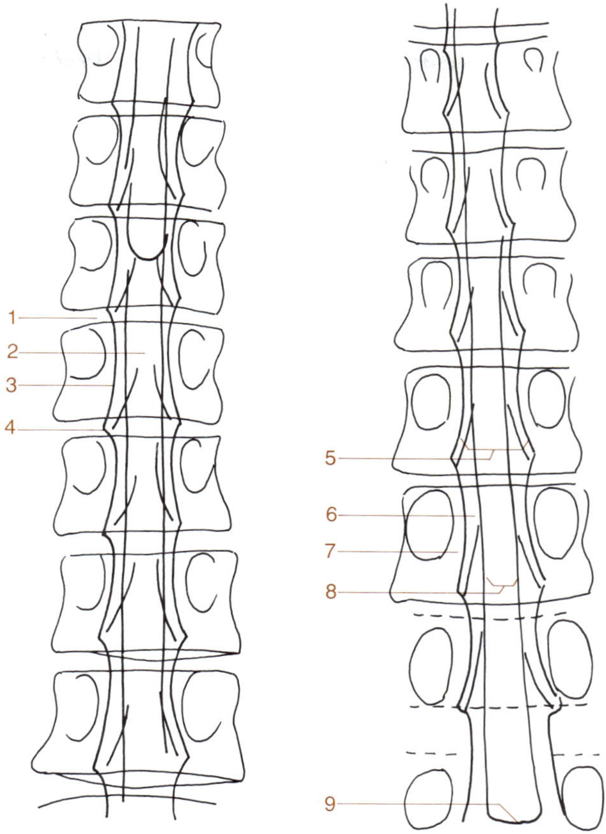

1 Intervertebral disk
2 Spinal cord
3 Lateral margin of the dural sac
4 Nerve root sleeve
5 Intradural space
6 Lateral subarachnoid space
7 Extradural space
8 Intramedullary region
9 Conus medullaris

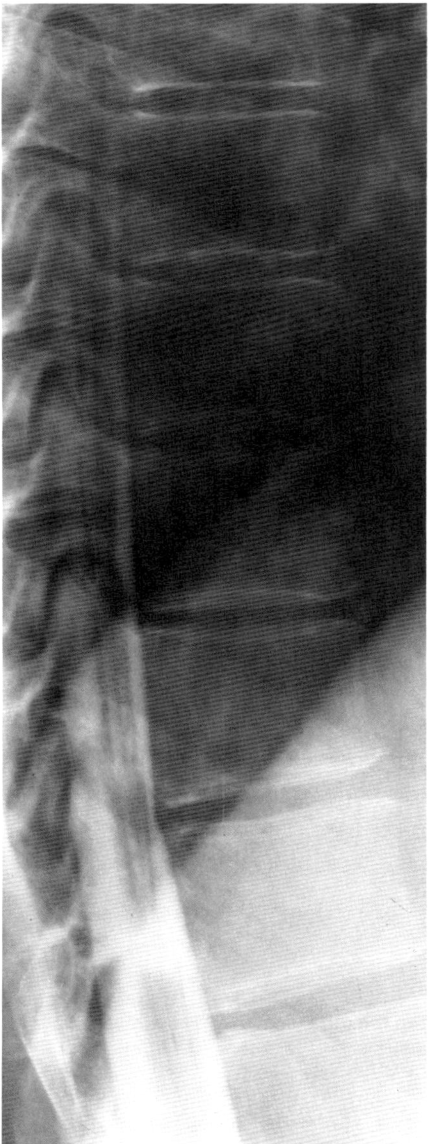

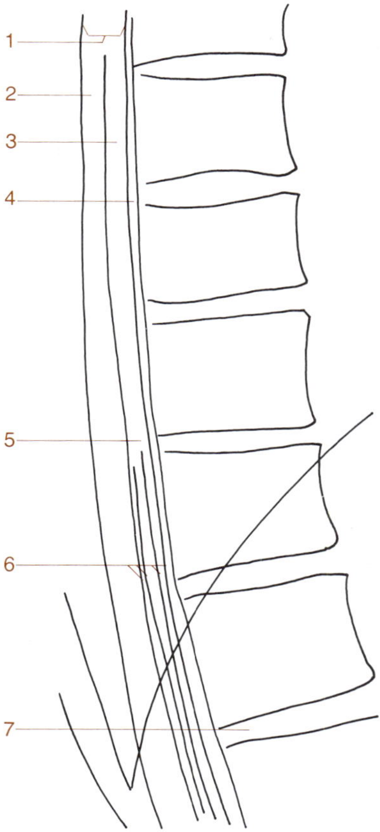

1 Dural sac
2 Posterior subarachnoid space
3 Spinal cord
4 Anterior subarachnoid space
5 Conus medullaris
6 Cauda equina
7 Intervertebral disk

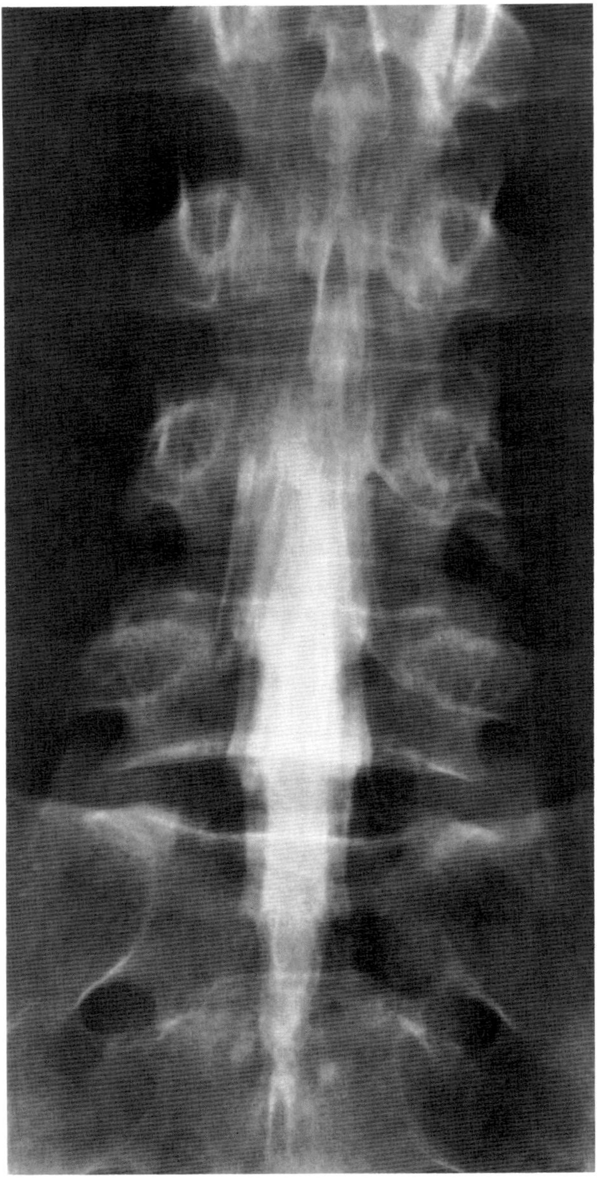

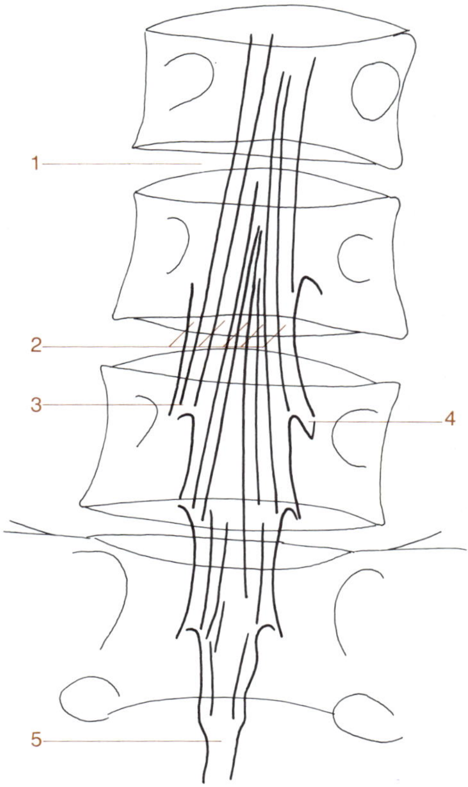

1 Intervertebral disk
2 Cauda equina
3 Spinal nerve root in the subarachnoid space
4 Nerve root sleeve
5 Distal end of the dural sac

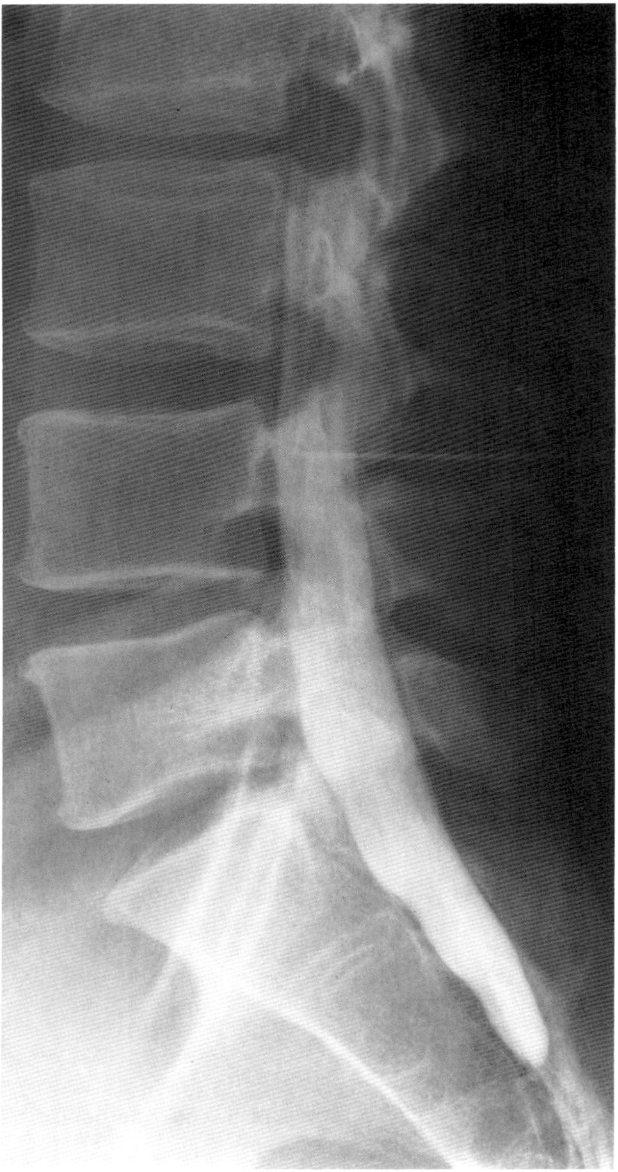

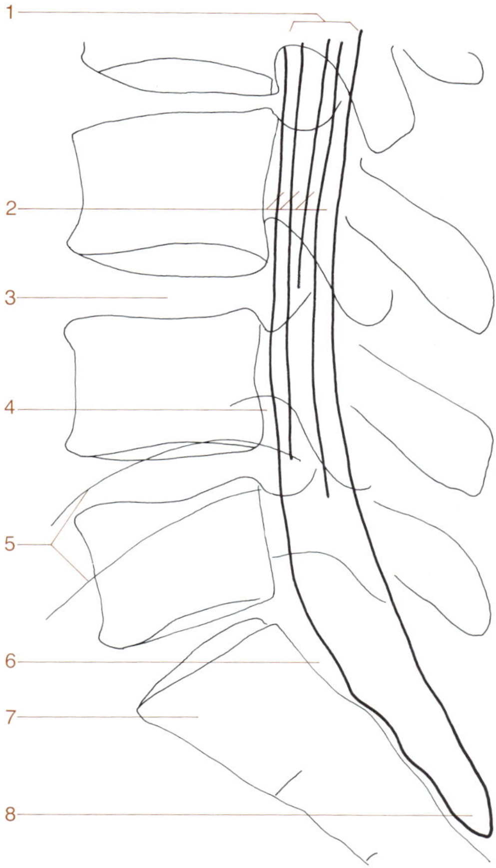

1 Dural sac
2 Cauda equina
3 Intervertebral disk
4 Intervertebral foramen
5 Iliac crest
6 Epidural fat
7 Sacrum
8 Distal end of the dural sac

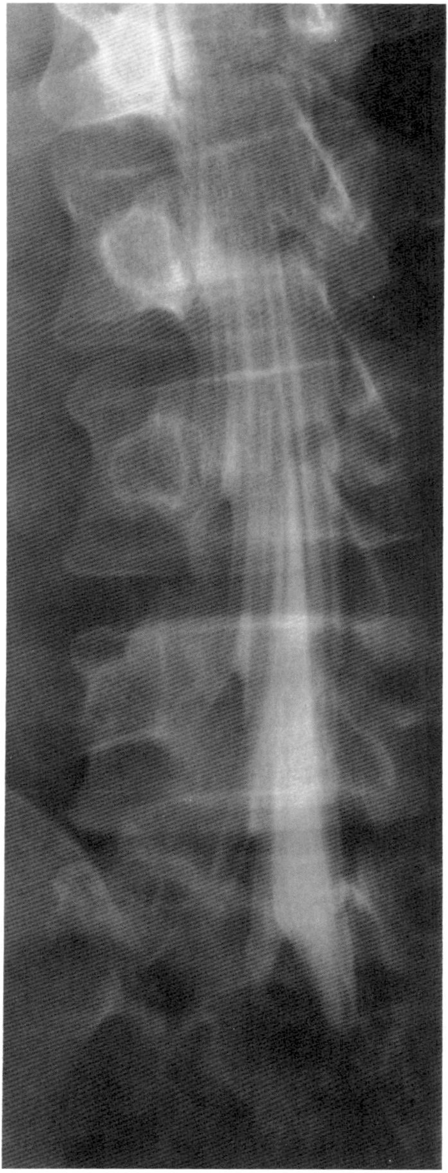

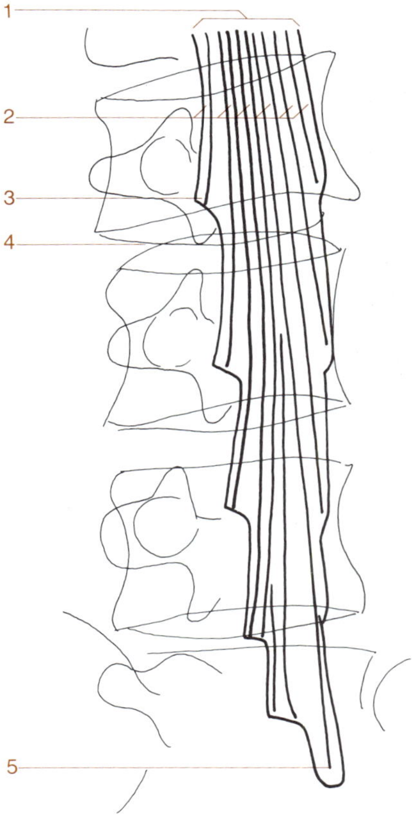

1 Dural sac
2 Cauda equina
3 Nerve root sleeve, L3
4 Intervertebral disk L3/L4
5 Distal end of the dural sac (at level of S1 or S2)

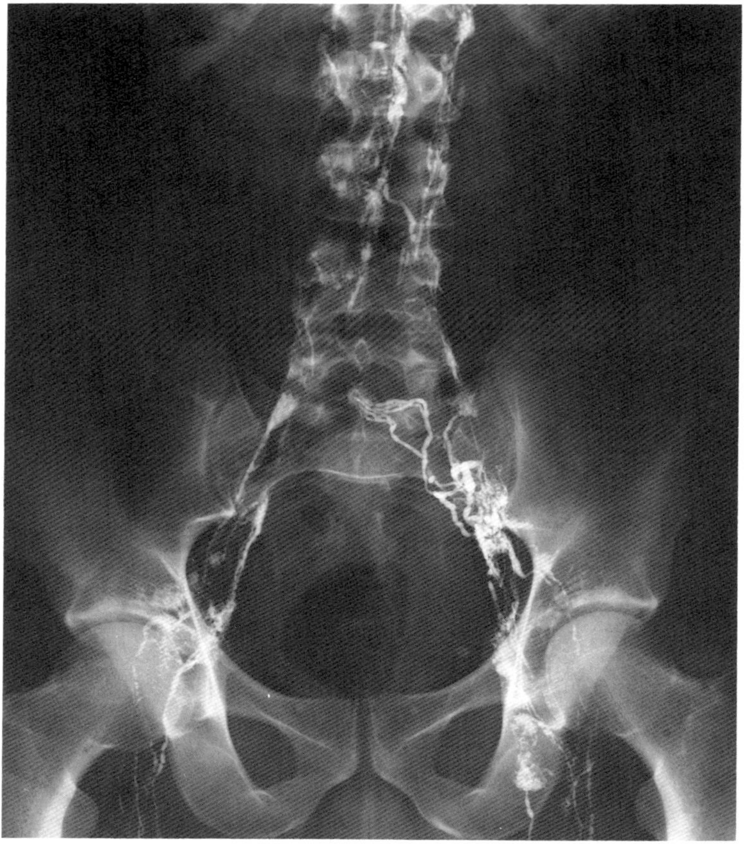

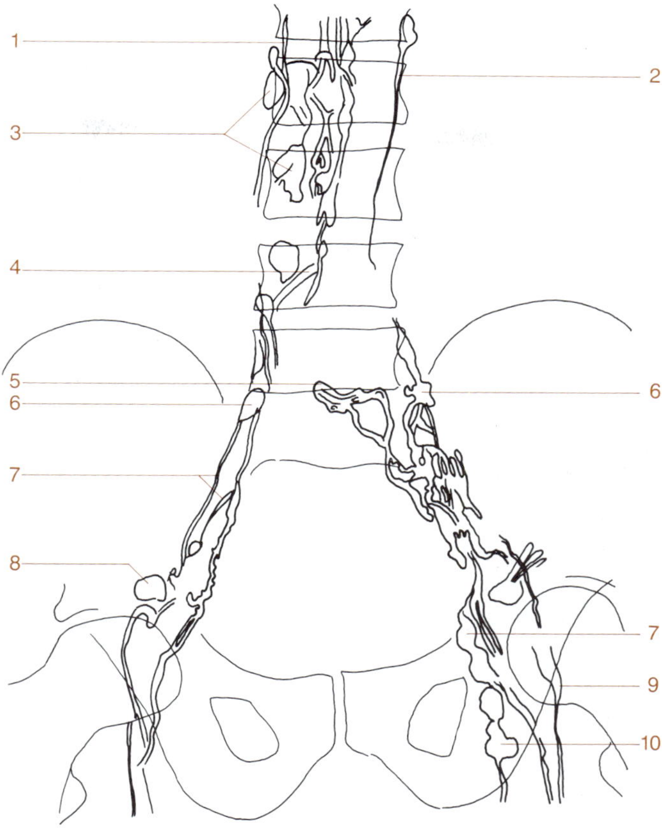

1 Right lumbar trunk
2 Left lumbar trunk
3 Lumbar lymph nodes
4 Cross-over
5 Promontory lymph nodes
6 Common iliac lymph nodes
7 Lymph tracts of the external iliac lymph-node group
8 Lateral lacunar lymph nodes
9 Superficial inguinal lymph nodes
10 Deep inguinal lymph nodes

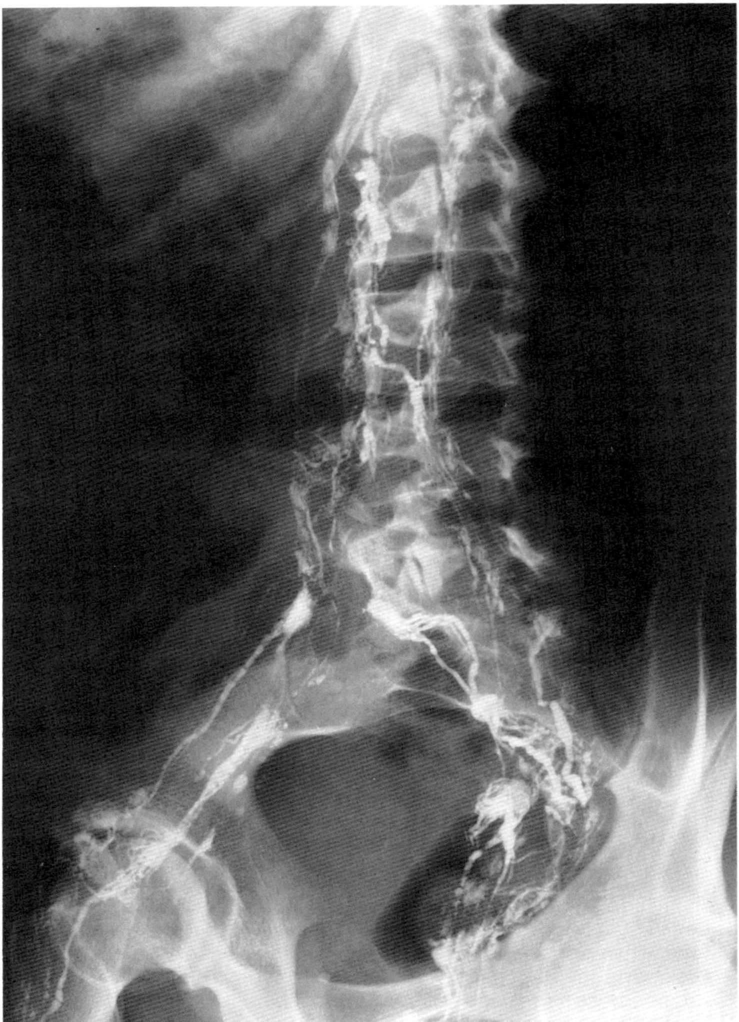

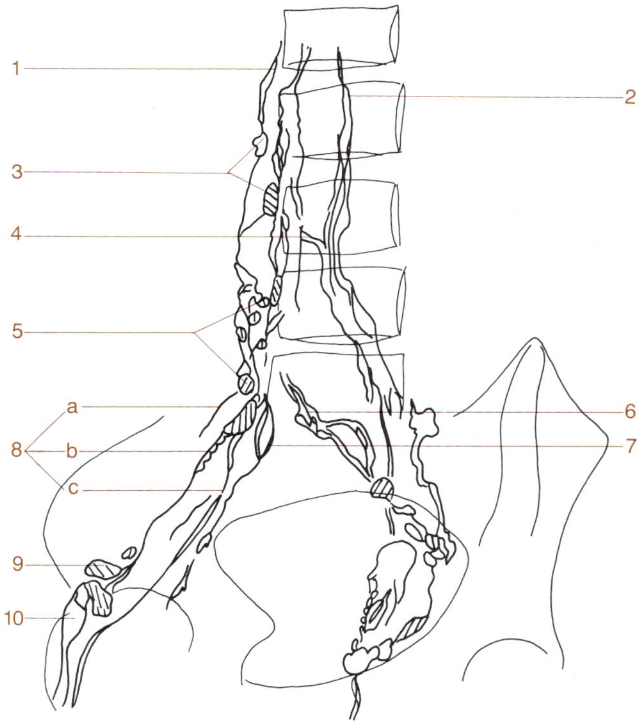

1 Right lumbar trunk
2 Left lumbar trunk
3 Lumbar lymph nodes
4 Cross-over
5 Common iliac lymph nodes
6 Promontory lymph nodes
7 Lymph tracts connecting the internal iliac lymph nodes with the external and common iliac lymph nodes
8 External and common iliac lymph nodes
  a External chain
  b Middle chain
  c Internal chain
9 Lacunar lymph node
10 Superficial inguinal lymph nodes

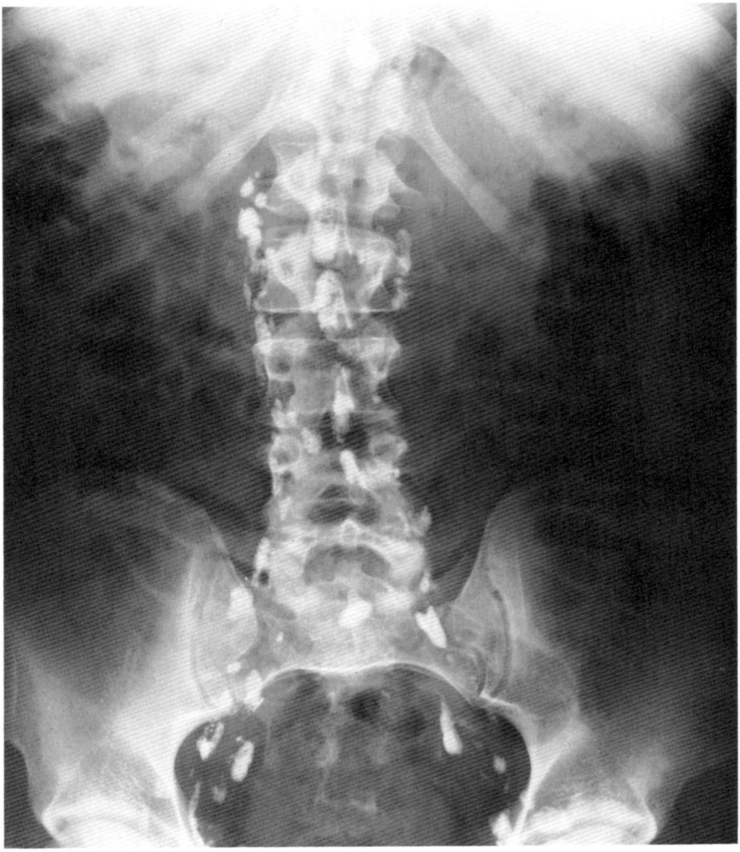

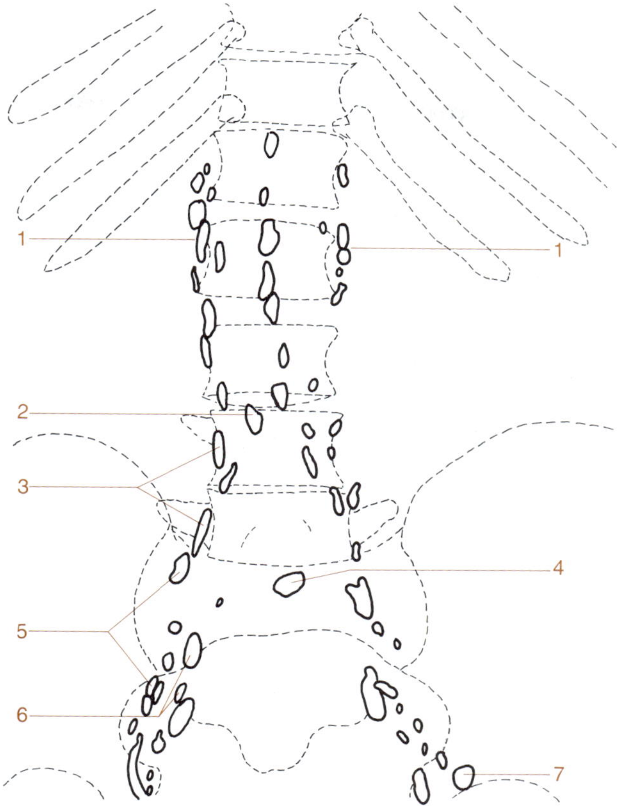

1 Para-aortal lymph nodes (lateral aortic, preaortic, and retroaortic)
2 Cross-over
3 Common iliac lymph nodes
4 Promontory lymph nodes
5 External iliac lymph nodes
6 Internal iliac lymph nodes
7 Lacunar lymph node

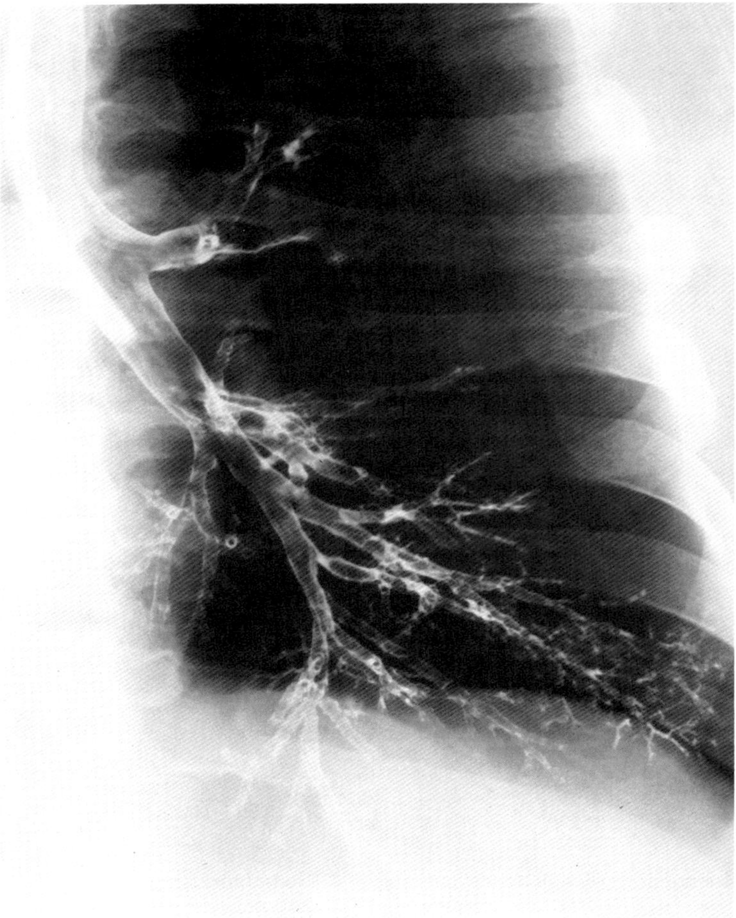

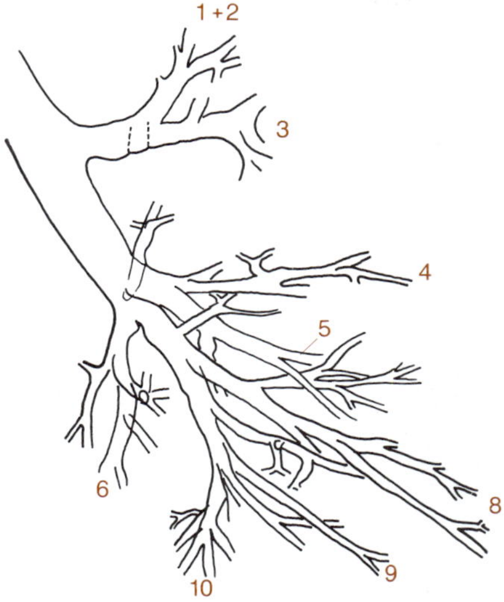

1 and 2 Apical-posterior segment, upper lobe
3 Anterior segment, upper lobe
4 Lingula, superior segment
5 Lingula, inferior segment
6 Superior segment of the lower lobe

7 Mediobasal segment, variable on left side
8 Anteromediobasal segment, left lower lobe
9 Laterobasal segment, lower lobe
10 Posterobasal segment, lower lobe

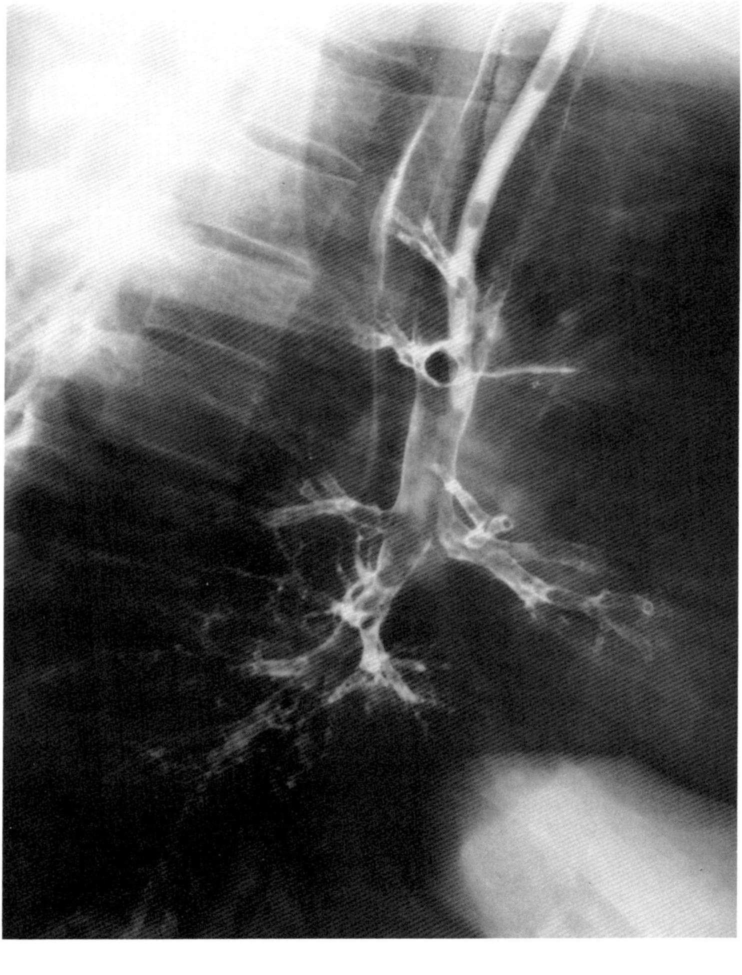

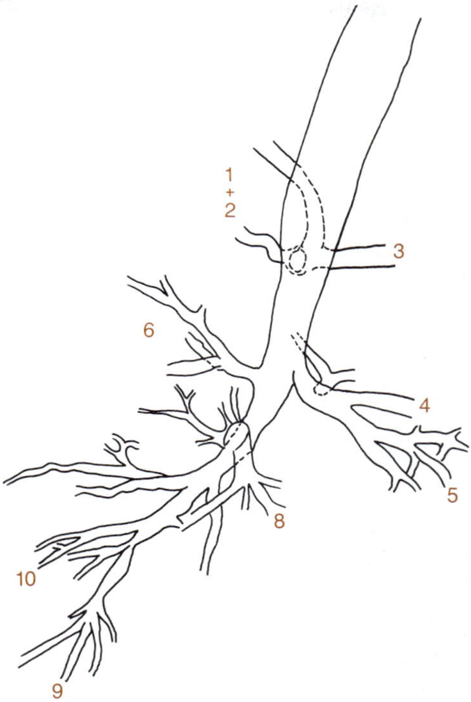

1 and 2 Apical-posterior segment, upper lobe
3 Anterior segment, upper lobe
4 Lingula, superior segment
5 Lingula, inferior segment
6 Superior segment, lower lobe
7 Mediobasal segment, variable on left side
8 Anteromediobasal segment, lower lobe
9 Laterobasal segment, lower lobe
10 Posterobasal segment, lower lobe

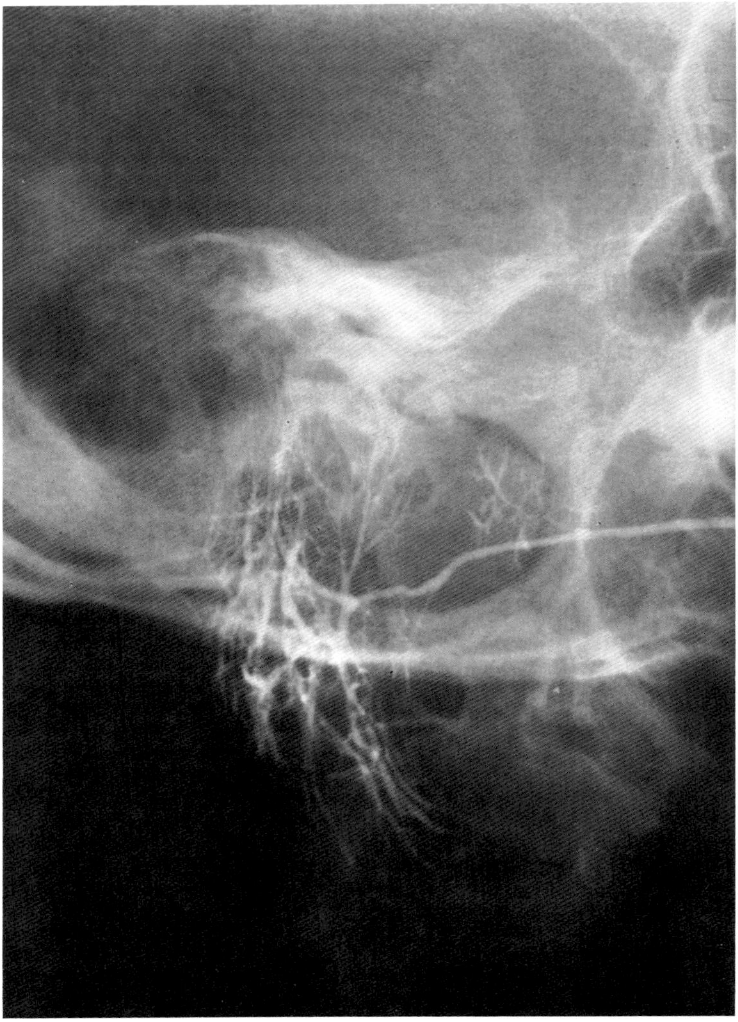

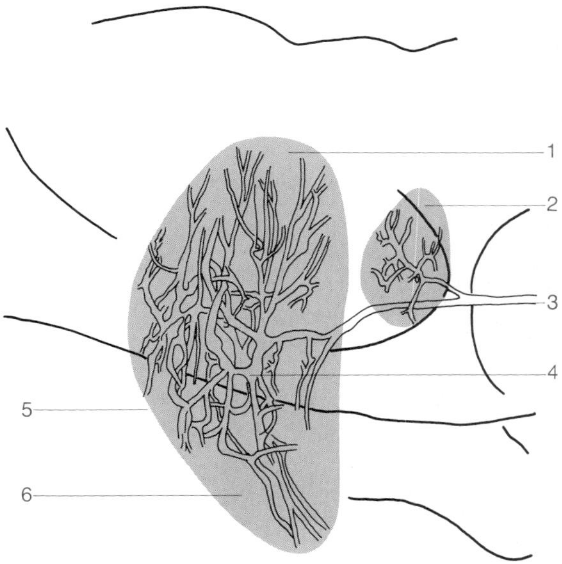

1 Superficial lobe of the parotid gland
2 Accessory parotid gland
3 Parotid duct (Stenson duct)
4 Intralobular ductal system
5 Parotid gland
6 Deep lobe of the parotid gland (lies deep to the facial nerve)

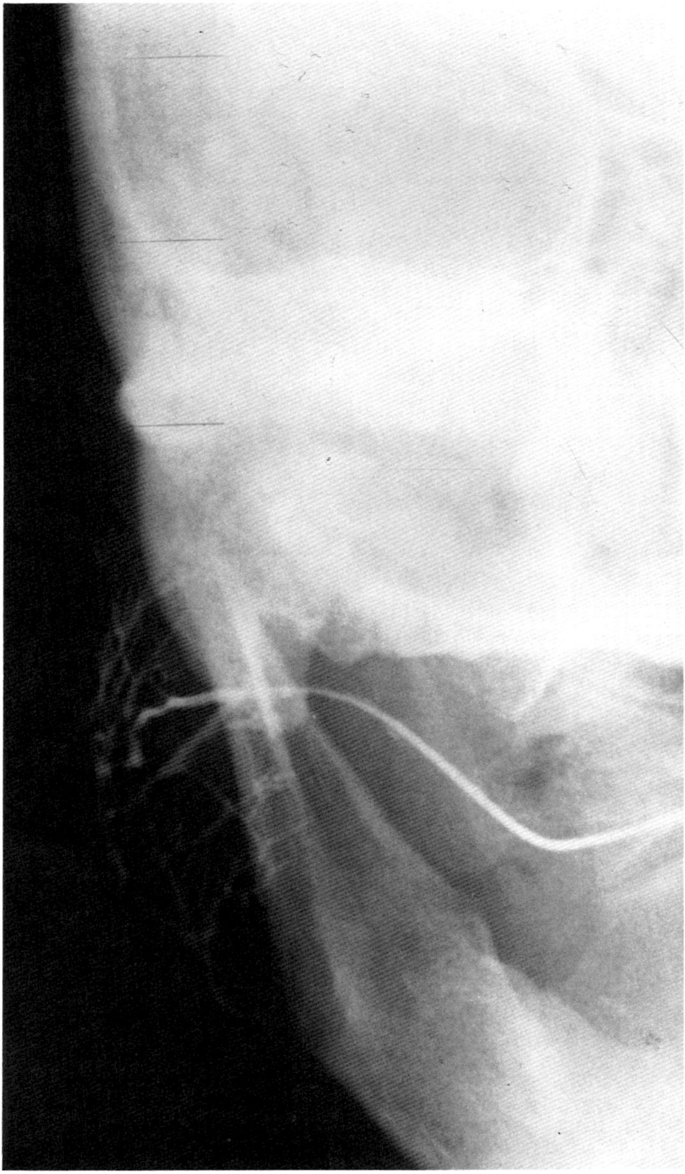

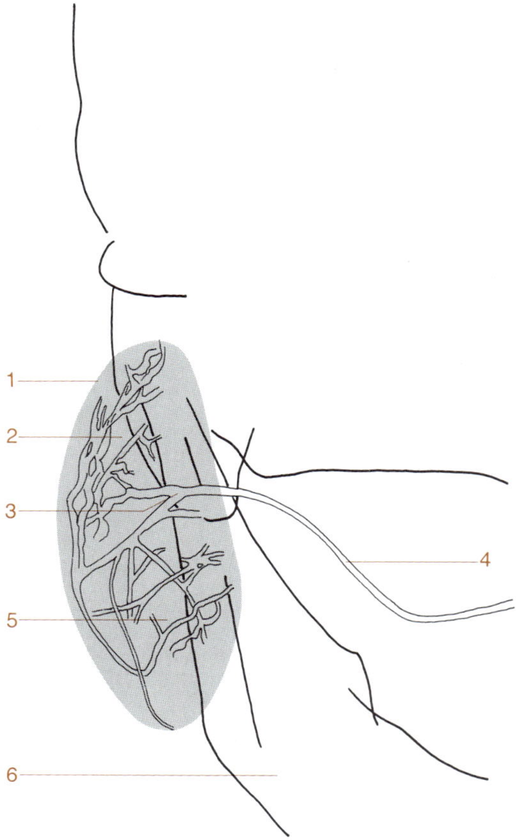

1 Parotid gland
2 Superficial lobe of the parotid gland (lies superficial to the facial nerve)
3 Intralobular parotid ductal system
4 Parotid duct (Stenson duct)
5 Deep lobe of the parotid gland (lies deep to the facial nerve)
6 Mandible

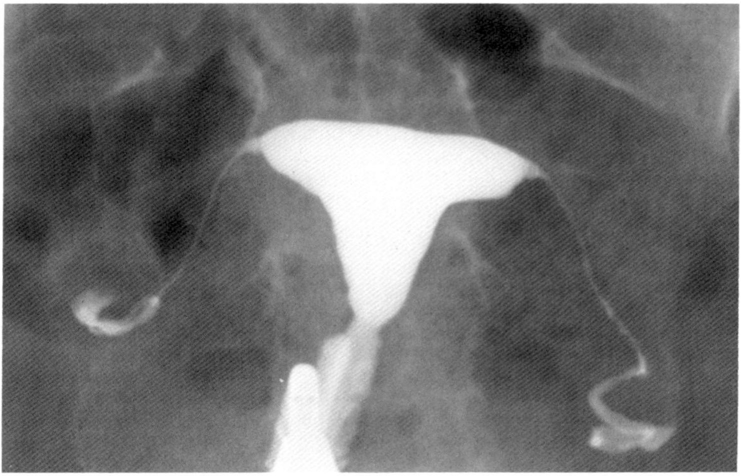

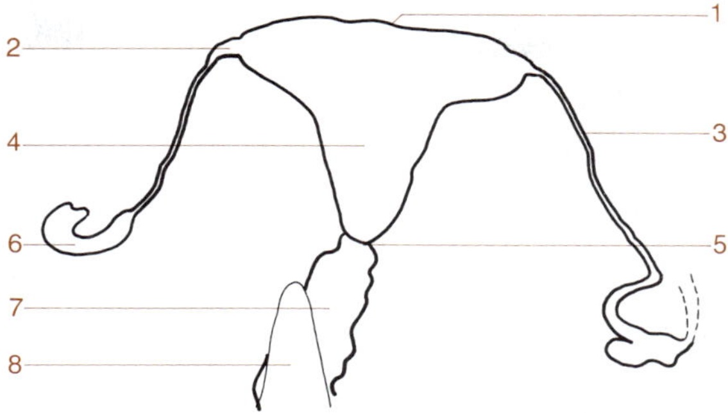

1 Fundus of the uterus
2 Uterine orifice of the tube
3 Tube
4 Uterine cavity
5 Isthmic canal
6 Ampulla
7 Vagina
8 Tenaculum

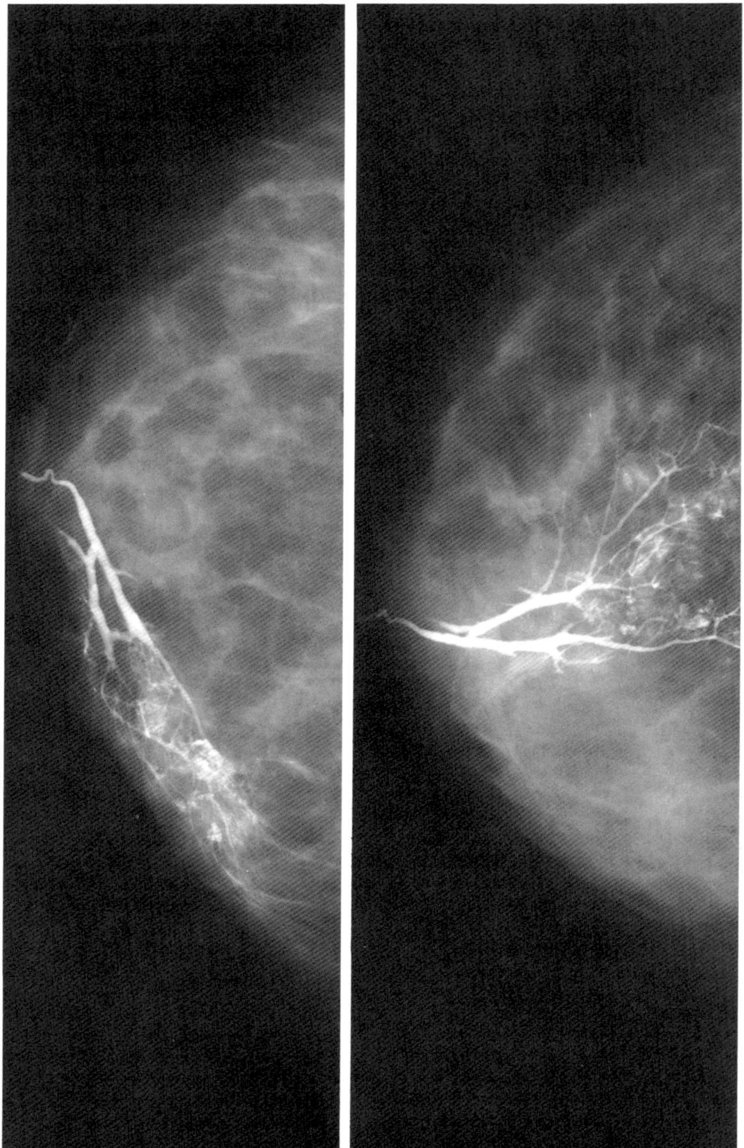

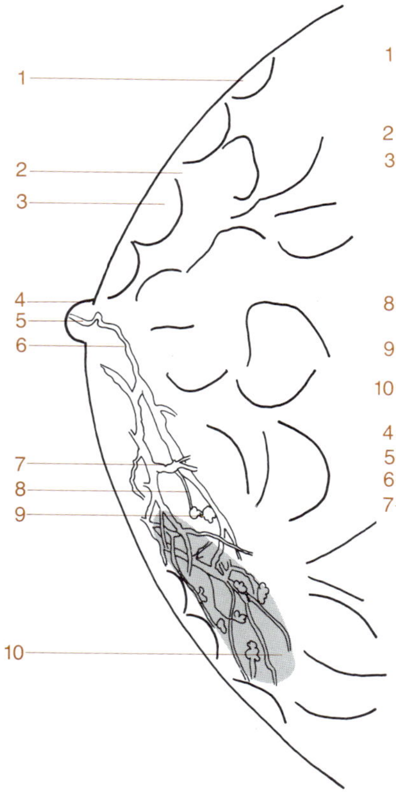

Mediolateral

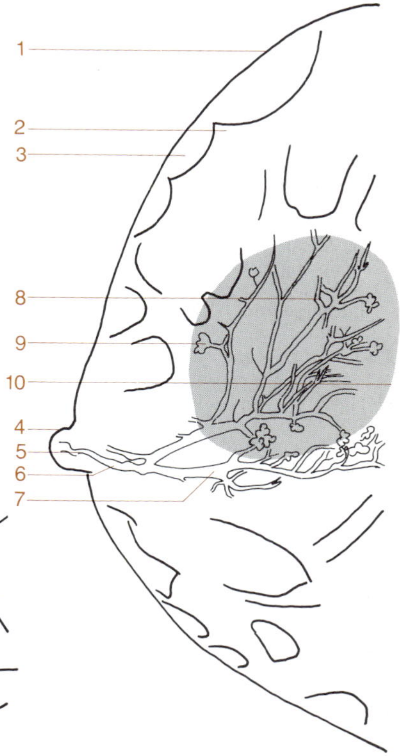

Craniocaudal

1 Skin
2 Cooper's ligament
3 Subcutaneous fatty tissue
4 Nipple
5 Areolar ducts
6 Mammary duct
7 Areolar duct
8 Mammary ductule
9 Lobules of the mammary gland
10 Lobules of the mammary gland

Dihlmann, W.: Gelenke, Wirbelverbindungen, 3. Aufl. Thieme, Stuttgart 1987

Fischedick, O.: Arthrographie des Kniegelenkes. In Diethelm, L., et al.: Handbuch der medizinischen Radiologie, Bd. V/2. Springer, Berlin 1973

Fischedick, O., H. Haage: Die Kontrastdarstellung der Schultergelenke. In Diethelm, L., et al.: Handbuch der medizinischen Radiologie, Bd. V/2. Springer, Berlin 1973

Gmelin, E., I. P. Arlart: Digitale Subtraktionsangiographie. Thieme, Stuttgart 1987

Haage, H.: Arthrographie des Handgelenkes. In Diethelm, L., et al.: Handbuch der medizinischen Radiologie, Bd. V/2. Springer, Berlin 1973

Haage, H., O. Fischedick: Arthrographie des Sprunggelenkes. In Diethelm, L., et al.: Handbuch der medizinischen Radiologie, Bd. V/2. Springer, Berlin 1973

Hach, W.: Phlebographie der Bein- und Bekkenvenen. Schnetztor, Konstanz 1985

Hoefken, W., M. Lanyi: Erkrankung der Brustdrüse. In Schinz, H. R., et al.: Lehrbuch der Röntgendiagnostik, 6. Aufl., Bd. II/2. Thieme, Stuttgart 1981

Kahle, W., H. Leonhardt, W. Platzer: Taschenatlas der Anatomie, 6. Aufl. Thieme, Stuttgart 1991

Klemencic, J., E. Willich: Konventionelle Röntgendiagnostik der Lungen. In: Conscientia Diagnostica. Byck, Konstanz 1986

Köhler, A., E. A. Zimmer: Grenzen des Normalen und Anfänge des Pathologischen im Röntgenbild des Skeletts, 13. Aufl. Thieme, Stuttgart 1989

Krayenbühl, H., M. G. Yasargil: Zerebrale Angiographie für Klinik und Praxis, 3. Aufl. Thieme, Stuttgart 1979

Lange, S.: Radiologische Diagnostik der Lungenerkrankungen. Thieme, Stuttgart 1986

Langlotz, M.: Lumbale Myelographie mit wasserlöslichen Kontrastmitteln. Thieme, Stuttgart 1981

Lusza, G.: Röntgenanatomie des Gefäßsystems. Barth, München 1972

Mahieu, P., J. Pringot, P. Bodart: Defecography: I. Description of a new procedure and results in normal patients. Gastrointest. Radiol. 9, 1984

Meschan, I.: Analyse der Röntgenbilder. Enke, Stuttgart 1981

Meschan, I.: Röntgenanatomie. Enke, Stuttgart 1987

Möller, T. B.: Röntgennormalbefunde. Thieme, Stuttgart 1987

Müller, K. H. G.: Lymphographie. Springer, Berlin 1979

Nadjmi, M.: Digitale Subtraktionsangiographie in der Neuroradiologie. Thieme, Stuttgart 1986

Neufand, K. F. R., D. Beyer: Der rechte paratracheale Streifen – Bedeutung für die Analyse oberer Mediastinalprozesse. Röntgen-Bl. 35, 1982

Pasler, F. A.: Zahnärztliche Radiologie, 2. Aufl. Thieme, Stuttgart 1989

Rochlin, D. G., E. Zeitler: Röntgendiagnostik der Hand und Handwurzel. In Diethelm, L., et al.: Handbuch der medizinischen Radiologie, Bd. IV/2. Springer, Berlin 1968

Rohen, J. V., Ch. Yokochi: Anatomie des Menschen. Schattauer, Stuttgart 1988

Schnitzlein, H. N., F. Reed Murtagh: Imaging Anatomy of the Head and Spine. Urban & Schwarzenberg, München 1990

Snell, R. S., A. C. Wyman: An Atlas of Normal Radiographic Anatomy. Little, Brown, Boston 1976

Sobotta, J., H. Becher: Atlas der Anatomie des Menschen. Urban & Schwarzenberg, München 1972

St. John, J. N., J. C. Palmaz: The cubital tunnel in ulnear entrapment neuropathy. Radiology 158, 1986

Thurn, P., E. Bücheler, Einführung in die radiologische Diagnostik, 8. Aufl. Thieme, Stuttgart 1986

Treichel, J.: Doppelkontrastuntersuchung des Magens, 2. Aufl. Thieme, Stuttgart 1990

Tristant, H., M. Benmussa: Atlas der Hysterosalpingographie. Enke, Stuttgart 1984

Weigand, H., D. Sarfert, W. Kurock: Diagnostik und Einteilung der Hüftpfannenbrüche. Unfallchirurgie 3, 1977

Wicke, L.: Atlas der Röntgenanatomie. Urban & Schwarzenberg, München 1980